Physiological Pharmaceutics

For Alexander and Sarina

With all our love

Physiological Pharmaceutics

Barriers to drug absorption

Second Edition

Neena Washington, Clive Washington and Clive G. Wilson

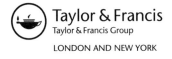

Taylor & Francis
Taylor & Francis Group

LONDON AND NEW YORK

First edition 1989
Second edition first published 2001 by Taylor and Francis
11 New Fetter Lane, London EC4P 4EE

Simultaneously published in the USA and Canada
by Taylor and Francis Inc,
29 West 35th Street, New York, NY 10001

Reprinted 2002, 2003

Taylor and Francis is an imprint of the Taylor & Francis Group

Publisher's Note
This book has been prepared from camera-ready copy provided by the
authors.

Printed and bound in Great Britain by TJ International Ltd, Padstow,
Cornwall

British Library Cataloguing in Publication Data
A catalogue record is available for this book from the British Library

Library of Congress Cataloging in Publication Data
Washington, Neena, 1961-
Physiological pharmaceutics: barriers to drug absorption/ Neena
Washington, Clive Washington, and
Clive George Wilson.—2nd ed.
p. cm.
Previous ed. Physiological pharmaceutics: biological barriers to drug
absorption/Clive George Wilson, Neena Washington.
"Simultaneously published in the USA and Canada."
Includes bibliographical references and index.
1. Drugs—Bioavailability. 2. Drugs—Dosage forms. 3. Drugs—Physiological
transport. 4. Absorption (Physiology) I. Washington, Clive, 1957- . II. Wilson,
Clive George. III. Wilson, Clive George. Physiological pharmaceutics: biological
barriers to drug absorption. IV. Title.

RM301.6.W54 2000
615´.7—dc21

ISBN 0-748-40610-7 (hbk)
ISBN 0-748-40562-3 (pbk)

PREFACE

Considering the variety in the human race, height, weight, temperament, enzymatic capacity, it is amazing that pharmaceuticals work at all. Add environmental factors, and personal preferences, and suddenly you begin to realise the scale of the problem. Some years ago I ran a clinical trial in patients with ulcerative colitis. When I was recruiting the subjects, I asked people to keep a diary of everything that they ate. Even within the catchment area of Queen's Medical Centre in Nottingham, the diversity of food eaten, let alone the frequency of eating, was beyond comprehension. This led me to think about the world outside Nottingham, eating habits within the UK, the north/south divide (which we are assured by the Government does not exist) let alone what people eat in Africa, China, Fiji......?? Then remember that medication is designed for sick people, who by definition have a physiology disordered in some way. So how can one pill fit all?

The development work is aimed at the "average" patient. Is there such a thing as an average patient? Is the "average" person really a 70 kg man? In the U.K. 41% of males and 20% of females are overweight. Even the "average" healthy woman may be excluded from pharmacokinetic trials not only due to the risk of potential genetic damage to reproductive tissue but also a tacit admission that the menstrual cycle may affect not only gastrointestinal transit, but also a wide range of physiological processes. This leaves basic data concerning the behaviour of drugs in women largely undiscovered until they are treated as patients.

The realisation that the USP dissolution test bore little resemblance to dosage form behaviour in the body, particularly for the new sophisticated dose forms, led to the first edition of this book being written ten years ago. Over the past 30 years, a predominant focus of drug delivery has been the development of sustained and controlled release formulations, whose interaction with the body is even more critical and complex than that of 'ordinary' tablets. In 1996 there were 35 pharmaceutical products based on advanced drug delivery with a worldwide sales of ten million US dollars each or higher; this was 11 more than in 1994. In these two years total sales had increased from 5.5 to 6.5 billion dollars. Four products were responsible for more than half of the total sales in 1996; these were ProcardiaXL (nifedipine), Lupron (leuprolide), Cardizem (diltiazem) and Zoladex (goserelin).

The primary goals are usually to minimise the dose of drug administered and to optimize the delivery of the drug, to achieve an 'ideal' plasma-concentration time profile. An added advantage is that simplification of the dosage regimen leads to increased patient compliance by reducing the number of daily doses. With the new requirement to deliver drugs to precise locations of the gastrointestinal tract came the need to study physiological variations in gastrointestinal transit, such as those brought about by eating, levels of physical activity and chronobiological effects. The focus on once-a-day dosing necessitated larger payloads of drugs per unit than conventional counterparts. Premature release of the drug could have potentially disastrous effects, so prediction of dosage form behaviour needs to be accurate.

With the leap in the number of sophisticated technologies reaching the market place the amount of literature which has become available since 1990 is considerable, and hence the second edition of "Physiological Pharmaceutics" is a complete re-write and not just an update. We are very aware that people placed advance orders for this book and we would like to thank them for buying it on faith. We also would like to thank them for their patience and we hope that they feel that the wait was worthwhile. We would like to thank our publishers, who I am sure, at times, thought the manuscript was a figment of the imagination (either theirs or ours). Ironically, the first draft of the manuscript was delivered to them 3 years *to the day* late. By way of an explanation for the tardiness of this book, I would like you to realise that this book was written in "our spare time", as if scientists with full time jobs and a young family have "spare time"! The university obsession with the research assessment exercise has made the production of textbooks a rather low priority, so much of the volume has been written after 11 at night!

For this very reason I would like to thank our children, Alex (9 years) and Sarina (4 years) for their patience whilst mummy was writing or daddy was drawing diagrams, and Alex for 'helping' with the diagrams… We are painfully aware that it is they who have suffered as we have had virtually no time for them, particularly over the last year. As I write this, they know that the "end of book" promised trip to LegoLand is coming closer!

I also must thank my friends and colleagues, Drs Caroline Herd, Mike Nassim, Gerry Hooper and Carol Astbury for their caring and support. I would also like to thank my husband, who saw the vast amount of work which needed to be done on the book and mucked in. In acknowledgement of his substantial contribution, we made him a full author on this edition. Without him, the book would probably have been 6 years late!

Neena Washington   14th February 2000

FIGURE ACKNOWLEDGEMENTS

Fig 1.13 is reprinted from Volkheimer G et al., Gut 1969;10:32-3. with the permission of the BMJ Publishing Group.

Fig 3.4 is reprinted from Sanford PA, Digestive System Physiology (1982) with the permission of Arnold.

Fig 3.5 is reprinted from Pimlott & Addy, Oral Surg. Oral. Med. Path. 1985;59:145-8. with the permission of Mosby.

Fig 3.6 is reprinted from Squier CA & Johnson NW, British Medical Bulletin 1975;31:169 with the permission of Christopher A Squier.

Fig 3.8 is reprinted from Wilson CG et al., Int J Pharm 1987;40:119-123 with the permission of Elsevier Science.

Fig 3.9 is reprinted from Davis SS et al, In: Modern Concepts in Nitrate Delivery Systems, Goldberg AAJ & Parson DG (eds) pp29-37 (1983) with the permission of Pharmaceutical Press.

Fig 4.6 is reprinted from Wilson CG et al., Int. J. Pharm. 1988;46:241-46 with the permission of Elsevier Science.

Fig 4.7 is reprinted from Kikendall JW et al., Dig. Dis. Sci. 1983;28:174-182 with the permission of Kluwer Academic/Plenum Publisher.

Fig 4.8 is reprinted from Weinbeck M et al, Bailliere's Clin. Gastroenterol. 1988;2:263-274 with the permission of Harcourt Publishers Ltd.

Fig 5.1 is reprinted from Sanford PA, Digestive System Physiology (1982) with the permission of Arnold.

Fig 5.6 is reprinted from Johnson LR (ed), Gastrointestinal physiology, 3rd edition (1985) with the permission of W. B. Saunders.

Fig 5.7 is reprinted from Sanford PA, Digestive System Physiology (1982) with the permission of Arnold.

Fig 5.11 is reprinted from Sanford PA, Digestive System Physiology (1982) with the permission of Arnold.

Fig 5.13 is reprinted with thanks to Dr Wright of the Department of Surgery, Queen's Medical Centre, Nottingham, UK.

Fig 5.15 is reprinted from Goo RH et al, Gastroenterol. 1987;93:515-518 with the permission of W. B. Saunders.

Fig 5.17 is reprinted from O'Reilly S et al., Int. J. Pharm. 1987;34:213-216 with the permission of Elsevier Science.

Fig 5.19 is reprinted from O'Reilly S et al., Int. J. Pharm. 1987;34:213-216 with the permission of Elsevier Science.

Fig 5.20 is reprinted from Meyer JH et al., Gastroenterol. 1985;88:1502 with the permission of W. B. Saunders.

Fig 6.1 is reprinted from Moog F., The lining of the small intestine. Scientific American 1981;245:154-158 with the permission of Carol Donner.

Fig 6.2 is reprinted from Weiner D, Chapter 43 in: Biological Foundations of Biomedical Engineering, Kline J (ed) (1976) with the permission of Lippincott Williams & Wilkins and D Weiner.

Fig 6.4 is reprinted from Sanford PA, Digestive System Physiology (1982) with the permission of Arnold.

Fig 6.5 is reprinted from Johnson LR (ed), Gastrointestinal Physiology, 3rd edition (1985) with the permission of W. B. Saunders.

Fig 6.7 is reprinted from Davis SS et al., Int. J. Pharm. 1987;34:253-8 with the permission of Elsevier Science.

Fig 6.8 is reprinted from Davis SS et al., Gut 1986;27:886-892 with the permission of the BMJ Publishing Group.

Fig 6.10 is reprinted from Fischer W et al, Pharm. Res. 1987;4:480-485 with the permission of Kluwer Academic/Plenum Publisher.

Fig 6.11 is reprinted from Bechgard H et al., J. Pharm. Pharmacol. 1985;37:718-721 with the permission of Pharmaceutical Press.

Fig 6.12 is reprinted from Schinkel AH, Adv. Drug Deliv. Rev 1999;36:179-194 with the permission of Elsevier Science.

Fig 7.1 is reprinted from Sanford PA, Digestive System Physiology (1982) with the permission of Arnold.

Fig 7.2 is reprinted from Krstic RV, Human Microscopic Anatomy (1991) with the permission of Springer-Verlag.

Fig 7.3 is reprinted from Stephen AM et al., Br. J. Nutr. 1986;56:349-361 with the permission of CABI Publishing.

Fig 7.4 is reprinted from Washington N et al., Moderation of lactulose induced diarrhoea by psyllium: effects on motility and fermentationAm. J. Clin. Nutr. 1998;67:317-321 with the permission of The American Society for Clinical Nutrition.

Fig 7.5 is reprinted from Davis et al., Relationship between the rate of appearance of oxprenolol in the systemic circulation and the location of an oxprenolol Oros 16/260 drug delivery system within the gastrointestinal tract as determined by scintigraphy. Br. J., Clin. Pharmacol. 1988;26:435-443 with the permission of Sage Publications Inc.

Fig 7.6 is reprinted from Hardy JG et al., J. Pharm. Pharmacol. 1985;37:874-877 with the permission of Pharmaceutical Press.

Fig 7.7 is reprinted from Hardy JG et al., J. Pharm. Pharmacol. 1985;37:874-877 with the permission of Pharmaceutical Press.

Fig 7.9 is reprinted from Tozer, T.N., Kinetic perspectives on colonic delivery. Proc. Int. Symp. Cont. Rel. Bioact. Mat. 1990;17:126 with the permission of the Controlled Release Society.

Fig 7.11 is reprinted from Tukker J, Ph.D thesis, University of Leiden 1983 with the permission of J Tukker.

Fig 7.12 is reprinted from Wood E et al., Int. J. Pharmaceut. 1985;25:191-197 with the permission of Elsevier Science.

Fig 7.13 is reprinted from van Hoogdalem E.J., de Boer A.G. and Briemer D.D., Pharmacokinetics of rectal drug administration. Part I – general considerations and clinical applications of centrally acting drugs. Clin. Pharmokinet. 1991;21:11-26 with the permission of Adis International Ltd.

Fig 7.14 is reprinted from van Hoogdalem E.J., de Boer A.G. and Briemer D.D., Pharmacokinetics of rectal drug administration. Part II – Clinical applications of periphereally acting drugs and conclusions. Clin. Pharmokinet. 1991;21:110-128 with the permission of Adis International Ltd.

Fig 9.3 is reprinted from Hussain A.A., Intranasal drug delivery. Advanced Drug Delivery Reviews 1998;29:39-49, with the permission of Elsevier Science.

Fig 9.4 is reprinted from Fisher A. et al, The effect of molecular size on the nasal absorption of water-soluble compounds in the albino rat. J. Pharm. Pharmacol. 1987;39:357-362 with the permission of Pharmaceutical Press.

Fig 9.5 is reprinted from Jackson SJ et al., J. Pharm. Pharmacol 1997;49:suppl 84 with the permission of Pharmaceutical Press.

Fig 9.6 is reprinted from Ridley D. et al., The effect of posture on the nasal clearance of starch microspheres. STP Pharma Sciences 1995;5:442-446 with the permission of Editions de Sante.

Fig 9.7 is reprinted from Hehar SS et al. Clin. Otolaryngology 1999;24:24-25 with the permission of Blackwell Science.

Fig 9.8 is reprinted from Huang C. et al., J. Pharm. Sci. 1985;74:550-552 with the permission of John Wiley & Sons.

Fig 9.9 is reprinted from Washington N et al., Int. J. Pharm. 2000;198:139-146 with the permission of Elsevier Science.

Fig 10.2 is reprinted from Bell GH, Emslie-Smith D and Paterson CR, Textbook of Physiology, 10th edn. (1980) with the permission of W. B. Saunders/Churchill-Livingstone.

Fig 10.3 is reprinted from Vander AJ, Sherman JH & Luciano DS, Human Physiology (1975) with the permission of Tata McGraw-Hill Publishing Company.

Fig 11.1 is reprinted from Mitra AK, Ophthalmic Drug Delivery Devices (P.Tyle ed) Marcel Dekker , New York (1993) with the permission of Marcel Dekker Inc.

Fig 11.5 is reprinted from Greaves JL and Wilson CG, Treatment of diseases of the eye with mucoadesive delivery systems. Advanced Drug Delivery Reviews 1993;11:349-383 with the permission of Elsevier Science.

Fig 12.3 is reprinted from Krstic RV, Human Microscopic Anatomy (1991) with the permission of Springer-Verlag.

The authors and publishers have made every effort to contact authors/copyright holders of works reprinted from in *Physiological Pharmaceutics 2nd ed*. This has not been possible in every case, however, and we would welcome correspondence from those individuals/companies we have been unable to trace.

Table of Contents

Contents

Contents

Chapter One

Cell Membranes, Epithelial Barriers and Drug Absorption

INTRODUCTION

All living things are made of cells - small individually functional units which, in higher organisms, are organised into collections called *tissues*. A typical cell consists largely of *cytoplasm*, an aqueous liquid in which a wide range of biochemical processes occur. The cytoplasm is held as an intact unit by a *cell membrane*, which surrounds it and prevents it from mixing with its surroundings. Depending on the cell type and function, a number of other structures may be present, particularly a *nucleus*, in which the cell genetic information is stored in the form of DNA. Provision must be made for the supply and retention of substrates from extracellular sources and for the secretion of waste products that would otherwise accumulate in toxic amounts. The outer membrane of the cell must therefore allow penetration of some substances and not others, i.e. it must be selectively permeable. This is one of the most important features of the cell membrane.

Organs and tissues are collections of cells surrounded by specialised cell structures called *epithelia*, which can be thought of as the organ's 'outer membrane' in an analogous fashion to the membrane that surrounds the individual cell. Like cell membranes, they not only bound the organ, but also are the site for a wide range of transport, barrier and secretory processes which vary widely with the particular organ. Many epithelia protect organs from hostile environments (for example the skin or the contents of the stomach) and such cells generally have a rapid turnover and numerous barrier features.

In order for a drug to reach a site of action it must pass from an 'external' site (for example the surface of the skin or the small intestine) to an 'internal' site (the bloodstream or the cytoplasm of a particular cell group). In doing so it will have to pass through a number of tissues and epithelia, either by going through the cells themselves (and thus penetrating their plasma membranes) or by finding pathways between the cells. Overcoming these barriers to absorption is one of the most important considerations in the drug delivery process, and requires a detailed knowledge of the structure and behaviour of the cell membranes and epithelial tissues.

THE PLASMA MEMBRANE

The plasma membrane retains the contents of the cell and acts as a permeability barrier. That is, it allows only certain substances to enter or leave the cell, and the rate of entry is strictly controlled. Early researchers recognised that hydrophobic materials entered cells easily and proposed that an oily or 'lipoidal' layer was present at the cell surface. Gorter and Grendel in 1925 estimated the thickness of this layer by extracting the oily membrane from erythrocytes with acetone and spreading it as a monomolecular film in a Langmuir trough[1]. By measuring the film area and calculating the surface area of the original red cells (chosen since their geometry is reasonably constant), they concluded that exactly two layers of molecules were present at the interface, and proposed a lipid bilayer as the major cell membrane element. We now know that their experiment was subject to a considerable number of errors[2], but fortunately these cancelled out in the final analysis and hence they obtained the correct answer by the wrong route. Electron micrographs indicate a double layered lipid membrane with bands approximately 3 nm in width and an overall thickness of between 8 to 12 nm. Although this is consistent with the lipid bilayer view, electron micrographic evidence was held in doubt for many years due to the difficulty of preparing the samples and the possibility of artefacts at so small a scale.

Subsequent discovery of the incorporation of proteins and polysaccharides led to the fluid mosaic model of Singer and Nicholson[3]. This model tended to suggest that the membrane was a sea of tightly packed phospholipids interspersed with proteins, leading to a rather ill-defined mixed membrane. However, studies during the last decade have demonstrated that the membrane is a highly organised structure; proteins in specific conforma-

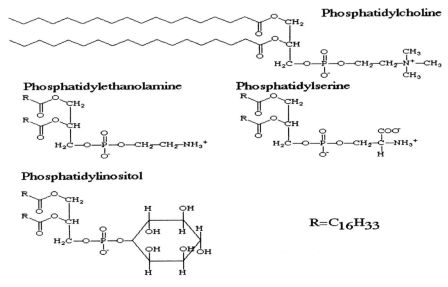

Figure 1.1 Common membrane phospholipids

tions act as structural elements, transport nutrients, and sample the cell environment. The bilayer is not a lipid 'sea' but a carefully designed liquid crystal whose composition is controlled by the cell to achieve a specific degree of fluidity and an optimum environment for the processes which occur within it.

The phospholipid bilayer

The detailed chemistry of the cell membrane was not worked out for many years due to the very large number of components that occur in membranes from varying organs. The development of chromatography was pivotal in allowing the lipid mixtures to be separated into their numerous components for detailed analysis. We now know that the main 'scaffolding' of the bilayer consists of a range of surfactant molecules, of which *phospholipids* are the most important. Most membranes also contain other materials, most notably proteins and sterols, but the surfactant lipids themselves are sufficient to form the lipid bilayer.

Phospholipids are compounds of glycerol (propane-1,2,3-triol) in which two of the alcohol groups are joined to fatty acids, and the third to phosphoric acid (Figure 1.1). The phosphate group can additionally form a bond to a smaller organic molecule (generally a hydrophilic one). The resultant molecule thus has two oily tails, usually of 12-24 carbon atoms' length, and a hydrophilic region around the charged phosphate ester, called the *headgroup*. Common headgroup molecules are choline, ethanolamine, serine and inositol, and the resulting phospholipids are termed phosphatidylcholine, phosphatidylethanolamine, phosphatidylserine and phosphatidylinositol respectively. Due to the cumbersome names these are normally abbreviated to PC, PE, PS and PI. These molecules have a typical surfactant structure. In water surfactants usually aggregate to form *micelles*, small clusters in which the oily tails are turned towards a common centre, since it is energetically unfavourable for the oily tails to be surrounded by water molecules. However, in phospholipids and other membrane-forming surfactants, the molecules aggregate to a bilayer sheet in which the tails are in the centre of the bilayer and the polar headgroups are in contact with the external aqueous environment (Figure 1.2). Phospholipids are not the only surfactants that behave in this way; the distinction between whether a surfactant forms a closed micelle or a

Aqueous Phase

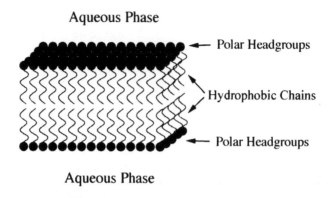

Aqueous Phase

Figure 1.2 The phospholipid bilayer

bilayer sheet depends purely on the geometry of the molecule. Phospholipids form bilayers spontaneously when dispersed in water, as this is their thermodynamically most stable configuration, that is, it has the lowest free energy. However the bilayers do not form infinite planar sheets, but generally close in on themselves to form spherical structures in which one layer is on the outside of the sphere, and the other on the inside, enclosing an aqueous space. Simply shaking phospholipids in water results in the formation of these microscopic structures, which are termed liposomes.

Dynamic behaviour of membranes

Although membranes are often depicted as regular structures, as in Figure 1.2, the reality is that the bilayer is much more disordered and dynamic. The most important dynamic processes are *lateral diffusion*, in which the lipid molecules can move in the plane of the bilayer, and *transverse diffusion* or *flip-flop*, where a lipid molecule switches from one side of the membrane to the other. Since this involves moving the headgroup through the oily core of the bilayer, this is an extremely slow process, and in natural systems is generally catalysed when required by specialised membrane proteins.

The most important factor in determining the dynamic behaviour of the membrane is the *transition temperature* of the bilayer. At low temperatures the lipid tails are held in a relatively ordered array in the bilayer core. As the temperature is raised, little movement takes place until the transition temperature is reached. At this point the lipid spacing increases slightly and the tails become much more disordered in arrangement. The transition is often thought of as a gel-liquid melting of the bilayer, and in the fluid state the lipid molecules are relatively mobile to lateral diffusion; they diffuse at a speed of several microns a second and can move around a typical cell membrane on a timescale of seconds. The transition temperature depends mainly on the structure of the fatty acid chains attached to the glycerol backbone, with unsaturated chains causing low transition temperatures (generally below 0°C) and saturated chains having higher transition temperatures. For example, when the fatty chains in PC are both formed from palmitic acid (C16 saturated fatty acid) the lipid bilayer melts at 42°C. It is thus evident that the cell can control the fluidity of its membrane by varying the fatty acid composition of the phospholipids.

Modulation of membrane fluidity by sterols

Although cell membrane fluidity can be regulated by altering the phospholipid fatty acid content, this is not the organism's only means of control. Most cell membranes contain varying amounts of sterols. In plants the primary membrane sterol is sitosterol; in animals, cholesterol, and in fungi ergosterol, although many other similar compounds also occur. Sterols alter the fluidity of the cell membrane by 'broadening' the melting transition so that the membrane melts over a much wider temperature range than that observed for the lipid alone. This is illustrated in Figure 1.3, which is a thermogram for the melting of a typical lipid membrane, in this case dipalmitoyl phosphatidylcholine. A thermogram is a plot of the energy absorbed as the temperature of the system is raised; the peak is caused by the absorption of energy required to melt the lipid bilayer. In the absence of sterols the bilayer melts over a small temperature range, causing a sharp peak in the thermogram. In the presence of cholesterol the melting transition is much broader, and the thermogram peak spans several degrees. The membrane begins to melt at a lower temperature than in the absence of sterol, and retains some structure up to a temperature above the transition temperature of the pure lipid. The effect of this is to 'smear out' the melting of the membrane, so that the fluidity is not so dependent on temperature. Obviously, this is of considerable importance in allowing the cell to function over a range of temperatures.

Models of cell membranes

Cell membranes are extremely complex structures, and it is difficult to untangle all the aspects of their behaviour by studying whole cells. Consequently, most of our understanding of membrane function has arisen from a study of membrane models, systems which display certain aspects of membrane behaviour without the complexity of the whole cell. We have already mentioned liposomes, which are the spherical structures formed when

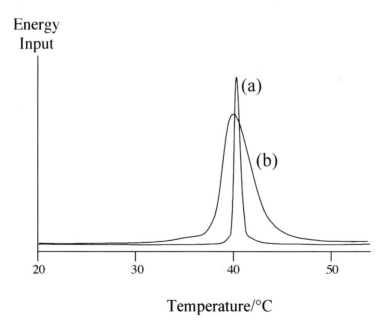

Figure 1.3 Melting transition in DPPC bilayers (a) DPPC (b) DPPC + cholesterol. Note the broadening of the peak due to the inclusion of the sterol.

phospholipids are dispersed in water. Liposomes made in this way are actually multilay-ered, in a concentric 'onion-like' structure, and unlike cells do not have a large central aqueous space. They are termed large multilamellar vesicles or MLVs. Exposure to shear fields (normally by ultrasound) breaks them into small unilamellar vesicles or SUVs which are, however, rather smaller than single cells. Better membrane models are provided by giant unilamellar vesicles (GUVs) which can be made by careful injection of ethanolic lipid solutions into water.

Although liposomes can be made from well-characterised lipid mixtures, it is often useful to study natural membranes which have a more 'natural' structure, without the com-plexity added by the cell contents. The most widely used model in this respect is the *eryth-rocyte ghost*, which is the membrane surrounding a red blood cell from which the contents have been removed. These are prepared by placing the cells in hypertonic saline, which causes pores to form in the membrane. The cell contents then equilibrate with the suspend-ing medium, and since this is normally much larger in volume than the total cell interior, the cells effectively become washed clean. Markers such as dyes or radiolabels can then be added, and will equilibrate with the solution inside the cells. If the tonicity is then adjusted to normal, the cell pores will re-seal and the cells, now labelled in their inner space, can be washed free of unentrapped marker by repeated centrifugation. There have been several attempts to place drugs inside the cells which are then returned to the donor, the idea being that they will then not be recognised as foreign, the outer membrane having the donor's correct antigen profile[4]. This has proven only partly successful, the cell surfaces being easily damaged during the labelling process.

The most serious problem with these membrane models is that it is only possible to access the outside of the membrane, the interior being sealed, unless an invasive technique such as the insertion of a microelectrode is used. This problem can be avoided by the use of *black lipid films*, a technique in which a lipid bilayer is formed across a small hole in the partition of a two-compartment vessel (Figure 1.4). The technique allows access to both sides of the membrane so that electrical measurements can be made, and the composition of the fluid on either side of the membrane can be readily altered. Using this method it is, for example, possible to measure the ion current across the membrane caused by pore-forming antibiotics, and study the operation of ion pump proteins.

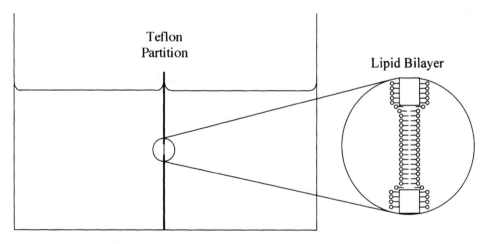

Figure 1.4 The black lipid film between 2 aqueous compartments

Membrane proteins

The cell membrane is home for a number of types of proteins, which are generally divided into integral proteins and peripheral proteins. Integral proteins contain a sequence of hydrophobic groups that are embedded in the lipid bilayer, while peripheral proteins are adsorbed on to the surface of the cell, generally attached to an integral protein. The majority of functional proteins are integral, the most important peripheral proteins being the spectrin and ankyrin proteins. These bind to the inside of the plasma membrane to form the cytoskeleton, a network of proteins which runs throughout the cell, and is involved in a range of structural and transport functions.

One of the most important groups of integral membrane proteins from a pharmacological viewpoint is the transport proteins. These are responsible for moving substances into and out of the cell; for example, ATPase proteins pump ions across the cell membranes to maintain the required Na^+/K^+ electrolyte imbalance, and secrete H^+ from the gastric parietal cells. Proteins also recognise and transport nutrients such as small carbohydrates and amino acids into the cell, each protein transporting a small group of structurally similar compounds.

A second important group of membrane proteins are the cell surface receptors. Although many biochemical receptors are present in the cytosol, a number of important materials are recognised by membrane proteins. These include a range of pituitary hormones, histamine receptors on mast cells, prostaglandins, and gastric peptides in the intestine.

Glycoproteins are a group of integral proteins carrying polysaccharide chains which are responsible for cell recognition and immunological behaviour. The segment of the protein chain, which is external to the cell, consists of hydrophilic protein residues, many of which carry small carbohydrate groups such as sialic acid. In many cells, these hydrophilic oligosaccharides form a continuous coat around the cell, together with polysaccharides attached to lipids (glycolipids). This layer is termed the *glycocalyx*. A common component of this layer is a peripheral protein called fibronectin, which contains binding sites for many membrane proteins, extracellular structural proteins such as collagen, and polysaccharides, and is thus an important component in intercellular binding and tissue formation.

Membrane asymmetry

Although liposomes are normally made with a similar lipid composition on both the inside and outside, living cells are much more asymmetric since they perform a range of processes which are obviously directional. The phospholipid composition of the inside and outside layers of the membrane is different in most cells; for example in the erythrocyte membrane phosphatidylcholine occurs predominantly on the outside of the cell and phosphatidylethanolamine predominantly on the inside. Glycolipids are normally oriented so that the polysaccharide segment is outside the cell, since it is responsible for immunogenicity and tissue adhesion. Integral proteins always have a specific orientation in the membrane that depends on their function; all molecules of the protein point in the same direction.

EPITHELIA

With a few exceptions, all internal and external body surfaces are covered with epithelium. This consists of a layer of structural protein, normally collagen, called the *basal lamina*, on which sit one or more layers of epithelial cells. There are several morphologically distinct common epithelial types (Figure 1.5):

a) Simple squamous epithelium. This forms a thin layer of flattened cells and consequently is relatively permeable. This type of epithelium lines most of the blood vessels.

(a)   (b)

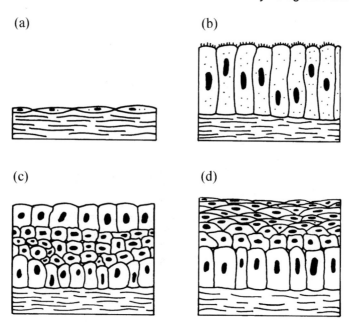

(c)   (d)

Figure 1.5 Common epithelial membrane types (a) simple squamous (b) simple columnar (c) transitional (d) stratified squamous epithelium

b) Simple columnar epithelium. A single layer of columnar cells is found in the epithelium of organs such as the stomach and small intestine.

c) Transitional epithelium. This is composed of several layers of cells of different shapes and it lines epithelia which are required to stretch.

d) Stratified squamous epithelium. These membranes are several cells thick and are found in areas which have to withstand large amounts of wear and tear, for example the inside of the mouth and oesophagus, and the vagina. In the skin the outer cells become filled with keratin, and then die and slough off from the outside. This type of epithelium is termed *keratinized* and provides a major permeability barrier as well as protection from the environment.

Epithelial cells are said to be polarised due to the asymmetric distribution of transport proteins on the opposite ends of their plasma membranes. This causes the transport activity of the apical membrane of the cell to be different to that of the basolateral membrane. For example, nutrients absorbed across the intestinal epithelium have to cross two types of barrier to enter the blood from the lumen. At the apex of the cell, nutrients are actively transported into the cell by carrier-mediated mechanisms. At the base of the cell they are resecreted out of the cell and into the bloodstream by different transport proteins.

Cell junctions

In the vast majority of tissues the cell membranes are not in close contact, but have an irregular intermembrane space of approximately 20 nanometres. Between this space lies the glycocalyx of the cells and a collection of glycoproteins and binding proteins such as fibronectin. In many tissues this space is bathed by the extracellular fluid and so is relatively permeable to small molecules. Drugs injected into a tissue of this type can diffuse with relative freedom. A typical example of this behaviour is the diffusion of drugs from an intramuscular injection, which rapidly spreads through the local muscle cells and into the

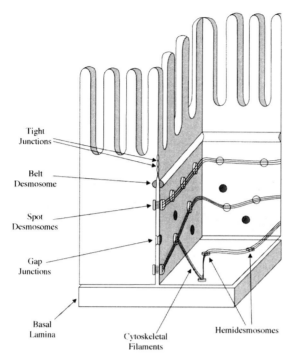

Figure 1.6 Intestinal epithelium illustrating the various types of junction

bloodstream. In epithelial tissues there is a need for a more effective chemical and physical barrier, and as a result the epithelial cells are bonded together by a number of different types of junctions which prevent diffusion of solutes around the cells. The primary types are (Figure 1.6):

      a) tight junctions or zonulae occludens
      b) gap junctions
      c) desmosomes or zonulae adherens.

Tight junctions

Tight junctions are formed when specific proteins in two adjacent plasma membranes make direct contact across the intercellular space (Figure 1.7). A belt-like structure composed of many protein strands completely encircles each cell in the epithelium, attaching it to its neighbours and sealing the outer (luminal) space from the interior of the tissue or organ. At a tight junction, the interacting plasma membranes are so closely apposed that there is no intercellular space and the membranes are within 2Å of each other. As these junctions can be disrupted either by treatment with proteolytic enzymes or by agents that chelate Ca^{2+} or Mg^{2+}, both the proteins and divalent cations are thought to be required for maintaining their integrity. Beneath the tight junction, the spaces between adjacent cells are wider[5]. The structure of the epithelium has been likened to "a six-pack of beer extended indefinitely in 2 dimensions"[6].

Tight junctions play a critical part in maintaining the selective barrier function of cell sheets. For example, the epithelial cells lining the small intestine must keep most of the gut contents in the lumen. Simultaneously, the cells must pump selected nutrients across the cell sheet into the extracellular fluid on the other side, from which they are absorbed into

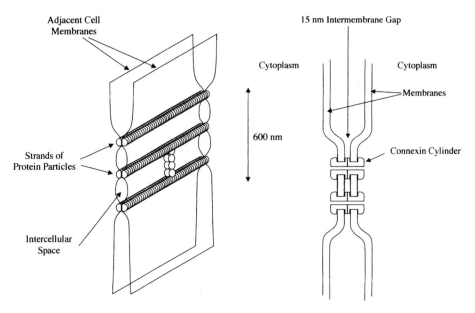

Figure 1.7 The tight junction   Figure 1.8 The gap junction

the blood. Studies have shown that the tight junctions are impermeable to colloidal particles, small molecules and ions, and possibly even to water. Electron microscopy shows that
the junction consists of protein particles which are partly embedded in the membranes of
both cells, so that the membranes become a single fused unit. As well as sealing the cells
together, this prevents membrane proteins from the apical side of the cell diffusing to the
basal side, maintaining the polarization of the cell.

Gap junctions

The commonest type of cell junction is the gap junction, which is widely distributed
in tissues of all animals (Figure 1.8). It is not so much an adhesion point between cells as a
means by which cells may communicate via the exchange of cytoplasmic materials. Gap
junctions consist of regions in which the gap between adjacent cell membranes narrows to
approximately 2 to 3 nm, over a cross-sectional area of several hundred square nanometres.
In this region both cell membranes contain a specialised protein called connexin, which
forms tubular hexameric clusters with a central pore. These clusters are aligned in both
membranes so that they form a path from one cell to another, through which cytoplasm and
its solutes can be transferred.

Molecules up to 1200 Daltons can pass freely through the gaps but larger molecules
cannot, suggesting a functioning pore size for the connecting channels of about 1.5 nm.
Coupled cells share a variety of small molecules (such as inorganic ions, sugars, amino
acids, nucleotides and vitamins) but do not share their macromolecules (proteins, nucleic
acids and polysaccharides). ATP can pass between the cells, as can cyclic AMP, which
mediates many types of hormonal control. Consequently, hormonal stimulation in just one
or a few epithelial cells will initiate a metabolic response in many cells. Gap junctions
close in the presence of high concentrations of Ca^{2+} ions, so that if a cell is damaged, the
influx of extracellular calcium will seal the cell's gap junctions and prevent the leak extending through the tissue.

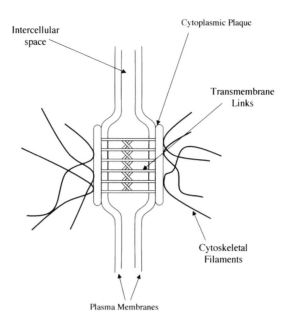

Figure 1.9 The desmosome

Desmosomes

Desmosomes are small structures which bond adjacent cells together, and are most abundant in tissues that are subject to severe mechanical stress, such as cardiac muscle, skin epithelium and the neck of the uterus (Figure 1.9). They are widely distributed in tissues, and enable groups of cells to function as structural units. Desmosomes can be divided into three different types: spot desmosomes, belt desmosomes and hemidesmosomes, all three of which are present in most epithelial cells.

Belt desmosomes form a continuous band around each of the cells in an epithelial sheet, near the cell's apical end, typically just below the tight junction. The bands in adjacent cells are directly apposed and are separated by a poorly characterised filamentous material (in the intercellular space) that holds the interacting membranes together. Within each cell, contractile bundles of actin filaments run along the belts just under the plasma membrane and connect the structure to the cytoskeleton.

Spot desmosomes act like rivets to hold epithelial cells together at button-like points of contact. They also serve as anchoring sites for actin filaments which extend from one side of the cell to the other across the cell interior, forming a structural framework for the cytoplasm. Since other filaments extend from cell to cell at spot desmosomes, the actin filament networks inside adjacent cells are connected indirectly through these junctions to form a continuous network of fibres across the entire epithelial sheet.

Hemidesmosomes or half-desmosomes resemble spot desmosomes, but instead of joining adjacent epithelial cell membranes together, they join the basal surface of epithelial cells to the underlying basal lamina. Together spot desmosomes and hemidesmosomes act as bonds that distribute any shearing force through the epithelial sheet and its underlying connective tissue.

TRANSPORT ACROSS CELL MEMBRANES

In order to function correctly a cell must be able to take up and release a wide range of materials; for drug therapy to be successful it must also be possible to get therapeutic substances into cells and across layers of cells such as epithelia. There are a number of possible mechanisms for transport across membranes; substances may simply diffuse across, or be carried by a range of more selective processes, depending on the substance involved.

Passive diffusion

Studies using model membranes have revealed that the phospholipid bilayer itself is remarkably impermeable to all but very small molecules such as water and ethanol, and gases such as oxygen and carbon dioxide. These compounds move across the membrane by *passive diffusion,* a process driven by the random motion of the molecules. Diffusion is described by Fick's law, which states that the diffusion rate R (in moles s^{-1}) is proportional to the concentration gradient $\Delta c/\Delta x$:

$$R = -D \, A \, \Delta c/\Delta x$$

Where Δc is the concentration difference between the outside and inside of the membrane, and Δx is the thickness of the membrane. A is the area of membrane over which diffusion is occurring, and D is a constant (for a specific molecule in a specific environment) called its *diffusion coefficient.* Since the area and thickness of the membrane are usually outside our control, it is evident that uptake of a molecule into a cell by passive diffusion can only be influenced by either increasing the external concentration of the drug, or by selecting our molecule so that D is large.

The diffusion coefficient of a drug is determined by a number of factors, but two are particularly important. These are the *solubility* of the drug, and its *molecular weight.* For a molecule to diffuse freely in a hydrophobic membrane it must be soluble in it, and conversely if it is to also diffuse in the extracellular fluid it must also be soluble in aqueous systems. The relative solubility of molecules in aqueous or oily environments is described by their *partition coefficient,* labelled P, which describes how the drug distributes itself between a pair of solvents (usually water and an oily solvent such as octanol). Hydrophobic molecules dissolve mainly in the oil and have a high partition coefficient, while hydrophilic molecules dissolve mainly in the water and have a low partition coefficient. Only for intermediate values of the partition coefficient will the drug be soluble in both the membrane and the extracellular fluid, and be free to diffuse from the extracellular fluid, across the membrane, and into the cell. Drugs which have a very low partition coefficient are poorly absorbed because they cannot dissolve in the oily membrane; conversely drugs which have a high partition coefficient cannot dissolve in the extracellular fluid and so cannot reach the membrane. Such drugs are said to be *solubility-limited.*

The diffusion coefficient, and hence rate of absorption, is also influenced by the molecular weight of the drug. Small molecules diffuse rapidly and so will cross the membrane more quickly than large, slowly-diffusing molecules. These concepts are illustrated in Figure 1.10, which shows how absorption depends on partition coefficient for drugs of different molecular weights. This is not based on specific drugs but is intended to illustrate the concepts. The drug with a molecular weight of 400 is rapidly absorbed for intermediate partition coefficients (P of approximately 100 or Log P = 2). However, it is absorbed more slowly for larger values of P as its aqueous solubility falls, or for smaller values of P as its membrane solubility falls. The smaller drug with a molecular weight of 250 is subject to the same influence of P, but is generally absorbed more quickly due to its more rapid diffusion.

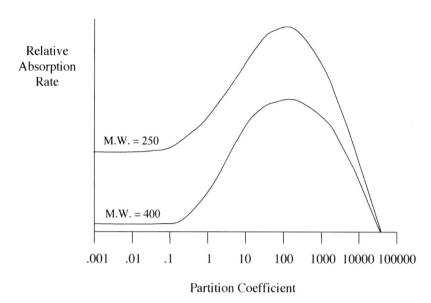

Figure 1.10 Absorption as a function of drug partition coefficient

Figure 1.10 shows how the diffusion of drug across a pure lipid membrane will vary depending on the properties of the drug. However, drug diffusion across real cell epithelia takes place not only through membranes, but also through small aqueous pores between cells (the *paracellular* route), and this enhances the absorption of hydrophilic molecules which are small enough to pass through the pores. The drug with a molecular weight of 250 can pass through these pores, but that with a higher molecular weight of 400 cannot.

The pH-partition hypothesis

Drug molecules are predominantly weakly ionizable species containing groups such as amine, carboxyl, phenyl, etc. These materials are absorbed across plasma membranes in their unionised forms, since these are non-polar; the ionised forms of the drug cannot pass through the membrane due to its hydrophobic character. Consequently, the pH of the extra-cellular environment is critical in determining the absorption across the membrane. Thus, for example, an acidic drug is absorbed from acidic solution if the pH is lower than the drug pK, since it will be in its unionised form. This is the basis of the pH-partition hypothesis, stressed in most classical texts of pharmacology, which discuss the absorption of drugs based on the relative degrees of ionization in the lumen and the blood.

The pH-partition hypothesis provides an indication of drug absorption, but suffers from many shortcomings. The most notable of these can be seen in the widely quoted example of the absorption of an acidic drug from the stomach, in which the drug is in its unionised state at pH 2 and so passes across the membrane. In the blood (at pH 7.4) the drug is ionized, and so cannot pass back across the membrane. This effect is referred to as ion-trapping. The conclusion is that pH and ionization are highly important in determining drug absorption. This example is logically correct but suffers from a number of errors. The gastric epithelium represents the most extreme example available of a pH gradient *in vivo,* but drug absorption from the stomach is minimal and most absorption takes place in the small intestine, which is normally close to pH 7. Here the ionisation of the drug in the lumen is similar to that in the blood and little ion-trapping can occur. Gastric contents delivered into the duodenum make the first few centimetres of the intestine acidic, until the chyme has been neutralised by bicarbonate. The duodenal absorptive capacity is high, but transit through this region is extremely rapid and so no significant absorption occurs.

The biggest failing of this hypothesis is to attempt to calculate absorption from equilibrium drug distributions, when in practice the absorbed drug is swept away by the circulation. Absorption is a dynamic process involving dissolution, ionization, partition and blood flow, and consequently the correlation of pH-partition predictions with experiment is often poor.

Facilitated and carrier mediated diffusion

Despite the hydrophobic nature of the cell membrane, it is necessary for a number of hydrophilic materials to enter and leave the cell. Typical examples are small amino acids and carbohydrates, which the cell requires in quantity for metabolism. Ions are also required, as the cell maintains an ion imbalance with the surroundings, with the cell having substantially more potassium and less sodium than the extracellular fluid.

Since these molecules cannot diffuse freely across the cell membrane, they are transported by a range of membrane proteins collectively called *permeases*. These proteins fall into two broad groups, those which allow molecules to pass into the cell down a concentration gradient, and behave like passive but selective pores, and those which actively pump molecules into cells against a concentration gradient. The former group contains transporters that allow nutrients such as glucose into the cell; this *hexose transporter system* is present in most mammalian cells. Since the glucose is utilized inside the cell rapidly, the internal concentration is low and the diffusion always occurs down a concentration gradient. Consequently, no input of energy is required to drive this transport system.

The second group of proteins actively accumulate materials in cells even if their concentration is higher inside the cell than outside. This requires an input of energy, usually derived from the hydrolysis of intracellular ATP, and consequently the carriers are called ATPases. The best known examples are the Na^+/K^+ ATPase that pumps potassium into the cell and sodium out, and the H^+/K^+ ATPase which pumps hydrogen ions out of the gastric parietal cells, thus acidifying the stomach contents.

An important characteristic of carrier-mediated absorption is that it is *saturable*. If the external concentration of the molecule being transported is extremely high, the carrier will be fully utilized and will become rate limiting. Under these conditions, increasing the external concentration of the transported molecule will have no effect on the transport rate. The maximum transport rate will be determined by the concentration of carrier molecules and the speed with which they can shuttle material across the membrane, and not by the concentration of the molecules being transported.

A number of drugs are thought to be absorbed by carrier-mediated processes rather than passive diffusion. These include amoxycillin and cyclacillin[7], which show saturable kinetics, and cardioglycosides such as digitalis. The actual carrier mechanism is unclear since these materials are xenobiotics and are presumably being transported by a protein which normally serves some other purpose.

Cotransport

Energy must be expended in order to pump any molecule up a concentration gradient, and this is ultimately derived from ATP hydrolysis. The only transport systems that are directly coupled to ATP are those which pump ions such as Na^+ and Ca^{2+}. However, cells often have to accumulate other materials, such as amino-acids and carbohydrates, at high concentrations. This is performed by cotransport, in which the cells' ion concentration

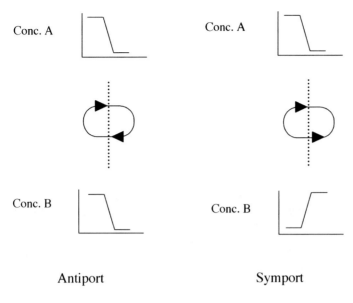

Antiport   Symport

Figure 1.11 Cotransport across membranes

gradient is used as a secondary energy source (Figure 1.11). The transport proteins are systems which couple the transport of an ion to that of another molecule, so that, in allowing an ion to move out of the membrane to a lower concentration, the protein also moves a different molecule from lower to higher concentration. If the ion and molecule move across the membrane in the same direction, the process is called symport, while if they are exchanged in opposite directions it is called antiport.

An important example of this process is the absorption of glucose from the intestinal lumen by the intestinal epithelial cells. In most cells glucose is actively metabolized, so its concentration is low and it can be transported by passive transport. However, the intestinal epithelium is responsible for absorbing molecules like glucose, so it is often necessary to pump them up a concentration gradient into the epithelial cells before they can be passed into the bloodstream. This is accomplished by a sodium-glucose symport protein which couples the inward movement of a glucose molecule to that of a sodium ion. The intracellular sodium concentration is lower than in the intestinal lumen, so the inward movement of sodium is energetically favourable. A glucose molecule is simultaneously transported into the epithelial cell up a concentration gradient.

Uptake of macromolecules and particles

Membrane transport by diffusion or by transport proteins is only feasible for small molecules, since there is a limit to the size of pore that can be opened and closed by the conformational change of a membrane protein. Consequently, larger objects, such as macromolecules and particles, are internalized by a completely different mechanism, in which a portion of the membrane extends and envelops the object, drawing it into the cell to form a vacuole. This process is called *cytosis* and there are a number of variants which occur in different cells.

Endocytosis occurs when a small cavity forms on the membrane surface, which is gradually enclosed by membrane movement and finally taken within the cell (Figure 1.12). The process may be spontaneous in certain cells, and causes a small amount of extracellular

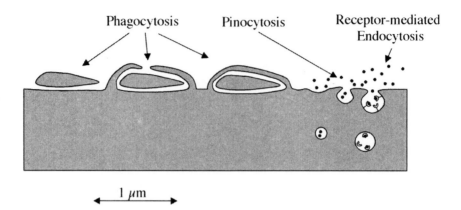

Figure 1.12 Uptake of particles and solutes by cytosis

fluid to enter the cell. This is called *pinocytosis*. More commonly the process is triggered by the binding of a particular macromolecule to a surface receptor on the membrane, a process termed *receptor-mediated endocytosis*.

Phagocytosis occurs when a particle is taken inside a cell. The most important example of this occurs when a white blood cell called a macrophage engulfs a foreign body such as a bacterium or virus. The foreign body first adheres to the cell membrane, which then gradually extends over it until it is internalized to form a vacuole within the cell. This then normally fuses with lysosomes and is degraded. The vacuoles formed in this process are much larger than those involved in endocytosis.

INTERCELLULAR ROUTES OF ABSORPTION

As well as being absorbed through the epithelial cells, molecules can pass through tissues via the intercellular or paracellular route through junctional gaps between cells. There has been much discussion regarding the importance of this process in transport across the gastrointestinal mucosa. There is considerable variation in the integrity of the tight junctions along the gastrointestinal tract, with the membranes of the stomach and large intestine having the highest transepithelial resistance. Norris and coworkers suggested that molecules with a greater molecular radius than 1.1 nm cannot permeate the intestinal paracellular space[8]. The pore size has been calculated to be 0.8 nm in the jejunum and 0.3 nm in the ileum and colon, so it unlikely that molecules of a significant size could be absorbed from the intestine by this route.

PERSORPTION

There is a special mode of permeation across the intestinal wall in which the cell membranes are not involved. Intestinal cells are continuously produced in the crypts of Lieberkühn and migrate towards the tip of the villus. During digestion the cells are sloughed off leaving a temporary gap at the cell apex, and through this gap large particles can slip into the circulation through the intercellular gaps. This process has been termed persorption. The observation that large objects such as starch grains can be found in the blood after a meal of potatoes or corn is often quoted as the prima facie evidence of persorption (Figure 1.13). Volkheimer and coworkers[9] hypothesised that a "kneading" action of the villus on the luminal contents allowed particles of up to 100 μm diameter to enter the lamina propria

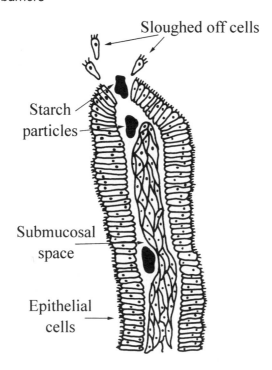

Figure 1.13 Persorption in the intestinal villus

of the intestinal mucosa near the apex of the villus. Metallic iron particles of up to 52 μm were identified in both portal venous blood and thoracic duct lymph of dogs after the animals were fed 200 g of iron powder suspended in milk and cream. There is also some evidence that very small numbers of polymer particles can pass from the intestinal lumen into the bloodstream in this way[10]. Large foreign particles should be expected to enter intestinal lymph vessels in preference to mucosal blood vessels and it is remarkable that such large particles should appear at all in portal venous blood without finding their way to the lung capillary filter. It is possible that potentially harmful materials such as asbestos fibre can be absorbed in this way, but a detailed understanding of these effects is still lacking, and artefacts in many of the published experiments cannot be discounted.

MUCUS

Most epithelia consist of a number of different cell types with different functions. One cell that is common in many epithelia is the mucosal cell, which secretes mucus. An epithelium containing mucosal cells is called a mucosal epithelium or simply mucosa.

Mucus has several functions. It restricts the penetration of large molecules, and prevents the tissue from dehydrating. It keeps the tissue surface clean by its continuous removal, and lubricates the passage of materials such as food through the gastrointestinal tract. Its most important property is its viscoelasticity, which enables it to act as a locally rigid mechanical barrier which can flow under the influence of peristalsis. The primary component of mucus is a large polysaccharide called mucin built up in subunits of 500,000 Daltons or larger. It consists of a protein backbone approximately 800 amino acids long, rich in serine and threonine, which are hydroxylated amino acids. Most of the hydroxy-residues are linked to oligosaccharide side chains which serve to stiffen the backbone, and which carry an extensive layer of water of hydration. The oligosaccharide chains are generally up to 18 residues in length and are composed of N-acetylgalactosamine, N-acetylglucosamine, galactose, fucose or N-acetylneuraminic acid.

Mucus is 95% water and so makes intimate contact with hydrophilic surfaces. Small particles less than ~600 μm (the average thickness of a mucus layer) may be buried in the surface and held securely due to the stickiness of the mucus, but since the mucus is continually secreted the particles move further away from the mucosa and are ultimately sloughed off. Small molecules pass easily through mucus due to its high water content; larger molecules diffuse through the mucus more slowly and remain in contact for longer periods.

Many research groups have attempted to develop mucoadhesive materials, the idea being to bind a drug carrier to a mucous membrane in order to optimize drug delivery. However, mucus turnover can be rapid and there seems little point in attaching a drug to a surface which is to be sloughed off in a short time.

CONCLUSIONS

The absorption of drugs, although dependent on the site of absorption, is often controlled by similar types of barriers. These are mucus, hydrophobic membranes, transport processes and cell junctions. In the following chapters we will see how these barriers manifest themselves in different organs according to the form and function of the tissue involved, and how they determine the success or failure of drug delivery technology.

REFERENCES

1. Gorter E, Grendel F. Bimolecular layers of lipoids on chromatocytes of blood. *J. Exp. Med.* 1925;41:439-443.
2. Bar RS, Deamer DW, Cornwell DG. Surface area of human erythrocyte lipids: reinvestigation of experiments on plasma membrane. *Science* 1966;153:1010-1012.
3. Singer SJ, Nicholson GL. The fluid mosaic model of the structure of cell membranes. *Science New York* 1972;175:720-731.
4. Bax BE, Bain MD, Talbot PJ, Parker Williams EJ, Chalmers RA. Survival of human carrier erythrocytes *in vivo. Clin. Sci.*1999;96:171-178.
5. Esposito G. Polarity of intestinal epithelial cells: permeability of the brush border and basolateral membranes. In *Pharmacology of Intestinal Permeation Vol. 1* ed. Csáky T.Z. Springer Verlag, Berlin 1984:283-308.
6. Diamond JM. The epithelial junction: bridge, gate and fence. *Physiologist* 1977;20:10-18.
7. Csáky TZ. Intestinal permeation and permeability: an overview. In *Pharmacology of Intestinal Permeation Vol. 1* ed. Csáky T.Z. Springer Verlag, Berlin 1984:51-59.
8. Norris DA, Puri N, Sinko PJ. The effect of physical barriers on the oral absorption of particulates. *Adv. Drug Deliv. Rev.* 1998;34:135-154.
9. Volkheimer G, Schulz FH, Lindenau A, Beitz U. Persorption of metallic iron particles. *Gut* 1969;10:32-33.
10. Jani P, McCarthy DE, Florence AT. Nanosphere and microsphere uptake via Peyer's patches: observation of the rate of uptake in the rat after a single oral dose. *Int. J. Pharmaceut.* 1992;86:239-246.

Chapter Two

Parenteral Drug Delivery

INTRODUCTION

The term parenteral drug delivery covers a number of administration routes, which have little in common other than the fact that they generally involve the use of a hypodermic needle to inject the drug into the body. This route bypasses a number of physiological barriers and hence the constraints on the composition and formulation of the medicine are much more rigorous than for less invasive routes such as oral or transdermal delivery. Despite this a surprising range of materials can be injected into various tissues if the appropriate precautions are taken. We will examine the constraints for specific formulations with respect to the appropriate physiological route, but a number of general principles are common to all routes. The most important is that the formulation must be sterile, since the major defence mechanisms of the body (the skin and mucous membranes) are bypassed, and so any infective agent in the formulation may cause major disease. It is not only necessary to remove live microorganisms; parts of dead organisms can elicit an immune response, and polysaccharides from the bacterial cell wall, known as pyrogens, can cause a substantial increase in body temperature.

The most important routes of parenteral delivery are intravenous and intramuscular, with subcutaneous being widely used for small volumes and for vaccination. There are a number of less important routes, since it is generally possible to inject materials into virtually any part of the body in an attempt to gain a rapid local action. Thus we also have relatively specialized routes such as intrathecal, intraarticular and intracardiac.

INTRAVENOUS DELIVERY

Physiology

Intravenous delivery involves the direct injection of the formulation into the venous circulation. To understand the behaviour of intravenous drugs it is essential to consider the function of the circulatory system. This is shown in diagrammatic form in Figure 2.1. Although the heart is normally described as a pump, it is in fact two pumps, one of which circulates the blood around the tissues, and one which circulates it specifically around the lungs in a separate loop. Oxygenated blood is pumped by the left side of the heart through the aorta and arteries into a network of capillaries which allow transfer of oxygen and nutrients into the tissues, and remove waste products. The blood is then collected by a network of veins and passes into the right side of the heart. It is then passed through the pulmonary circulation into the lungs, where it loses carbon dioxide produced by tissue respiration, and is reoxygenated. It then passes back to the left side of the heart for the cycle to repeat.

Not all of the circulation from the tissues returns directly to the heart. A fraction, in particular that which perfuses the gastrointestinal tract, is pumped to the liver first. The liver performs a wide range of metabolic processes, but for drug delivery it can be rather more of a hindrance since it absorbs a fraction of the drug from the bloodstream and begins the cycle of metabolism and excretion. Consequently drugs which are administered orally will visit the liver before they have the opportunity to reach the target tissue; this effect is called first pass metabolism and can remove a significant and often unpredictable fraction of the dose. When the drug is injected into a vein it passes directly into the heart, and is carried to the tissues before passing on to the liver. Consequently first pass metabolism is avoided and the drug has an opportunity to act on the tissues before it passes to the liver on subsequent cycles around the circulation.

The capillaries are, in general, designed to retain their contents, and so in most tissues the capillary endothelial cells are in close contact without gaps, and a continuous basement membrane underlies them. Capillaries of this type can allow only relatively small solutes, such as water, low molecular weight drugs, and small proteins (maximum molecular weight

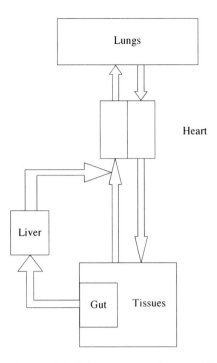

Figure 2.1 Schematic circulation of the blood

<10 KDa) to diffuse into the surrounding tissues. This mixture forms the interstitial fluid which bathes the tissues, and under normal conditions there is a slow outflow of this fluid from the capillaries, driven by the blood pressure within the circulation and the osmotic pressure of its solutes. If this fluid accumulated continuously, oedema would result, so it is drained into highly permeable blind-ending capillaries which are the termini of the lymphatic system. These capillaries combine to form the lymph ducts which empty into the bloodstream again in major veins. In certain specialised or diseased areas the capillaries are more permeable and allow larger solutes and particles to leave the circulation. These will be discussed shortly.

Advantages and disadvantages of intravenous delivery

Intravenous delivery of drugs offers significant advantages which cannot easily be achieved by other routes. The most important of these is the rapidity of action which results from the drug being presented directly to the circulation without the need for release from a formulation or absorption through an epithelium. As a result it is possible for the physician to titrate the dose of drug to obtain a desired response, a procedure which is rarely possible with other routes owing to the time lag between administration and action. Dye and tracer experiments have demonstrated that liquids injected into an arm of a human subject appear in the leg within 20-30 seconds, attesting to the rapidity with which the formulation becomes spread around the body.

The second advantage of intravenous administration is a much more predictable response than is obtained from other routes. The uncertainty of poor or incomplete absorption and its variability is eliminated, so that blood levels are more predictable and pharmacokinetics is much simpler, being confined to elimination pathways alone. As a result new drugs (new chemical entities or NCEs in the trade) are usually studied firstly as intravenous formulations to elucidate their pharmacokinetics and metabolism before oral formulations are developed. Many drugs cannot be usefully administered by any other route because they are degraded in the stomach (for example, peptides) or are unabsorbed due to their insolubility, size, or molecular properties (for example the antifungal amphotericin B). In these cases parenteral delivery is one of the few available options. Finally it should be noted that intravenous delivery can be used when the patient cannot be fed orally (for example they may be comatose or have had gastric resection) or is uncooperative, as in the case of psychiatric patients.

Despite being the most direct and rapid route of delivery, the intravenous route is paradoxically one of the safest for the testing of new drugs. If the drug under test is infused over a period of several minutes, delivery can be stopped instantly should any adverse reaction develop. In comparison, if the drug under test was administered using an oral formulation, the material in the gastrointestinal tract would be absorbed over a period of hours. Hence combating a serious adverse effect would be much more difficult since the unadsorbed material in the small intestine would be almost impossible to remove; absorption would persist and the adverse effect would be more difficult to terminate.

There are a number of disadvantages which generally confine intravenous delivery to situations where its specific advantages are vital. Foremost among these is the need for extensive training of medical staff so that the correct amount of drug goes into the right place with the right technique. As a result this is an expensive procedure and generally only used within a clinic or hospital where appropriate facilities are available. Sterility must be maintained, so the formulation must be prepared and handled in a sterile fashion, although the availability of radiation-sterilized disposable syringes, needles and ancillary equipment has done much to ease this burden. Dosages must always be checked; even so there are still occasional incidences of errors in dosing leading to serious injury or death. There are a number of complications which can have serious consequences. These include:

i) Air embolism, or the injection of air into a vessel. Small air bubbles may be absorbed in the blood but larger amounts (a few ml) of air can prove fatal, particularly if it reaches the brain. To prevent this most infusion pumps are designed to stop pumping and sound an alarm if air is present in the line.

ii) Thrombosis, the formation of a clot in a blood vessel, can be particularly dangerous if the clot circulates in the bloodstream. Certain disease states, or old age, can predispose to thrombosis, but it can also be caused by irritant formulations which are injected too rapidly.

iii) Haemolysis, the breakdown of red cells with the release of haemoglobin, can cause kidney damage if severe. This is normally a problem with strongly hypotonic injections, although certain membrane-active drugs such as amphotericin B can also cause this problem.

iv) Phlebitis is the inflammation of the vein wall due to irritation from the formulation; it can be caused by the formulation itself, or may be due to precipitation of the drug if injection is too rapid.

v) Extravasation, or the leakage of the injection from the vein into the surrounding tissue, can lead to extensive damage since there may be no mechanism to rapidly clear it fom the injection site. This is a particular problem for cytotoxic materials, (e.g. methotrexate or mitomycin) as it can lead to ulceration and necrosis which is slow to heal[1].

Methods for studying these effects have been reviewed by Yalkowsky[2]. As a result of these problems it is essential that injection sites be used with care, particularly if patients are to be maintained on long-term therapy, since it is possible to run out of usable sites over the lifetime of the patient, and maintaining a viable site is essential. The use of implanted catheters helps considerably; patients undergoing permanent parenteral nutrition have cannulae which must be maintained for several years before replacement. In such cases it is possible to perform treatment in a home setting if the patient can be sufficiently educated in the techniques of sterile handling of total parenteral nutrition mixtures[3].

Formulation considerations

We have already noted that intravenous formulations must be sterile in order to avoid causing an infection. The preferred method of achieving this is by terminal sterilization using an autoclave, but this may not be possible if the formulation is heat sensitive. In this case it can be filtered through a 0.22 μm filter which removes all bacteria and spores, or in some cases it may be possible to sterilize using gamma radiation. If all else fails, the formulation can be prepared in a fully aseptic environment, but this is extremely expensive. Particulate material, such as small fragments of dust, glass, or pieces of rubber closures, must also be rigorously excluded. Pharmacopoeial specifications generally require that no particle larger than 5 μm be present in the formulation; this is largely an unverifiable requirement, but the occurrence of particles in modern infusion fluids is extremely rare.

It might be imagined that the formulation must be very similar in pH and tonicity to blood, but in fact there is considerable latitude, depending on the volume of the formulation and the injection site. Small volume parenterals, defined as those below 100 ml in volume, can be formulated at a pH ranging from 4 to 10, and be considerably hypotonic or hypertonic. Large volume parenterals must be more closely matched to the properties of the blood, and the pH is rarely outside the limits 6-8. Plasma extenders, which are often infused through a peripheral vein, are closely matched in tonicity, but parenteral nutrition mixtures may have a tonicity up to around twice that of blood. Such mixtures are usually administered through an indwelling catheter which empties into the subclavian vein[4]. In this case the infusion is very rapidly diluted, so that variations in its properties are of lesser importance. There is increasing interest in the use of peripheral sites for parenteral nutrition, and in these cases the mixtures should be close to isotonic in order to avoid damage at the infusion site[5].

Ideally all injections would be formulated at pH 7.4 and be isotonic with blood; however it is often necessary to use less physiologically acceptable solvents, especially to aid the solubility of a drug which may be poorly soluble near neutral pH, or to control stability. In certain cases it may also be necessary to add cosolvents such as ethanol or propylene glycol, or surfactant-based solubilizing agents (for example deoxycholate, which is used to solubilize amphotéricin B in the injectable Fungizone®). These injections are far from physiological and it is wise to infuse them slowly over several minutes, or ideally with an infusion pump, to ensure that they are rapidly diluted as they enter the blood. However, their use poses an additional problem. If the injection has been formulated under extreme conditions to enhance the drug solubility, when it is injected it becomes diluted in the bloodstream, and the drug may precipitate. This can lead to unpredictable pharmacokinetics as submicron drug particles are processed by the reticuloendothelial system (see below), and cause pain and damage at the injection site. The situation becomes even less predictable if the formulation is added to a concurrent intravenous fluid by an inexperienced clinician, and precipitates in the infusion bag.

Devices and technologies

A wide range of technologies have been developed to reduce the effort and training, and associated cost, of intravenous delivery. In its simplest form the use of sterile disposables minimizes the possibility of infection, and the cost of resterilizing syringes is far greater than that of disposables, even when the cost of proper disposal is taken into account.

Long term infusions are generally administered through catheters, which range in length from a few inches for peripheral use, to much longer devices which can be implanted so that they reach the subclavian vein for the infusion of hypertonic solutions, for example in TPN. Catheters are generally made of PVC, Teflon, polyethylene, silicones or polyurethane, with the latter being preferred for long-term use[6].

Although small volumes are often infused manually, mechanical pumps are used if a low infusion rate is required. These can be used to drive conventional syringes, or to infuse larger volumes from bags. For long-term administration of small volumes, implantable pumps can be used, and there is now considerable interest in allowing the patient a degree of control over the infusion rate, as in patient-controlled analgesia.

A major source of cost and effort in intravenous therapy is associated with the preparation of the material for administration, particularly if complex mixtures are required. As a result a large number of packaging systems have been devised, including prepacked minibags, premixed drugs in intravenous fluids, and frozen premixes. Reconstitution systems such as the Abbott Add-Vantage and Lilly Faspak allow the drug to be administered from the container in which it was reconstituted, avoiding a transfer step. The increased cost of novel packagings like this can often be justified since it may avoid major expenditure on skilled labour and sterile compounding facilities.

Injected particulates

Although pharmacopoeial specifications generally require parenterals to be free of particles, there are occasions in which we need to understand the behaviour of particulate materials in the bloodstream, not least because they may form the basis of potentially useful drug delivery systems. Particles present in intravenous fluids will pass through the heart and circulate around the pulmonary circulation. This represents the first stage of filtration in which any material with a particle size larger than around 5 μm will be trapped in the small pulmonary capillaries. Large amounts of such materials will cause dangerous pulmonary embolisms, although smaller amounts of materials may be used as a useful way of targeting drugs to the lung. This has also been explored as a possible means of targeting tumours, particularly hepatic tumours[7]. Embolisms can also be caused by smaller particles if they aggregate together. There is an extensive body of science concerning the dispersion and aggregation of colloidal particles[8], but despite this it is possible to formulate an injected colloid (for example, a fat emulsion) which while stable alone, becomes unstable in plasma, the large aggregates of droplets depositing in the lungs[9].

Particles which are sufficiently small to pass through the pulmonary capillaries return to the heart, after which they are circulated to the tissues. Large particles which have escaped the pulmonary filter may deposit in the capillaries by blockage but they are more likely to be captured by macrophages. This is particularly important if tissues are inflamed, as extensive macrophage activity can result in considerable uptake of particles in such areas, and has been explored as a possible mechanism of targeting sites of inflammation[10]. Small pores called fenestrae, of diameter 50-60 nm, are present in the exocrine glands, but the capillary basement membrane is continuous in these regions and particles cannot pass through into tissues. Only in a few regions, specifically the liver and spleen, are there pores which are sufficiently large to allow particles to escape the circulation. In these regions particles of size smaller than 100 nm can leave the circulation to be taken up by hepatocytes. However the capillaries in these regions are lined with active macrophages called Kupffer cells, which remove most circulating particles. The majority of injected colloidal particles will end up in the Kupffer cells rather than the hepatocytes. As a result of these combined processes, injected colloids are efficiently removed, largely irrespective of their size (Figure 2.2).

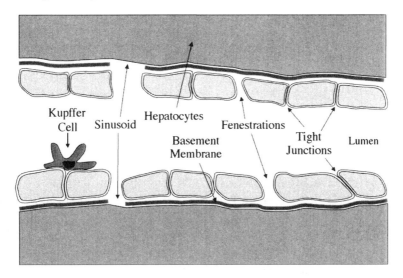

Figure 2.2 Structure of the hepatic blood vessels

This uptake and clearance by the system commonly termed the reticuloendothelial system is a major barrier in the application of colloidal particles for intravenous targeting applications, and considerable effort has been expended in trying to defeat this mechanism. One of the few promising approaches is the use of long-chain hydrophilic polymers (primarily polyethylene glycol) to form a heavily hydrated layer around the particle[11]. The method by which this coating escapes phagocyte surveillance is still uncertain but is thought to be due to the prevention of absorption of serum recognition factors or opsonins which mediate the uptake process. Initally experiments were performed using simple non-degradable polystyrene particles coated with an adsorbed layer of ill-characterized industrial polymer, and much of the early literature in this area is confused and irreproducible. The current state of the art involves the use of highly characterized self-assembling materials such as poly(d,l lactide) - poly (ethylene glycol), and phospholipids with poly(ethylene glycol) grafted to the headgroup to form 'stealth'[12]. Despite the interest these advanced materials, our understanding of their behaviour is largely incomplete.

Intravenous oxygen carriers

There has been a great deal of effort into the possibility of replacing or supplementing blood with an alternative oxygen transport fluid, for example in major trauma, where matched blood may not be available. The increase in AIDS also prompted a transient increase in interest in this area until screening processes were introduced for blood products. There are two main technologies under development:

i) Fluorocarbon emulsions. Fluorocarbons are inert water-immiscible oils which dissolve large quantities of respiratory gases; a well-known demonstration by Clark (1966)[13] showed a hamster breathing while submerged in liquid perfluorodecalin. There have been a number of attempts to develop water-miscible fluorocarbon emulsions which could be used as blood substitutes, of which the Green Cross Fluosol® and the Alliance Oxygen® are the most well-known. The possibility of developing a large-volume blood replacement with this technology seems remote due to the extensive immunological problems which may ensue, coupled with the reticuloendothelial load involved in clearing the emulsion;

however a number of indications for smaller doses, such as myocardial oxygenation during coronary angioplasty, show some promise. The field has been recently reviewed by Krafft and coworkers (1998)[14].

ii) Haemoglobin-based products. Free haemoglobin resulting frim lysis of erythrocytes is cleared rapidly from the circulation; large amounts of haemoglobin will cause kidney damage. Two approaches are being studied to prevent renal excretion; modification and encapsulation. The modified route uses polymerized or cross-linked haemoglobin, usually treated with glutaraldehyde or coated with polyethylene chains[15]. Rabinovici and coworkers[16] and others have studied the possibility of encapsulating haemoglobin in liposomes to make an artificial red cell.

INTRAMUSCULAR DELIVERY
Physiology

Intramuscular delivery involves the injection of the dose form into a muscle, from where it is absorbed due to the perfusion of the muscle by blood. The formulation forms a local depot which is partly mixed with interstitial fluid, and partly forms a bolus within the muscle, particularly if the injected volume is large. As a result it is important to realize that the injection is made into abnormal tissue; this may be particularly important if the formulation is intended to reside in the body for a significant length of time.

The structure of a typical muscle is shown in Figure 2.3. The muscle is wrapped in a connective sheath called the epimysium, within which are bundles of individual fibres, each surrounded by a connective membrane termed the perimysium. A finer matrix of connective fibrous tissue, the endomysium (omitted from Figure 2.3 for clarity), surrounds the muscle fibres, and the blood capillaries run within the endomysium, largely in a longitudinal manner, with numerous cross-connections. As a result the whole muscle is extremely well perfused. There are also numerous lymphatic vessels, but these lie in the epimysium and perimysium.

The preferred sites for injection are the gluteal, deltoid, triceps, pectoral and vastus lateralis. The deltoid muscle is preferred due to its greater perfusion rate compared to the other muscles, although the vastus lateralis has the advantage of having fewer major blood vessels into which the injection might accidentally be placed. When an intramuscular injection is administered, it is normal practice to withdraw the syringe plunger briefly to see if blood can be withdrawn. Blood indicates that the needle may be in a vessel, and the injection should be repositioned. There is also a minor danger of damaging a nerve fibre during the injection.

Pharmacokinetics

The most significant advantage of intramuscular delivery is the ease with which a wide range of drugs can be administered in a variety of dosage forms, which not only provide rapid absorption, but can also be used for sustained therapy. Intramuscular delivery involves a number of steps (Figure 2.4); i) release of the drug from the dose form into the intercellular fluid (ICF), ii) absorption from the ICF into the blood and lymphatics, iii) transport from the local blood volume into the general circulation, and iv) metabolism. The concentration of drug and kinetic profile are determined by the relative rates of these processes, and we should note that the capillary membrane is highly permeable and in general will not be rate-limiting, but perfusion of the muscle by the blood may be significantly slower. We can distinguish two particular limiting cases of interest:

i). Injection of a bolus of soluble drug. In this case the drug is immediately available in the ICF and is rapidly absorbed into the capillaries. In this case the rate-limiting absorption step is the perfusion of the muscle by the blood. Any factor which influences muscle perfusion (such as movement or exercise) will change the rate of absorption. In particular,

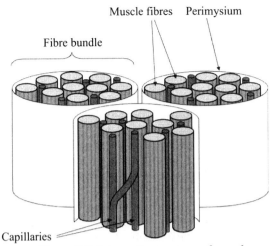

Figure 2.3 Schematic structure of muscle

if cardiac failure has occurred, absorption will be extremely low since the muscle perfusion rate will be small. For this reason intramuscular delivery is contra-indicated if cardiac function is poor.

ii) Injection of the drug in sustained-release form (e.g a solid depot or crystal suspension). In this case release from the formulation is slower than absorption or perfusion, and so the behaviour of the device becomes the rate-limiting step, and the effects of muscle perfusion are not evident. Under these conditions the concentration of drug in the plasma remains approximately constant until the delivery device is exhausted, a period which can be designed to last from several hours to several months.

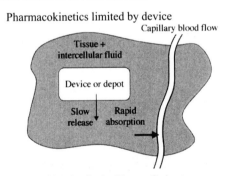

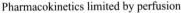

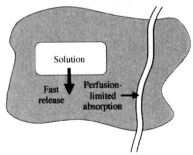

Figure 2.4 Absorption of drugs from intramuscular injections

Formulation considerations

Since the formulation does not have to be miscible with water, it is possible to inject a much wider range of materials than those which can be administered intravenously. The possible formulations include aqueous solutions, aqueous suspensions, oily solutions, oil in water emulsions, water in oil emulsions, oily suspensions, and dispersions in polymer or solid implants. These are listed approximately in order of release rate, as aqueous solutions can be absorbed in minutes, while implants can deliver drugs for several months.

In addition a range of other factors can influence the absorption rate. If the drug is extremely hydrophobic it will not dissolve in the ICF, while if it is strongly ionized or extremely water soluble it will not be able to cross the capillary membrane. Drugs which are strongly protein-bound will also be slowly absorbed since their activity in solution will be reduced. A number of drugs administered in solutions may be absorbed anomalously slowly if the composition of the formulation changes after injection. For example, phenytoin is formulated as an injection at pH 12 due to its low solubility. On injection the ICF quickly reduces the pH to normal levels, and the drug precipitates. As a result it may then take several days for the dose to be fully absorbed.

SUBCUTANEOUS DELIVERY

Physiology

A subcutaneous injection (SC) is made into the connective tissue beneath the dermis, and should be contrasted with an intradermal injection which is made into the dermal layer, often between the dermis and the epidermis (Figure 2.5). This is a critical distinction because the subcutaneous tissues have a significant volume of interstitial fluid into which the drug can diffuse, while the epidermal tissue has relatively little available fluid, nor is it well perfused by blood. As a result an intradermal injection persists at the site for a long period and the available volume for injection is small; it is normally used for antigens (e.g. tuberculin) and vaccines (smallpox).

Drugs injected subcutaneously dissolve in the interstitial fluid and gain entry to the bloodstream by two routes. They may be absorbed directly into blood vessels, but the subcutaneous tissues are often adipose and poorly perfused. Alternatively the interstitial

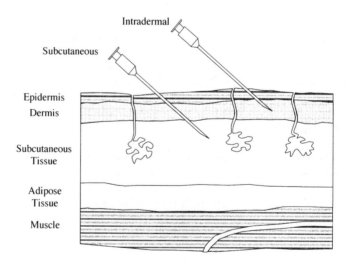

Figure 2.5. Physiology of parenteral administration routes

fluid is collected by lymphatic capillaries and these drain into the regional lymph nodes and then into the bloodstream. These pathways are both relatively slow and depend on the local vasculature, so absorption from subcutaneous sites can be slow and unpredictable. To some extent this allows a sustained release effect to be obtained; however it is not particularly satisfactory to design a dose form in this way because of the inherent variability of the pharmacokinetics. A better strategy is to make the release from the dose form rate-limiting (as is the case for intramuscular depot delivery systems) so that biological variation then has little influence on the drug pharmacokinetics. A large number of delivery systems have been devised which work in this way; probably the best known being Zoladex® (AstraZeneca) which releases the hormone goserelin, a chemical castrating agent used in the treatment of androgen-dependent tumours. The hormone is incorporated into a small rod of biodegradable poly (D,L lactide) polymer about 5mm long and implanted subcutaneously in the abdomen. A single injection lasts for 28 days; the cost (over £100 per injection at the time of writing) reflects the difficulty of manufacturing the device in a totally aseptic environment. Technology of this type is particularly suited to peptide hormones in which the dose is small and the size of the device can be minimized. A number of other interesting examples of this depot technique can be found in the literature, including the use of emulsion depots for methotrexate[17], hydrogels[18] and block copolymer gels[19].

Subcutaneous colloidal delivery systems

It has already been indicated that materials injected subcutaneously may be carried by the lymphatic flow into the regional lymph nodes and then into the blood. Colloidal particles which are injected subcutaneously can follow the same route, although their large size (tens to hundreds of nanometres) relative to drug molecules will reduce their diffusion rate considerably. On reaching the lymph nodes they will be taken up by macrophages rather than passing to the bloodstream.

Most of the work in this area has been performed in rats, with the foot and footpad being the most closely studied injection sites. Ousseren and Storm[20] used this technique to study the lymphatic uptake of liposomes from SC injection, and found relatively high lymphatic localization (60% of injected dose). However, injections into the flank produced only a slight uptake, and the suspicion is that footpad injections cause a large increase in local interstitial pressure due to the small volume of the site, and that this drives the injection into the lymphatic vessels. Consequently the targeting effect may not be so pronounced if the technique were used in man. The same study showed that the liposomes needed to be small (> 0.2 µm) or they could not be moved from the injection site, and that highly charged liposomes were taken up more efficiently than weakly charged ones. Interestingly, liposomes made from the 'stealth phospholipid' with grafted PEG-chains were taken up to a similar extent to normal liposomes of the same size. Although this study was performed exclusively with liposomes there seems to be no reason why the results should not broadly apply to other colloidal particles.

TISSUE DAMAGE AND BIOCOMPATABILITY

With any injected formulation damage occurs to the surrounding tissues. In the case of an intravenous injection, this usually has little consequence for drug absorption, but in the case of intramuscular and subcutaneous systems the drug or device is inherently present in a wound site and the body will react accordingly. The reaction depends on the size and composition of the device. Small isolated particles less than 10 µm will be engulfed by macrophages without any major reaction occurring, but larger objects in a microsphere form will gather a layer of macrophages and giant cells adhering to the surface of the particles. Larger devices with large surface areas will elicit a foreign body reaction which begins with inflammation and the formation of a layer of macrophages and giant cells, and is followed by the formation of granulation tissue. Ultimately a fibroid capsule consisting of fibroblasts and collagen will surround the device. The consequences of these changes for drug delivery have not been widely explored but at present it is thought that they make little difference to drug release and absorption unless the reaction is severe.

DRUG DISTRIBUTION FOLLOWING PARENTERAL ADMINISTRATION

The blood transports the drug to the tissues, however the drug concentration in the tissues is usually not equal to that in the blood. A number of factors influence the drug concentration in tissues, one of the most important being the blood flow per unit mass of the tissue. Tissues can be broadly classified as poorly-perfused, adequately perfused and well-perfused on this basis as shown in Table 2.1. Note how organs with a relatively small mass, such as the heart and brain, only require a modest blood flow to perfuse them well. The blood flow to the heart musculature (not to be confused with the flow *through* the heart) is equal to that through the adipose tissue, but the heart has a much smaller mass and so is correspondingly better perfused.

The blood flow controls the rate at which the drug is supplied to the particular tissue, and will be reflected in the drug concentration profile in that tissue. If the tissue is well-perfused, the tissue pharmacokinetics will reach a maximum value at a similar time to that in the blood. However, if the tissue is less well perfused, the supply of drug to the tissue will be rate-limiting and so the concentration in the tissue will increasingly lag behind that in the blood, as shown in Figure 2.6.

The second important factor determining the tissue pharmacokinetics is the affinity of the tissue for the drug. This can take 2 forms; passive or active. Passive affinity is simply the partitioning of the drug. For example, the partitioning of a lipophilic drug into adipose tissues results in high drug concentrations in that tissue, although this is achieved slowly due to the poor perfusion of the adipose tissue.

Table 2.1 Blood flow through various human organs

Tissue	Blood flow (litres min^{-1})	Tissue mass as (% of body weight)
Blood	5.4	8.0%
Poorly perfused		
Skeleton	0.2	17%
Adipose tissue	0.25	14-20%
Adequately perfused		
Skin	0.4	7%
Muscle	0.8	48%
Well perfused		
Kidneys	1.2	0.5%
Heart	0.25	0.5%
Liver	1.55	3.5%
Brain	0.75	2.0%

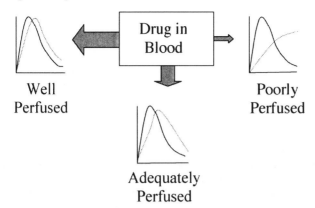

Figure 2.6. Pharmacokinetic profiles of drugs in tissues of varying perfusion. Solid line: concentration in blood; dotted line: concentration in tissue

Active affinity occurs if the drug is taken up by the tissue by a specific transport mechanism. An example of this is guanethidine, which is used in the treatment of hypertension. This drug reaches its site of action by active transport into the heart and skeletal muscle. As a result the drug concentrations in these tissues are much higher than would be expected on the basis of partition from the blood, and due to the affinity of the tissue for the drug, are sustained for a much longer period than those in the bloodstream (Figure 2.7).

PROTEIN BINDING

One of the underlying principles of clinical pharmacology is that only the unbound, free drug is pharmacologically active and that only in this form can a drug cross a biological membrane or interact with a receptor. Interaction with the receptor results in a biochemical change leading to a physiological response.

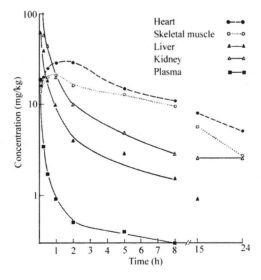

Figure 2.7. Concentrations of guanethidine in tissues following intravenous administration[21]

Drugs bind to a number of plasma proteins including albumin, lipoproteins, and gamma globulins, and the more extensively the drug is bound, the lower will be the drug activity available to exert a pharmacological effect. Since the concentrations of these proteins change in disease, and as a function of nutrition, the effect of the drug may be significantly and unpredictably modulated. For example, most antimicrobials bind primarily to albumin, while basic drugs including erythromycin, clindamycin, and trimethoprim bind to the "acute-phase" serum protein ([[alpha]]1-acid glycoprotein). Moreover, binding is not limited to proteins in the serum. Because albumin is the principal protein in interstitial fluid, substantial binding to this protein and to other tissue constituents, takes place. Differential concentrations of these proteins, and cell debris, leads to marked alterations in peripheral drug concentrations around an inflamed area such as a wound or abscess.

THE BLOOD-BRAIN BARRIER

Physiology

The ventricles of the brain lie within the ventricular compartment and are surrounded by approximately 150 ml of cerebrospinal fluid (CSF) which is secreted by the choroid plexi and circulates around the brain before being absorbed into the venous circulation. The entire fluid volume surrounding the brain is replaced every five hours in normal subjects. As a result it is rarely practical to deliver drugs by injection of a bolus into the ventricular space, since they are efficiently cleared before they can diffuse into the brain tissue. As a result the only practical means of delivering a drug effectively to the whole brain volume is via the systemic circulation. A significant feature of the blood flow in the brain is that capillaries are very close together (of the order of 40 micrometres), so that any substance passing into the brain from the circulation will equilibrate within seconds through the whole of the brain tissue.

Unfortunately, delivery of drugs to the brain from the systemic circulation is difficult due to the presence of the so called *blood brain barrier*. This is not so much a physical structure as the absence of the usual mechanisms which allow drugs to be transferred across the capillary wall in other tissues. The junctions separating the capillary endothelial cells are extremely tight, eliminating the possibility of paracellular transport, and there is an almost complete absence of pinocytosis across the endothelial membrane. It also appears that there is a specific transport molecule, P-glycoprotein, which actively back-transports a wide range of drugs out of the apical cells, preventing their passage into the brain tissues[22]. A number of workers have attempted to open channels through the endothelium by infusing osmotic agents such as mannitol. Although this does lead to an increase in permeability, extensive side effects are observed, including seizures in experimental animals, and the practicality of this method seems limited. It is also possible to increase the permeability of the endothelium pharmacologically using bradykinin[23]. However, the most widely studied pathways for drug absorption are those which are part of the normal endothelial function, i.e. simple diffusion in the lipid membrane, and receptor-mediated active transport.

Uptake by diffusion

In order for a molecule to cross the endothelial capillary by diffusion, it must have two properties; it must be highly lipid soluble, and of relatively low molecular weight. A number of studies have examined the dependence of uptake on molecular weight, and an upper limit between 400 and 700 Daltons is generally accepted[24][25]. The absorption of hydrophilic molecules can be increased by administering them as hydrophobic prodrugs. A good example of this is provided by the absorption of morphine, codeine (methylmorphine) and heroin (diacetylmorphine) which have LogP (calculated) of 0.24, 1.14 and 1.86 respectively. Codeine has a blood-brain permeability of approximately 10 times that of morphine, while that of heroin is 10 times greater still.

Receptor-mediated transport

The brain capillary endothelium possesses a number of receptors which allow the transport of specific materials. These include small molecule nutrient receptors, such as those for hexose, amino acids, amines, and a number of peptide and protein receptors, including those for insulin, transferrin and IGF-II[26]. It is possible to take advantage of these pathways for the delivery of mimetic drugs; for example, dopamine is poorly transported through the blood brain barrier, and its administration is of no direct therapeutic value, but the amino-acid analogue L-DOPA is transported through the phenylalanine receptor and can thus exert a useful pharmacological effect[27].

A number of reserchers have attempted to make use of these active pathways to develop blood brain barrier vectors which can improve drug uptake. A typical example is the OX26 monoclonal antibody to the endothelial transferrin receptor[28]. The antibody binds efficiently to the receptor, and is actively transported across the endothelium. The drug can be attached to the antibody using conventional avidin-biotin methods which do not degrade the activity of the drug. This technique has been used to deliver vasoactive intestinal peptide (VIP) attached to OX26 to the brain, resulting in a significant increase in hemispheric brain blood flow; the peptide alone was not significantly absorbed and showed no pharmacological effect[29]. It has also been used in an attempt to deliver antisense gene therapy agents to the brain[30]. Antisense oligonucleotide-OX26 conjugates were not delivered efficiently since they bound to plasma proteins, but peptide nucleic acid - OX26 conjugates did not suffer from this problem and were efficiently transported into the brain. More recently the antibody has been grafted to the surface of liposomes containing daunomycin and successfully used to produce elevated drug levels within the brain tissue.

The most significant difficulty with these vector methods is that the receptors being used in the target tissue occur in a wide range of organs; for example transferrin receptors are present on most cells since they are required for the active uptake of iron. It is thus important to distinguish between brain uptake and brain targeting; vector based conjugates may improve brain uptake but will not produce targeting, with the drug being absorbed in a wide range of organs. Many published studies are particularly vague on this point and one is led to suspect that it is a significant problem.

A number of polyionic macromolecules are also actively transported into the brain capillary endothelium by absorptive transcytosis. This mechanism is distinct from the receptor-mediated pathways discussed above since it involves the physical adsorption of the macromolecule (usually a polycation) to the negatively charged membrane by charge interactions, after which internalization occurs. Molecules transported in this way include lectins such as wheat germ agglutinin and polycationic proteins such as cationized albumin[31]. This approach has been used to deliver radiolabelled antibody diagnostics; for example a monoclonal antibody to the amyloid protein which is characteristic of Alzheimers disease. The antibody itself was not significantly taken up by brain tissue, but localized in the brain in dogs after it had been converted into a polycationic protein by reaction with hexamethylene diamine[32].

Colloidal delivery

We have already mentioned the use of liposomes coated with the OX26 transferrin antibody which successfully increased brain levels of daunomycin. In this case, it was unclear whether or not the liposomes were internalized in the endothelial cells or simply adhered to the surface, thus providing a greater concentration gradient to assist passive diffusion. It has also been found that cyanoacrylate microspheres coated with polysorbates can be used to deliver a number of hydrophilic analgesic peptides[33][34]. The mechanisms of this effect are also uncertain but may be due to a surface receptor recognizing the sorbate block of the surfactant.

REFERENCES

1. Comas D, Mateu J. Treatment of extravasation of both doxorubicin and vincristine administration in a Y-site infusion. *Ann. Pharmacother.* 1996;30:244-246.
2. Yalkowsky SH, Krzyzaniak JF, Ward GH. Formulation-related problems associated with intravenous drug delivery. *J. Pharm. Sci.* 1998;87:787-796.
3. Puntis JWL. The economics of home parenteral nutrition. *Nutr.* 1998;14:809-812.
4. Chung DH, Ziegler MM. Central venous catheter access. *Nutr.* 1998;14:119-123.
5. Macfie J. Infusion phlebitis and peripheral parenteral nutrition. *Nutr.* 1998;14:233-235.
6. Plusa SM, Webster N, Horsman R, Primrose JN, Kendall-Smith S. Fine-bore cannulas for peripheral intravenous nutrition: polyurethaneor silicone? *Ann. Royal College Surg. England* 1998;80:154-156.
7. Brown KT, Nevins AB, Getrajdman GI, Brody LA, Kurtz RC, Fong YM, et al. Particle embolization for hepatocellular carcinoma. *J. Vasc. Intervent. Radiol.* 1998;9:822-828.
8. Hunter RJ. *Foundations of colloid science*. New York: Oxford University Press, 1997.
9. Washington C. The stability of intravenous fat emulsions in total parenteral-nutrition mixtures. *Int. J. Pharmaceut.* 1990;66:1-21.
10. Kellaway IW, Seale L, Spencer PSJ. The *in vitro* characterization and biostability of Tc-99m-dextran and its accumulation within the inflamed paws of adjuvant-induced arthritic rats. *Pharm. Res.* 1995;12:588-593.
11. Illum L, Davis SS. The organ uptake of intravenously administered colloidal particles can be altered using a non-ionic surfactant (Poloxamer-338). *Febs Letters* 1984;167:79-82.
12. Woodle MC, Newman MS, Collins LR, Martin FJ. Efficient evaluation of long circulating or stealth liposomes by studies of *in vivo* blood-circulation kinetics and final organ distribution in rats. *Biophys. J.* 1990;57:A261.
13. Clark LC, Gollan F. Survival of mammals breathing organic liquids equilibrated with oxygen at atmospheric pressure. *Science* 1966;152:1755-1756.
14. Krafft MP, Reiss JG, Weers JG. The design and engineering of oxygen-delivering fluorocarbon emulsions. In: Benita S, ed. *Submicron Emulsions in Drug Delivery and Targeting*. Netherlands: Harwood Academic Publishers, 1998:235-333.
15. Chang TMS. Recent and future developments in modified hemoglobin and microencapsulated hemoglobin as red blood cell substitutes. *Artif. Cells Blood Substit. Immobiliz. Biotechnol.* 1997;25:1-24.
16. Rabinovici R, Rudolph AS, Vernick J, Feuerstein G. Lyophilized liposome-encapsulated hemoglobin - evaluation of hemodynamic, biochemical, and hematologic responses. *Crit.Care Med.*1994;22:480-485.
17. Bonetti A, Chatelut E, Kim S. An Extended-Release Formulation of methotrexate for subcutaneous administration. *Cancer Chemotherap. Pharmacol.* 1994;33:303-306.
18. Kuzma P, MooYoung AJ, Moro D, Quandt H, Bardin CW, Schlegel PH. Subcutaneous hydrogel reservoir system for controlled drug delivery *Macromol.Symp.*1996;109:15-26.
19. Jeong B, Bae YH, Lee DS, Kim SW. Biodegradable block copolymers as injectable drug-Del. systems. *Nature* 1997;388(6645):860-862.
20. Ousseren C, Storm G. Targeting to lymph nodes by subcutaneous administration of liposomes. *Int. J. Pharmaceut.* 1998;162:39-44.
21. Schanker LS, Morrison AS. Physiological disposition of guanethidine in the rat and its uptake by heart slices. *Int. J. Neuropharmacol.* 1965;4:27-39.
22. Schinkel AH. P-Glycoprotein, a gatekeeper in the blood-brain barrier. *Adv. Drug Del. Rev.* 1999;36:179-194.
23. Kroll RA, Neuwelt EA. Outwitting the blood-brain barrier for therapeutic purposes: osmotic opening and other means. *Neurosurg.* 1998; 42:1083-1099.
24. Levin VA. Relationship of octanol-water partition coefficient and molecular weight to rat brain capillary permeability. *J. Med. Chem.* 1990;23:682-684.

25. Greig NH, Soncrant TT, Shetty HU, Momma S, Smith QR, Rapoport SI. Brain uptake and anticancer activities of vincristine and vinblastine are restricted by their low cerebrovascular permeability and binding to plasma constituents in rat. *Cancer Chemotherap. Pharmacol.* 1990;26:263-268.

26. Tsuji A, Tamai I. Carrier-mediated or specialized transport of drugs across the blood-brain barrier. *Adv. Drug Del. Rev.* 1999;36:277-290.

27. Wade LA, Katzman R. Synthetic amino-acids and the nature of L-dopa transport at the blood-brain barrier. *J. Neurochem.* 1975;25:837-842.

28. Pardridge WM, Buciak JL, Friden PM. Selective transport of an antitransferrin receptor antibody through the blood brain barrier *in vivo*. *J. Pharmacol. Exp. Therapeut.* 1991;259:66-70.

29. Bickel U, Yoshikawa T, Landaw EM, Faull KF, Pardridge WM. Pharmacological effects *in vivo* in brain by vector-mediated peptide drug delivery. *Proc. Nat. Acad. Sci. USA* 1993;90:2618-2622.

30. Boado RJ, Tsukamoto H, Pardridge WM. Drug delivery of antisense molecules to the brain for treatment of Alzheimer's disease and cerebral AIDS. *J. Pharm.Sci.*1998;87:1308-1315.

31. Pardridge WM. *Peptide Drug Delivery to the Brain*. New York: Raven Press, 1991.

32. Bickel U, Lee VMY, Trojanowski JQ, Pardridge WM. Development and *in vitro* characterization of a cationized monoclonal-antibody against Beta-A4 protein - a potential probe for Alzheimers disease. *Bioconj. Chem.* 1994;5:119-125.

33. Kreuter J, Petrov VE, Kharkevich DA, Alyautdin RN. Influence of the type of surfactant on the analgesic effects induced by the peptide dalargin after its delivery across the blood-brain barrier using surfactant-coated nanoparticles. *J. Cont. Rel.* 1997;49:81-87.

34. Schroeder U, Sommerfeld P, Ulrich S, Sabel BA. Nanoparticle technology for delivery of drugs across the blood-brain barrier. *J. Pharm. Sci.* 1998;87:1305-1307.

Chapter Three

Drug Delivery to the Oral Cavity
or Mouth

ANATOMY AND PHYSIOLOGY
The oral cavity

The oral cavity or mouth is the point of entry of food and air into the body and the mouth and lips are essential to humans to allow speech by modifying the passage of air. This structure is also referred to as the buccal cavity, but strictly speaking this should be confined to the inner cheek area. The mouth extends from the lips to the oropharynx at the rear and is divided into two regions: (a) the outer oral vestibule, which is bounded by the cheeks and lips, and (b) the interior oral vestibule, which is bounded by the dental maxillary and mandibular arches. The oral cavity proper is located between the dental arches on which the teeth are situated. It is partly filled by the tongue, a large muscle anchored to the floor of the mouth by the frenulum linguae (Figure 3.1). At the back of the oral cavity are large collections of lymphoid tissue forming the tonsils; small lymphoid nodules may occur in the mucosa of the soft palate. This tissue plays an important role in combating infection.

The palate

The palate is located in the roof of the mouth. It separates the nasal and oral cavities. It consists of an anterior hard palate of bone and, in mammals, a posterior soft palate that has no skeletal support and terminates in a fleshy, elongated projection called the uvula. The hard palate, which composes two-thirds of the total palate area, is a plate of bone covered by a moist, durable layer of mucous-membrane tissue, which secretes small amounts of mucus. This layer forms several ridges that help grip food while the tongue agitates it during chewing. The hard palate provides space for the tongue to move freely and supplies a rigid floor to the nasal cavity so that pressures within the mouth do not close off the nasal passage. The soft palate is composed of muscle and connective tissue, which give it both mobility and support. This palate is very flexible; when elevated for swallowing and sucking, it completely blocks and separates the nasal cavity and nasal portion of the pharynx from the mouth and the oral part of the pharynx. While elevated, the soft palate creates a vacuum in the oral cavity, which keeps food out of the respiratory tract.

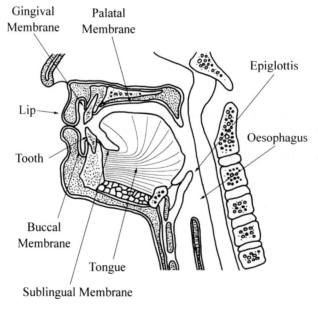

Figure 3.1 Cross section through the oral cavity

The tongue

In humans, the tongue aids in creating negative pressure within the oral cavity that enables sucking, and it is an important accessory organ in chewing, swallowing and speech. The tongue consists of a mass of interwoven, striated muscles interspersed with glands and fat and covered with mucous membrane. The ability of the tongue to touch the lips and teeth aids swallowing and speech. The top surface, or dorsum, contains numerous projections of the mucous membrane called papillae. They contain taste buds sensitive to food flavours and serous glands that secrete some of the fluid in saliva. The base, or upper rear portion, of the tongue has no papillae, but aggregated lymphatic tissue (lingual tonsils) and serous and mucus-secreting glands are present. The inferior, or under surface leads from the tip of the tongue to the floor of the mouth; its mucous membrane is smooth and purple in colour from the many blood vessels present. The root, the remainder of the underside that lies on the floor of the mouth contains bundles of nerves, arteries, and muscles that branch to the other tongue regions. Nerves from the tongue receive chemical stimulation from food in solution which gives the sensation of taste. There are four fundamental taste sensations: salt and sweet, the receptors for which are primarily located at the tip of the tongue, bitter at the base, and acid or sour along the borders. The flavour of a food comes from the combination of taste, smell, touch, texture or consistency, and temperature sensations.

The teeth

Teeth cut and grind food to facilitate digestion. A tooth consists of a crown and one or more roots. In humans, they are attached to the to the tooth-bearing bone of the jaws by a fibrous ligament called the periodontal ligament or membrane. The neck of the root is embedded in the fleshy gum tissue. Cementum is a thin covering to the root and serves as a medium for attachment of the fibres that hold the tooth to the surrounding tissue (periodontal membrane). Gum is attached to the alveolar bone and to the cementum by fibre bundles.

Caries, or tooth decay, is the most common disease of the teeth among humans. Tooth decay originates in the build-up of a yellowish film called plaque on teeth, which tends to harbour bacteria. The bacteria that live on plaque ferment the sugar and starchy-food debris found there into acids that destroy the tooth's enamel and dentine by removing the calcium and other minerals from them. Alkali production from urea by bacterial ureases in the oral cavity is thought to have a major impact on oral health and on the physiology and ecology of oral bacteria[1]. Another common dental disorder is inflammation of the gum, or gingivitis. It usually commences at or close to the gum margin, often between adjacent teeth. Pockets form between the gum and the adjacent teeth, sometimes penetrating deeply into the tissues. This leads to further infection, with inflammation and bleeding from the infected gums. A principal cause of gingivitis is the build-up of plaque on teeth, which causes irritation of the gums and thus leads to their inflammation and infection.

Organisation of the oral mucosa

The oral cavity and vestibule are entirely lined by relatively smooth mucous membranes containing numerous small glands (Figure 3.2). It is divided into a) the oral epithelium, b) the basement membrane, which connects the epithelium to the connective tissue, c) the lamina propria, which is underlying connective tissue and d) an area which contains loose fatty or glandular connective tissue and major blood vessels and nerves. It is often referred to as the muco-periostium. These tissues are laid over a layer of muscle or bone. To a certain extent, the structure of the oral mucosa resembles that of the skin.

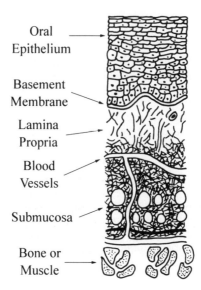

Oral Epithelium

Basement Membrane

Lamina Propria

Blood Vessels

Submucosa

Bone or Muscle

Figure 3.2 Cross section through the oral mucosa

The epithelial lining of the oral mucosa is composed of squamous cells with a characteristic layered structure formed by the process of cell maturation. The composition and thickness of this layer varies according to the tissue functions; the hard palate and tongue, for example, is composed of keratinized epithelium whilst the lining of the cheek is distensible and non-keratinized (Table 3.1). Keratinised tissue is dehydrated, tough and resistant to chemical damage and it covers approximately 50% of the surface. Non-keratinised tissue is more flexible and occupies about 30% of the surface area. The oral mucosa has a turnover time of 3-8 days.

Sebaceous glands are found in the mucosa of 60 to 75% of adults and are seen as pale yellow spots in the upper lip and buccal mucosa. The openings of minor salivary glands are evident in many areas. In general, the oral mucosa has a more concentrated network of vessels than is present in the skin. Almost all venous return from the oral mucosa enters the internal jugular vein. Lymphatic capillaries are also present in the lamina propria and arise as "blind" beginnings in the papillae.

Table 3.1   Characteristics of the mucosae found in the oral cavity

Tissue	Location	Thickness mm	Type
Gingival	Gums	0.2	Keratinized / nonpolar
Palatal	Roof of mouth	0.25	Keratinized / nonpolar
Buccal	Cheek	0.55	Nonkeratinized / polar
	Upper and lower lip		
Sublingual	Frenulum	0.15	Nonkeratinized / polar
	Floor of mouth		

Functions of the oral mucosa

The oral mucosa has similarities to both skin and intestinal mucosa. It has a protective role during the process of mastication, which exposes the mucosa to compression and shear forces. Areas such as the hard palate and attached gingiva have a horny surface to resist abrasion and are tightly bound to the underlying bone to resist shear forces. The cheek mucosae, on the other hand, are elastic to allow for distension.

The oral cavity contains the greatest variety of micro-organisms present within the human body. The entry into the body of these organisms and any potential toxic waste product is limited by the oral epithelium, which is not, as is often suggested, a highly permeable membrane.

The oral mucosa responds to the senses of pain, touch, and temperature in addition to its unique sense of taste. Some physiological processes are triggered by sensory input from the mouth, such as the initiation of swallowing, gagging and retching.

In some animals the oral mucosa is used to aid thermoregulation, for example, panting in the dog. The human skin possesses sweat glands and a more highly controlled peripheral vasculature, so this role is thought to be minimal, although in sleep, dehydration can result from prolonged breathing through the mouth.

Salivary secretion

Salivary glands

The major salivary glands are the parotid, submandibular (submaxillary) and sublingual glands (Figure 3.3). Minor salivary glands are situated in or immediately below the oral mucosa in the tongue, palate, lips, and cheeks. The major glands are situated some way from the oral cavity, but open into it by a long duct. The parotid salivary glands, the largest of the three, are located between the ear and ascending branch of the lower jaw. Each gland is enclosed in a tissue capsule and is composed of fat tissue and secretory cells and the major duct (Stensen's duct) opens near the second upper molar. The second pair, the sub-

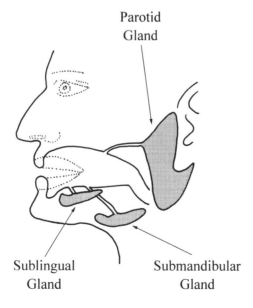

Figure 3.3 Position of the salivary glands

maxillary glands, is located along the side of the lower jawbone. The major duct of each (Wharton's duct) opens into the floor of the mouth at the junction where the front of the tongue meets the mouth's floor. A capsule of tissue also surrounds each of these glands. The third pair, the sublingual glands, is situated beneath the mucous membrane of the floor of the mouth, near the chin region. They are not covered by a capsule and are therefore more dispersed throughout the surrounding tissue. They have many ducts (Rivinus's ducts) that empty near the junction of the tongue and the mouth's floor; several unite to form Bartholin's duct which empties into or near the submaxillary duct. The parotid and sub-maxillary glands produce watery secretion, while the buccal and sublingual glands produce mainly viscous saliva.

Saliva

One to two litres of fluid are excreted daily into the human mouth and there is a continuous, low basal secretion of 0.5 ml min^{-1} which will rapidly increase to more than 7 ml min^{-1} by the thought, smell or taste of food. Control over salivary secretion is exerted primarily via the parasympathetic system. Small amounts of saliva are continually being secreted into the mouth, but the presence of food, or even the smell or thought of it, will rapidly increase saliva flow. Saliva is viscous, colourless and opalescent, hypotonic compared to plasma (between 110 and 220 milliOsmoles per litre), with a specific gravity of about 1003. The pH varies between 7.4 and 6.2 (low to high rates of flow), but the action of bacteria on sugar can reduce the pH to between 3 and 4 around the teeth.

Saliva can be detected in the oral cavity soon after birth. Salivary secretion increases up to the age of 3 to 5 years, but then sharply declines, reaching a steady state by the age of 8 years. In adult females, the flow rate of saliva is somewhat lower than in males[2].

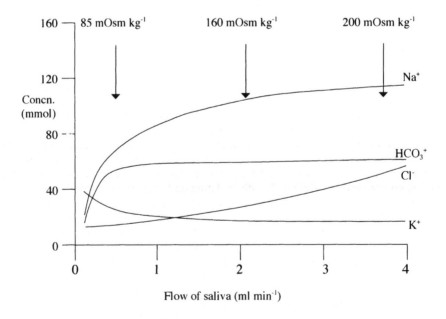

Figure 3.4 Influence of flow on saliva composition

Saliva is primarily composed of water, mucus, proteins, mineral salts, and amylase[3]. As it circulates in the mouth cavity it picks up food debris, bacterial cells, and white blood cells. The composition of saliva depends upon the rate at which the different cell types contribute to the final secretion. The two types of secretion are mucous secretion, which is thick due to a glycoprotein called mucin, and watery secretion which contains salivary amylase. The major ions are Na^+, K^+, Cl^- and HCO_3^-. In the ducts of the salivary glands, sodium and chloride are reabsorbed, but potassium and bicarbonate are secreted (Figure 3.4) and hence the electrolyte balance is altered depending upon the rate of flow of saliva.

Apart from the enzyme α-amylase, ptyalin is also present. This enzyme begins to hydrolyse polysaccharides such as glycogen and starch to smaller saccharides. The enzyme acts at an optimum pH of 6.9, but is stable within the range 4 to 11 and hence it will continue to act until the food is acidified by gastric acid. The time of contact in the mouth is too short for digestion to occur but the enzyme may prevent accumulation of starchy material in the gaps between teeth. Lingual lipase is responsible for hydrolysis of triglycerides. It is extremely hydrophobic and its digestive action continues in the stomach. A variety of esterases, mainly carboxylesterases are also present in the saliva and these may reduce the concentration of ester prodrugs or drugs containing susceptible ester groups[4].

Saliva lubricates and moistens the inside of the mouth to help with speech and to change food into a liquid or semisolid mass that can be tasted and swallowed more easily. The salivary film thickness is estimated to be between 0.07 and 0.10 mm[5]. It also helps to control the body's water balance; if water is lacking, the salivary glands become dehydrated, leaving the mouth dry producing a sensation of thirst thus stimulating the need to drink. The flow of saliva helps to wash away the bacteria and the food particles which act as their nutrient, into the acidic environment of the stomach where they are digested. Saliva also contains thiocyanate, and protein antibodies and lysozyme which destroy bacteria. In the absence of saliva, oral ulcerations occur and dental caries becomes extremely prevalent. This condition, xerostomia, can be treated with artificial saliva formulations, which are based on materials such as hydroxypropylmethylcellulose and more recently, pig gastric mucin.

MIGRATION AND CLEARANCE OF SUBSTANCES FROM THE ORAL CAVITY

Powdered charcoal placed under the tongue spreads through the oral cavity within a few minutes[6], but regional differences exist in the deposition, distribution and clearance of drugs which are dissolved in saliva[7]. This is of great importance if local treatment of the entire mucosa is required or the drug is absorbed preferentially from certain sites. Studying the pattern of fluoride concentration in the mouth arising from a slowly dissolving fluoride tablet revealed that when the tablet was placed in the lower mandibular sulcus, fluoride concentrations increased markedly in the region of the tablet, but there was no appreciable increase in salivary levels[8]. Relatively little had migrated to the opposite side of the mouth suggesting that the lower mandibular sulci are quite isolated from the remainder of the mouth. However, when the tablet was placed in the upper sulcus the fluoride migrated some distance from the site of administration. Glucose behaves in a similar fashion[9]. The pattern of fluoride distribution and the fluoride concentration are fairly consistent for any one subject, but a 20-fold intrasubject variation was observed. It is believed that the site specific differences are due to saliva movement and dilution of the test substance rather than the nature of the substance. The thickness of the salivary film will vary from place to place depending upon the proximity to the ducts of the major and minor salivary glands, separation of mucosal layers during speaking and mouth breathing.

ABSORPTION OF DRUGS ACROSS THE ORAL MUCOSA

The oral cavity is the point of entry for oral drug formulations but usually their contact with the oral mucosa is brief. In order to take advantage of some of the properties of the oral mucosa or to locally treat the mucosa, delivery systems have been designed to prolong residence in this area. The total surface area available for drug absorption is quite limited, being only approximately 100 cm^2.

Absorption of drugs through the buccal mucosa was first described by Sobrero in 1847 who noted systemic effects produced by nitroglycerin after administration to the oral mucosa[10]. The lingual route of administration became established in clinical practice in 1897 when William Murrell introduced nitroglycerin drops for the treatment of angina pectoris. Subsequently, nitroglycerin was formulated in tablets for sublingual use and was renamed glyceryl trinitrate.

The blood supply from the buccal mucosa and anal sphincter, unlike the remainder of the gastrointestinal tract, does not drain into the hepatic portal vein, since these peripheral areas are not specialised for the absorption of nutrients. Drugs which are absorbed through the oral mucosa enter the systemic circulation directly via the jugular vein, thereby initially avoiding passage through the liver where they might otherwise be metabolized. Drugs which are swallowed in the saliva do not avoid first pass metabolism and will be subjected to degradation by digestive juices.

The oral cavity is rich in blood vessels and lymphatics, so a rapid onset of action and high blood levels of drug are obtained quickly. In many cases buccal dose forms can result in the same bioavailability as intravenous formulations, without need for aseptic preparations. Finally, they share with transdermal systems the advantage that treatment can be rapidly stopped by removing the dose form, although the buccal epithelium can act as a reservoir for administered drug after the delivery system has been removed. Ideally the plasma concentration versus time profile should resemble a square wave, similar to that seen after skin application of a glyceryl trinitrate patch, but this is not always achievable.

In order to be absorbed orally, the drug must first dissolve in the saliva. Extremely hydrophobic materials (those with partition coefficients greater than approximately 2000) will not dissolve well and are likely to be swallowed intact unless a specialized delivery system is used to present them to the mucosa. Saliva containing dissolved drug is constantly being swallowed, and this process competes with buccal absorption. As described in Chapter 1, a balance must be found between good dissolution (implying a large ionized fraction of drug) and a large unionised fraction of drug (implying poor solubility but good absorption). A partition coefficient range of 40-2000 has been found to be optimal for drugs to be used sublingually. The importance of partition can be seen in the absorption of p-substituted phenylacetic acids, which have approximately the same pKa. The buccal absorption at pH 6 is (in order of increasing hydrophobicity): hydrogen - 1%, nitro - 1%, methoxy - 3%, methyl - 7%, ethyl - 10%, t-butyl - 25%, n-butyl - 34%, n-pentyl - 49%, cyclohexyl - 44% and n-hexyl - 61%[11].

Disadvantages of oral mucosal delivery

Not surprisingly, there are disadvantages to this route of administration. The buccal cavity, like the entire alimentary canal, behaves as a lipoidal barrier to the passage of drugs. Active transport, pinocytosis, and passage through aqueous pores play only insignificant roles in moving drugs across the oral mucosa, hence the majority of absorption is passive, and only small lipophilic molecules are well absorbed. Polar drugs, for example those which are ionized at the pH of the mouth (6.2-7.4), are poorly absorbed. Little intercellular absorption is possible across the cuboid squamous pavement epithelium of the oral cavity.

However, some amino acids such as glutamic acid and lysine[12] and some vitamins such as L-ascorbic acid[13], nicotinic acid[14] and thiamine[15] are reported to be transported via a carrier-mediated process.

Another major problem is that the dose form must be kept in place while absorption is occurring, since excessive salivary flow may wash it away. The total area for absorption is low compared to other routes, being in the region of 100-170 cm². The taste of the drug must be bland, otherwise it will not be acceptable. The drug must also be non-irritant, and it should not discolour or erode teeth. This may be partly overcome by using a drug delivery system which has a unidirectional drug outflow which is placed against the mucosa. However, these systems do have the potential for lateral diffusion and back partitioning of the drug into the oral cavity.

Effect of position on drug delivery

Within the oral cavity, delivery of drugs can be classified into four categories: (i) sublingual delivery in which the dosage form is placed on the floor of the mouth, under the tongue, (ii) buccal delivery, in which the formulation is positioned against the mucous membranes lining the cheeks, (iii) local oropharyngeal delivery to treat mouth and throat and (iv) periodontal delivery, to treat below the gum margin. Variations in epithelia thickness and composition will undoubtedly affect drug absorption. The permeability of the oral mucosa has been reviewed by Squier and Johnson[16]. The usual test of buccal absorption measures the average value of penetration of the drug through all the different regions of the oral mucosa, even though it is likely that regional differences in absorption occur. It has been suggested that drug absorption through the sublingual mucosa is more effective than through the buccal mucosa, even though both these regions are non-keratinized. The sublingual epithelium is, however, thinner and immersed in saliva, both of which will aid drug absorption (Figure 3.5).

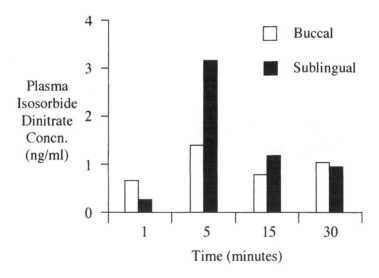

Figure 3.5 Comparison of isosorbide dinitrate absorption when drug is presented by the buccal and sublingual route

The rate of dissolution of the formulation may be position dependent, due to variations in its proximity to the major salivary gland and the water content of the saliva produced. The sublingual route is not suitable for the production of extended plasma concentration-time profiles, since absorption is completed quite quickly as the epithelium in the area is very thin (approximately 100 µm). This rapid absorption can lead to high peak plasma concentrations which may be overcome by delivering the drug to the thicker buccal mucosa which slows absorption. The metabolic activity of the oral mucosa and that of the resident population of bacteria can alter or degrade drugs[17].

The barrier function of the surface layers of the buccal epithelium depends upon the intercellular lipid composition. Epithelia which contain polar lipids (Table 3.1), notably cholesterol sulphate and glucosyl ceramides, are considerably more permeable to water than keratinized epithelia[18-20]. Intracellular lamellae, composed of chemically unreactive lipids, have been described in human buccal mucosa, and may be relevant to drug permeability[21].

During normal activities such as eating and drinking, the humidity and temperature in the oral cavity will be highly variable. The tongue is a highly sensitive organ and hence any device placed in the oral cavity will have to withstand being probed and explored by it, a process which the average patient will perform almost unconsciously. The sublingual area moves extensively during eating, drinking and speaking, so attachment of a delivery device to this region is likely to be impossible[22].

Intercellular junctions do not appear to affect the permeability of these tissues and it is possible that the presence of the intercellular barrier is not due to the distribution of the keratinized and non-keratinized layers, but rather to the presence of membrane-coating granules[16]. Membrane-coating granules are spherical or oval organelles, about 100-300 nm in diameter which are found in many stratified epithelia. These granules usually appear in the cells of the stratified spinosum in keratinized epithelia. As differentiation proceeds, they are discharged into the intercellular spaces by exocytosis. Membrane coating granules in keratinized epithelia have a structure of parallel lamination, whilst those in non-keratinized epithelia do not, but have an enclosed trilaminar membrane with finely granular contents which aggregate centrally. These organelles are absent from junctional epithelia and at the gingival margin, the areas of highest permeability. The barrier which the granules produce exists in the outermost 200µm of the superficial layer.

Two tracers which differ in size have been used to study the effective barrier produced by membrane-coating granules. These are horseradish peroxidase (m.w. 40,000 Dalton, 5-6 nm in size) and colloidal lanthanum (2 nm in size) which are both hydrophilic and hence would be confined to aqueous pathways[23]. When applied topically these tracers only penetrated the first three cell layers, but when introduced subepithelially, they extended through the intercellular spaces into the basal cell layers of the mucosal epithelium. In both keratinized and non-keratinized epithelia, the limit of penetration was related to the presence of the membrane-coating granules, implying that they cause a major barrier to penetration.

Gingival penetration

The gingival sulcus (Figure 3.6) is lined on its external surface by oral sulcular epithelium, which is continuous with the oral epithelium, but it is non-keratinized and has similar permeability to the oral epithelium. However, the "leakiest" area of the oral mucosa is the junctional epithelium in the gingival sulcus. This area has been studied extensively with respect to inflammatory periodontal disease. It is well documented that enzymes, toxins and antigens from plaque enter into the local tissue through this route and produce an immune inflammatory response in the tissue. Radioisotope and fluorescent compounds injected systemically can be detected at the surface. In healthy people, the sulcus is shallow

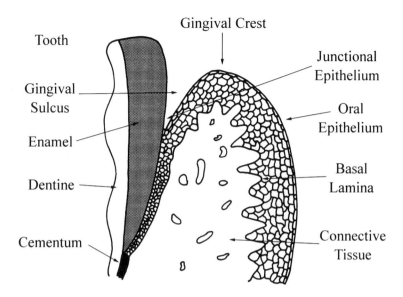

Figure3.6 The gingival margin

or non-existent, and its base is formed by junctional epithelium, which extends from the base of the sulcus. The intercellular spaces in the junction epithelium are considerably larger than in either the oral sulcular epithelium or the oral epithelium, and desmosome attachment is four times less common. The sulcus produces a fluid which is composed of an inflammatory exudate[24]. Mild mechanical agitation of the surface of the sulcular epithelium increases the flow of gingival fluid, and it is believed that no fluid flow occurs if the tissue is undisturbed, both in healthy and inflamed states.

Studies which have been carried out to examine the penetration of materials into the body via this route have rarely distinguished between junctional epithelium and oral sulcular epithelium. In addition many animals show differences in the way the epithelium is attached to the tooth in the sulcular region. Substances which have been claimed at various times to penetrate the sulcular epithelium are albumin, endotoxins, thymidine, histamine and horseradish peroxidase, which indicates a permeability of substances up to a molecular weight of 1 million[16]. Particulate material such as polystyrene microspheres with a 1 - 3 μm range of diameters have been reported to penetrate the epithelium[25]. It is possible that substances entering the gingiva do so through the intercellular spaces[26 27]. Topically applied peroxidase was found in the intercellular spaces after 10 minutes and application of hyaluronidase, which increases intercellular space, causes increased tracer uptake[28].

Gingival disease and ageing are likely to influence drug absorption through the buccal cavity, since the gum margin may recede or become inflamed. This may allow more access to the underlying connective tissues which have little barrier function to small molecules.

Improving penetration through the mucosa

There are three methods by which penetration of compounds through the oral mucosa can be achieved:

a) increasing the metabolic stability of the drug either by the use of pro-drugs or co-administration of enzyme inhibitors. For example, ketobemidone absorption was greatly increased when the phenolic hydroxyl group of the drug was derivatised into a carboxylic acid or carbonate ester[29]. This improved lipophilicity and resistance to saliva catalysed hydrolysis.

b) penetration enhancers, including chelators such as ethylenediaminepentaacetic acid or salicylates, surfactants (e.g sodium lauryl sulphate), bile salts (e.g sodium deoxycholate), fatty acids (e.g. oleic acid) and membrane fluidizers (e.g. Azone®).

c) physical enhancement, e.g. stripping layers from the epithelium using an adhesive strip, scraping the mucosa, or the application of an electric field across the epithelium (iontophoresis, see Chapter 8).

The use of penetration enhancers may be necessary to achieve adequate absorption of large molecules. However, their action is non-specific and care must be taken to ensure that toxins and bacteria are not allowed to enter the body in addition to drug. Currently no marketed buccal or sublingual products contain excipients registered as absorption enhancers.

MEASUREMENT OF ORAL MUCOSAL DRUG ABSORPTION

The original buccal absorption test was introduced by Beckett and Triggs in 1967[30]. An oral solution of the drug is held in the mouth without swallowing. After a measured period, the mouth is emptied and rinsed, and the amount of unabsorbed drug remaining is assayed. This method has several disadvantages, primarily that an absorption-time profile must be built up from several separate experiments. The drug concentration also changes due to salivary secretion[31] and swallowing; this latter can be compensated by using a non-absorbed internal marker[32]. More recently Tucker[33] has described a modification of the method which uses continuous oral sampling so that repeated experiments are not necessary. All these procedures suffer from the drawback that only absorption from the whole oral epithelia can be measured, and if the absorption is low, the precision of the method is poor.

To measure the absorption of drug from a specific region, a small filter paper disc soaked in drug can be applied to the mucosa. This technique has been used to measure the uptake or loss of water, sodium and potassium ions[34]. A more elegant method of measuring drug absorption from the various regions is a chamber through which drug solution can be circulated which can be applied to various regions of the mucosa[35]. This has the advantage that both plasma levels and effluent from the chamber can be analysed for drug content.

DOSAGE FORMS FOR THE ORAL CAVITY

Creams and ointments cannot be used successfully in the oral cavity since they will not adhere well and may be washed away by saliva, although the original mucosal delivery system Orabase® (E.R. Squibb and Sons Inc.) consisted of finely ground pectin, gelatin and sodium carboxymethylcellulose dispersed in a poly(ethylene) and mineral oil gel base. Generally, oral drug delivery devices have been adapted from traditional technology, for example tablets, but these do not adequately address the problems unique to the mouth. Formulations which have been specifically designed for oral delivery include gums, fast-dissolving dosage forms and mucoadhesive patches.

It is important that neither the drug nor the excipients stimulate saliva secretion since this will increase the amount of drug swallowed. Taste, irritancy and texture problems may discourage patients from taking dosage forms which are designed to reside in the oral cavity. In order to enhance patient compliance, the dosage form has to be unobtrusive

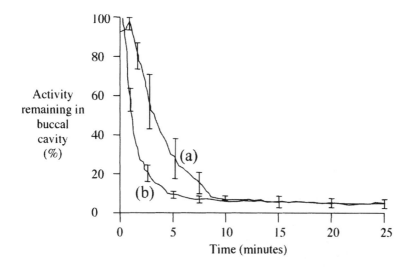

*Figure 3.7 Release of a radiolabelled marker from a chewable formulation when
(a) sucked and (b) chewed*

and pleasant to take: a maximum dimension might be no larger than 3 cm^2. Some formulations are keratinolytic and hence cannot be placed over the same site without the risk of ulceration.

Chewable formulations

Chewing gum was first patented in 1869[36] and medicated chewing gum containing aspirin (Aspergum®) was marketed in the USA in 1924. It was the discovery that smokers self-titrate the amount of nicotine which they are absorbing which led to the development of a nicotine gum to help people trying to withdraw from the habit. In theory the gum could be chewed until the correct amount of nicotine was absorbed, then the formulation could be discarded. It has been of some value as a tobacco substitute for people attempting to give up smoking [37].

Patients who have difficulty in swallowing tablets or capsules may prefer chewable systems, which also have the great advantage that they can be taken without water. The most important physiological variable which will markedly affect the release characteristics of a drug is whether a person sucks or chews the formulation since systems designed to be chewed will invariably be sucked and vice versa by a proportion of patients (Figure 3.7). The abuse potential of narcotic drugs is reduced in this type of formulation since it is much harder to extract the active ingredient from the base for subsequent intravenous administration.

The release of a drug from chewing gum is dependent upon its water solubility. Water-soluble substances are released rapidly and completely from chewing gum but it is possible to retard and extend their release. Slightly water-soluble drugs are released slowly and incompletely from chewing gum and require special formulation techniques to produce a satisfactory release profile[38]. The release of ^{99m}Tc-HIDA, a hydrophobic marker, was prolonged from a chewing gum compared to a sublingual tablet or lozenge[39]. Gums can be used to deliver drugs for the treatment of dental health and antifungal therapy e.g. nystatin[40] and miconazole[41]. The absorption of some substances such as vitamin C can be increased when administered in a gum compared to a conventional tablet[42]. Recently, mucin containing chewing gum has been used in the treatment of dry mouth[43].

Chewable formulations are used for the delivery of antacids where the flavouring agents give the sensation of relief from indigestion. Chewing antacid tablets prolongs the effect when compared to liquid antacids. Antacid tablets will react more slowly with gastric acid than liquids, even when thoroughly chewed, since the particle size will still be greater[44], but mixing the tablets with saliva also contributes to the prolonged duration of effect[45].

Fast-dissolving dosage forms

Fast dissolving dose forms for analgesics are well established as convenient systems for patient dosing, e.g. Solmin® (Reckitt and Colman Pharmaceuticals). These are solid dose forms which can be taken without water since they are designed to disperse on the tongue. They are also potentially useful where swallowing is difficult or oesophageal clearance is impaired.

Recently a new type of dosage form, Zydis™ (Scherer DDS), based on a freeze-dried mixture of drug and fast-dissolving excipients has been introduced to deliver sedative drugs such as benzodiazepines. Incorporation of ^{99m}Tc labelled micronised "Amberlite" CG400 resin during manufacture enabled the deposition and clearance of these formulations to be followed by gamma scintigraphy[46]. Two marker loadings were used, 2.5 mg and 10 mg, and the effect of incorporating the salivary stimulants talin and saccharin, and citrate, was investigated. Buccal clearance of the formulation containing the 10 mg resin was significantly faster than that containing 2.5 mg resin (Figure 3.8); however, calculation of the total activity remaining after dissolution showed that the amount remaining on the tongue was approximately 1 mg in each case. This probably represents the amount of resin trapped

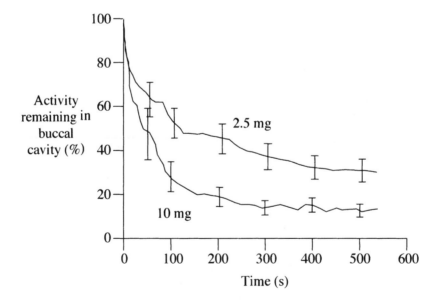

Figure 3.8 Clearance of a micronised resin from a Zydis™ formulation demonstrating trapping of resin between papillae on the tongue (mean clearance ± sd)

within the papillae of the tongue. There was little spread of the formulation laterally in the buccal cavity. Surprisingly, incorporation of salivary stimulants made little difference to the rate of dissolution of the formulation. Salivary stimulants increase the output of the submandibular and sublingual salivary glands, which discharge watery secretions onto the floor of the mouth, wetting the side of the tongue and cheek surfaces. The posterior third of the tongue surface contains mucus glands, but the quantity of secretion is relatively small. Thus increased salivary flow may not result in a more aqueous phase available for dissolution of the dosage form from the tongue surface. Delivery of drugs from a fast-dissolving formulation would not be expected to avoid first-pass metabolism since the unit disintegrates rapidly and the drug would be swallowed.

Bioadhesive dosage forms

Bioadhesion is a process which occurs when two materials, at least one of which is biological, are held together by interfacial forces. In pharmaceutics, bioadhesion is typically between an artificial material e.g. a polymer and/or a copolymer and a biological substrate. Where the biological substrate is covered with a mucus layer, the term "mucoadhesion" is used. It is described as a two-step process: first is the contact between two surfaces and second the formation of secondary bonds due to non-covalent bonding.

Many polymers can potentially be used in bioadhesive systems, including both water soluble and insoluble hydrocolloids, ionic and non-ionic and hydrogels. Appropriate materials for buccal delivery systems have to be mucoadhesive, have a sustained-release property and good feel in the mouth[47]. Bioadhesives have been formulated into tablets (e.g. Susadrin® (Pharmax Ltd.) which contains nitroglycerin[48]); gels and patches. Adhesive patches appear to be the most widely studied systems for buccal drug delivery. Patches vary in

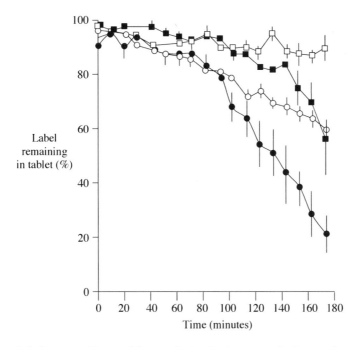

Figure 3.9 Inter- and intrasubject variation in the rates of release of a water soluble marker from a buccal mucoadhesive tablet

design and range from simple erodible systems, through non-erodible disks to laminated systems. Sizes vary from 1 to 15 cm^2, but smaller patches are much more comfortable. Patches will release drug both against the mucosa and into the oral cavity unless a backing layer is used to prevent release on the external face of the patch. Laminated systems permit local alteration of pH and inclusion of permeation enhancers which can markedly increase transport of drug. The use of the covered system removes luminal influences, such as saliva, mucus and enzymes, the presence of intercellular lipids, hence the mucosal thickness and the blood supply become rate limiting. The residence time of a bioadhesive system within the buccal cavity will depend on a variety of factors such as the strength of the mucoadhesive bond, the relative flexibility of both the system and the mucosa onto which it is adhered and the salivary flow. Hydrogels are currently being investigated extensively as bioadhesive vehicles for buccal drug delivery. They are swellable hydrophilic matrices that release a drug through the spaces in the polymer network by dissolution and disintegration.

Gamma scintigraphy was used to study the rate of release of ^{99m}Tc DTPA[49] from a buccal bioadhesive tablet (Figure 3.9). The tablet was designed to deliver glyceryl trinitrate and was based on a matrix of modified hydroxypropylmethylcellulose. The surface of the tablet quickly gels which serves both to anchor the tablet in position and to control the rate of diffusion of the drug[48]. The tablets are friable and the gel layer breaks on removal, and the in situ dissolution can be measured by gamma scintigraphy without disturbing the tablet. When the tablet was placed in the upper buccal pouch it was noted that between subjects there were marked differences in the rates of release, whereas within an individual measured on four occasions, the variation was quite small. This did not appear to be due to differences in saliva flow rate and the rate of dissolution, but interestingly may correlate with the extent to which the subject talked during the experiment. Articulation of the cheek surfaces during speech would increase the erosion of the tablet surface and hence the rate of release of the marker or drug into the buccal cavity. Drinking hot coffee or chewing gum did not affect the rate of release of marker. In general, when the tablet was placed behind the front incisors the rate of release of the marker was faster than when it was placed in the buccal cavity. The path of saliva flow in the human mouth can be monitored by measuring the distribution of charcoal particles placed at various locations in the mouth[6]. When the particles were placed under the tongue, the whole mouth became covered within 1 to 3 minutes, whereas administration to the lower right or left buccal vestibule covered that side of the tongue only. Hence, it is possible that salivary flow was responsible for the different rates of dissolution observed for the tablet.

Descriptions of a "semi-topical" buccal/gingival delivery system appeared in the literature about 12 years ago[50]. Lidocaine was delivered in an oral mucoadhesive tablet for the relief of toothache, or prostaglandin PGF2α into a gingival plaster for orthodontic tooth removal. Gingival absorption of lidocaine was poor due to the relatively low pH caused by the presence of carbopol-934, and more lipophilic derivatives such as dibucaine may be more suitable drug candidates. Studies in monkeys showed good results with the prostaglandin and limited clinical tests showed accelerated orthodontic tooth removal in 70% of patients studied.

Cydot™ (3M) is a flexible, mucoadhesive non-eroding disk which is placed on the gum. It has been used to deliver buprenorphene to volunteers and it is reported to remain in place for up to 17 hours regardless of food and drink consumed. The OTS (oral transmucosal system, TheraTech) is another commercially available device which has been used to deliver glucagon-like insulintropic peptide.

Dental systems

The use of antimicrobial agents in the treatment of chronic periodontal disease has utilised a variety of novel vehicles including hollow fibres, polymers (especially methacrylates) and oil-based vehicles to achieve sustained delivery of chlorhexidine, metronidazole and tetracycline. These materials are placed in the socket prior to occlusion with a dental appliance or wound dressing.

A controlled release compact containing tetracycline has been developed for treatment of severe forms of the diseases such as gingivitis, acute necrotising gingivitis, periodontitis and periodontosis[51]. The compacts (5 mm in diameter) were bonded to an upper molar and designed to release drug over a period of 10 days. The tetracycline reduced the quantity of plaque and gingival inflammation produced by the bacterial toxins around the gum margin. It is possible that similar systems can be developed to take advantage of the "leakiest" part of the buccal mucosa, the junctional epithelium.

A range of inflammatory, atrophic and ulcerative conditions occur in the mouth which justify the local application of corticosteroids[52]. The effect of the steroid reduces chemoattractants which in turn reduces the migration of white cells and prevents the increased permeability of small vessels at the site of damage. The use of mucoadhesive patches promotes transmucosal absorption and extends the duration of effective administration. Mucoadhesive tablets based on a mixture of hydroxypropylcellulose and carbopol have been used for the delivery of triamcinolone[53]. Following application to the mucosa, the formulation draws in water which helps promote adhesion to the lesions and more effective treatment. Restricting the distribution of the steroid may also be advantageous since it is known that the use of topical aerosol sprays in the mouth may induce fungal infection.

DRUGS ADMINISTERED VIA THE ORAL MUCOSA

Nitrates

The largest number of commercially available products for buccal and sublingual delivery are for organic nitrates (nitroglycerin (GTN), isosorbide dinitrate)[54-58]. GTN was rapidly and more effectively absorbed (30-60 s) from 2.5-5 mg buccal doses compared to a 10 mg transdermal patch. It was shown to be effective in prolonging the time to angina pectoris during exercise after a single dose, the effect lasting about five hours. Less convincing was its beneficial effect on heart failure in elderly patients in an open study over a minimum of fourteen days. Long-term therapy with buccal or transdermal glyceryl trinitrate may be associated with tolerance to drug action caused by sustained high plasma concentrations. Buccal nitroglycerin is reported to be a better prophylactic in the treatment of angina pectoris than sublingual nitroglycerin due to its longer duration of action, whereas both routes are comparable in the treatment of acute attacks[58].

Steroids

Steroids such as deoxycorticosterone are absorbed through the oral mucosa, but a threefold increase in dosage over intramuscular injections is required[59]. Testosterone and methyltestosterone are more efficiently absorbed when delivered buccally than by the peroral route[60 61]. Methyl testosterone for treating hypogonadism and delayed puberty is available commercially in devices which utilise this route for delivery. A range of inflammatory, atrophic and ulcerative conditions occur in the mouth for which topical treatment of corticosteroids is indicated[62].

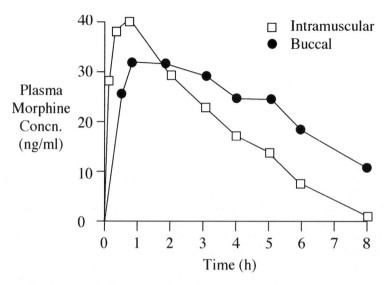

Figure 3.10 Plasma morphine concentration after intramuscular and buccal administration

Analgesics

Opioids (morphine, pethidine) are well absorbed with systemic availability and plasma concentrations which are similar to, or even higher than, that after intramuscular administration[63] (Figure 3.10). The reduction in post operative pain is comparable from both routes of administration[64]. Buccal morphine was reported not to be as effective as intramuscular morphine in relieving preoperative anxiety and wakefulness but this may have been produced by the lower bioavailability of the drug from the buccal dose form used[65 66]. A later study demonstrated that intramuscular administration of morphine produced an 8 fold increase in plasma levels compared to buccal administration. Buprenorphine is available as a sublingual commercial product for the treatment of analgesia.

Antibiotics

The oral cavity contains a diversity of microorganisms and over 300 different species of bacteria have been identified in the mouth. The density of microorganisms is high and saliva, which derives its flora from the oral surfaces contains 10^7-10^8 bacteria per ml. Most bacteria in the mouth are commensals and may have a protective role against pathogenic bacteria. Oral infections are categorized as primary, where bacteria cause diseases such as caries, chronic gingivitis, and inflammatory periodontal disease, and secondary, which aggravate existing damage associated with contaminated tissue. Antibacterial agents are used in the treatment of chronic gingivitis and effective agents, such as chlorhexidine, can persist for many hours. Antimicrobial plaque inhibitors are effective in preventing the formation of, rather than destroying, established plaque.

Antifungals

The predominant oral fungal pathogen belongs to the genus Candida, but in patients with HIV infection, less common species such as Crytococci, Histoplasma and Mucorales are often found[67]. Nystatin has been incorporated into a controlled delivery system for buccal use, but amphotericin B and clotrimazole are only available as a suspension or lozenge[68]. Two prolonged-release dosage forms have been devised for the treatment of oral candidiasis: chlorhexidine and clotrimazole, for therapy against Candida albicans, and also benzocaine and hydrocortisone to combat the pain and inflammation secondary to a candidal infection[69]. Interestingly only chlorhexidine and clotrimazole could be delivered in a controlled manner from the mucoadhesive patches, but release of all four drugs was controlled from the mucoadhesive tablets. Optimum release of the drugs over 24 h was achieved using sodium carboxymethylcellulose and polyethylene oxide combination tablets. Recently interferon-a has also been investigated for use against fungal infections of the oral cavity[70].

Others

Commercial products which deliver drugs either buccally or sublingually are available for lorazepam for anxiety and insomnia, nicotine for smoking cessation and ergotamine for migraine treatment. The buccal route has been tried with variable degrees of success for several other drugs, including metronidazole, metoclopramide, phenazocine, propranolol, timolol, salbutamol, fenoterol and insulin. Calcium channel blockers (nifedipine, verapamil) both produce effects similar to oral doses when administered sublingually or buccally[71 72]. The buccal route has also been explored for the delivery of peptides since the mucosa is reported to lack surface-bound peptidases, and preliminary work in dogs demonstrated significant absorption of a hydrophobic lauroyl derivative of a tripeptide[35]. Thyrotropin-releasing hormone, vasopressin analogues and insulin have been investigated as potential candidates for buccal and sublingual drug delivery. Oxytocin can be delivered by the buccal route, but this is now not often used since absorption was variable, and it was of real benefit only when the cervix was already ripe[73]. Its use was therefore largely abandoned in favour of the intravenous route. Most research groups are concentrating on using the nasal route to deliver peptides since it is more permeable than the oral cavity[74].

CONCLUSIONS

The attractiveness of the buccal route of dosing is the avoidance of first-pass metabolism of drugs. Drugs which can successfully be delivered by this route need to be highly active and able to produce a pharmacological response in small amounts. Absorption appears to be somewhat erratic due to an unpredictable salivary flow washing drug into the stomach, which is then available for absorption via the small intestine. Possibly the degree of plaque formation in the mouth and hence variability in junctional epithelium exposed also affects absorption to a degree.

REFERENCES

1. Chen YYM, Burne RA. Analysis of Streptococcus salivarius urease expression using continuous chemostat culture. *FEMS Microbiol. Letters* 1996;135:223-229.
2. Shannon IL, Prigmore JR. Physiologic chloride levels in human whole saliva. *Proc. Soc. Expt. Biol. Med.* 1958;97:825-828.
3. Schenkels L, Veerman ECI, Amerongen AVN. Biochemical composition of human saliva in relation to other mucosal fluids. *Crit. Rev. Oral Biol. Med.* 1995;6:161-175.
4. Lindqvist I, Noed CE, Soder PO. Origin of esterases in human whole saliva. *Enzyme* 1977;22:166-175.
5. Collins LMC, Dawes C. The surface area of the adult human mouth and thickness of the salivary film covering the teeth and mucosa. *J. Dent. Res.* 1987;66:1300-1302.
6. Jenkins GN, Krebsbach PM. Experimental study of the migration of charcoal particles in the human mouth. *Arch. Oral Biol.* 1985;30:697-699.
7. Weatherell JA, Robinson C, Rathbone MJ. Site-specific differences in the salivary concentration of substances in the oral cavity - Implications for the aetiology of oral disease and local drug delivery. *Adv. Drug Del. Rev.* 1994;13:23-42.

8. Weatherell JA, Robinson C, Ralph JP, Best JS. Migration of fluoride in the mouth. *Caries Res.* 1984;18:348-353.
9. Weatherell JA, Strong M, Robinson C, Nakagaki H, Ralph JP. Retention of glucose in oral fluids at different sites in the mouth. *Caries Res.* 1989;23:399-405.
10. Sobrero A. Surplusiers composé dé tonants produit avec l'acide nitrique et le sucre, la dextrine, la lactine, la mannite et la glycérine. *Comptes, Rendus Hebdomadaires des Séances de l'Academie des Sciences* 1847;24:247-248.
11. Beckett AH, Moffatt AC. The influence of substitution in phenyl acetic acids on their performance in the buccal absorption test. *J. Pharm. Pharmacol.* 1969;21:139S.
12. Gandhi RB. Some permselectivity and permeability characteristics of rabbit buccal mucosa. *Ph.D. Thesis, University of Wisconsin, Madison* 1990.
13. Sadoogh-Abasian F, Evered DF. Absorption of vitamin C from the human buccal cavity. *Br. J. Nutr.* 1979;42:15-20.
14. Evered DF, Sadoogh-Abasian F, Patel PD. Absorption of nicotinic acid and nicotimamide across the human buccal mucosa *in vivo*. *Life Sci.* 1980;27:1649-1661.
15. Evered DF, Mallett C. Thiamine absorption across the human buccal mucosa *in vivo*. *Life Sci.* 1983;32:1355-1358.
16. Squier CA, Johnson NW. Permeability of the oral mucosa. *Br. Med. Bull.* 1975;31:169-175.
17. Yamahara H, Lee VHL. Drug metabolism in the oral cavity. *Adv. Drug Del. Rev.* 1993;12:25-40.
18. Squier CA, Hall BK. The permeability of skin and the oral mucosa to water and horseradish peroxidase as related to the thickness of the permeability barrier. *J. Invest. Dermatol.* 1985;84:176-179.
19. Squier CA, Cox PS, Wertz W, Downing DT. The lipid composition of porcine epidermis and oral epithelium. *Arch. Oral Biol.* 1986;31:741-747.
20. Curatolo W. The lipoidal permeability barriers of the skin and alimentary tract. *Pharm. Res.* 1987;4:271-277.
21. Garza J, Swartzendruber DC, Vincent S, Squier CA, Wertz PW. Membrane structures in the human epithelium (abstract). *J. Dent. Res.* 1998;77:1502.
22. Harris D, Robinson JR. Drug delivery via the mucous membranes of the oral cavity. *J. Pharmaceut. Sci.* 1992;81:1-10.
23. Squier CA, Rooney L. The permeability of keratinised and non-keratinised oral epithelium to lanthanum *in vivo*. *J. Ultrastruct. Res.* 1976;54:286-295.
24. Cimasoni G. *Monographs in oral science, The crevicular fluid.* 3 Karger, Basel. 1974.
25. Fine DH, Pechersky JL, McKibben DH. The penetration of human gingival sulcular tissue by carbon particles. *Arch. Oral Biol.* 1969;14:1117-1119.
26. McDougall WA. Penetration pathways of a topically applied foreign protein into rat gingiva. *J. Periodontal. Res.* 1971;6:89-99.
27. McDougall WA. Ultrastructural localisation of antibody to an antigen applied topically to rabbit gingiva. *J. Periodontal. Res.* 1972;7:304-314.
28. Stallard RE, Awwa IA. The effect of alterations in external environment on dento-gingival junction. *J. Dent. Res.* 1969;48:671-675.
29. Hansen LB, Christrup LL, Bundgaard H. Ketobemidone prodrugs for buccal delivery. *Acta Pharmaceutica Nordica.* 1991;3: 77-82.
30. Beckett AH, Triggs ER. Buccal absorption of basic drugs and its application as an *in vivo* model of passive drug transfer through lipid membranes. *J. Pharm. Pharmacol.* 1967;19:31S-41S.
31. Dearden JC, Tomlinson E. Correction for effect of dilution on diffusion through a membrane. *J. Pharmaceut. Sci.* 1971;60:1278-1279.
32. Schurmann W, Turner P. A membrane model of the human oral mucosa as derived from buccal absorption performance and physicochemical properties of the beta-blocking drugs atenolol and propranolol. *J. Pharm. Pharmacol.* 1978;30:137-147.
33. Tucker IG. A method to study the kinetics of oral mucosal drug absorption from solutions. *J Pharm. Pharmacol.* 1988;40:679-83.

34. Kaaber S. Studies on the permeability of human oral mucosa. vi. The mucosal transport of water, sodium and potassium under varying osmotic pressure. *Acta Odont. Scand.* 1973;31:307-316.

35. Veillard MM, Longer MA, Martens TW, Robinson JR. Preliminary studies of oral mucosal delivery of peptide drugs. *J. Cont. Rel.* 1987;6:123-131.

36. Semple WF. Improved chewing gum. *U.S. Patent 98: 304* 1869.

37. Mulry JT. Nicotine gum dependency: a positive addiction. *Drug Intell. Clin. Pharm.* 1988;22:313-314.

38. Rassing MR. Chewing gum as a drug delivery system. *Adv. Drug Del. Rev.* 1994;13:89-121.

39. Christrup LL, Davis SS, Frier M, Melia CD, Rasmussen SN, Washington N, Disposition of a model substance 99m-Tc E-HIDA in the oral cavity, the oesophagus and the stomach during and following administration of lozenges, chewing gum and sublingual tablets, followed by gamma scintigraphy. *Int. J. Pharmaceut.* 1990;60:167-174.

40. Andersen T, Gramhansen M, Pedersen M, Rassing MR. Chewing gum as a drug delivery system for nystatin influence of solubilizing agents upon the release of water insoluble drugs. *Drug Dev. Indust. Pharm.* 1990;16:1985-1994.

41. Pedersen M, Rassing MR. Miconazole chewing gum as a drug delivery system application of solid dispersion technique and lecithin. *Drug Dev. Indust. Pharm.* 1990;16:2015-2030.

42. Christrup LL, Rasmussen SN, Rassing MR. Chewing gum as a drug delivery system. *Proc. 3rd Int Conf. Drug Absorpt. Edinburgh* 1988.

43. Aagaard A, Godiksen S, Teglers PT, Schiodt M, Glenert U. Comparison between new saliva stimulants in patients with dry mouth: A placebo-controlled double-blind crossover study. *J. Oral Pathol. Med.* 1992;21: 376-380.

44. Washington N. Antacids and anti-reflux agents. *CRC Press, Boca Raton* 1991.

45. Barnett CC, Richardson CT. *In vivo* and *in vitro* evaluation of magnesium-aluminium hydroxide antacid tablets and liquid. *Dig. Dis. Sci.* 1985;30:1049-1052.

46. Wilson CG, Washington N, Peach J, Murray GR, Kennerley J. The behaviour of a fast-dissolving dosage form (Expidet™) followed by gamma scintigraphy. *Int. J . Pharm.* 1987;40:119-123.

47. Nagai T, Machida Y. Buccal delivery systems using hydrogels. *Adv. Drug Deliv. Rev* 1993;11:179-191.

48. Schor JM. Sustained release therapeutic compositions. *U.S. Patent 4226849* 1980.

49. Davis SS, Kennerley JW, Taylor MJ, Hardy JG, Wilson CG. Scintigraphic studies on the *in vivo* dissolution of a buccal tablet. *In Modern Concepts in Nitrate Delivery Systems.* Eds Goldberg A.A.J and Parsons D.G. 1983:29-37.

50. Nagai T, Konishi R. Buccal/gingival drug delivery systems. *J. Cont. Rel.* 1987;6:353-360.

51. Collins AEM, Deasy PB, MacCarthy DJ, Shanley DB. Evaluation of a controlled-release compact containing tetracycline hydrochloride bonded to a tooth for the treatment of periodontal disease. *Int. J. Pharmaceut.* 1989;51:103-114.

52. Thorburn DN, Ferguson MM. Topical corticosteroids and lesions of the oral mucosa. *Adv. Drug Deliv. Rev.* 1994;13:135-149.

53. Nagai T, Machida Y. Advances in drug delivery - mucoadhesive dosage forms. *Pharm. Int.* 1985;6:196-200.

54. Naito H, Matsuda Y, Shiomi K, Yorozu T, Maeda T, Lee H, et al. Effects of sublingual nitrate in patients receiving sustained therapy of isosorbide dinitrate for coronary artery disease. *Am. J. Cardiol.* 1989;64:565-568.

55. Yukimatsu K, Nozaki Y, Kakumoto M, Ohta M. Development of a trans-mucosal controlled-release device for systemic delivery of antianginal drugs pharmacokinetics and pharmacodynamics. *Drug Develop. Indust. Pharm.* 1994;20:503-534.

56. Wagner F, Siefert F, Trenk D, Jahnchen E. Relationship between pharmacokinetics and hemodynamic tolerance to isosorbide-5-mononitrate. *Europ. J. Clin. Pharmacol.* 1990;38(Suppl 1):S53-S59.

57. Nyberg G. Onset time of action and duration up to 3 hours of nitroglycerin in buccal, sublingual and transdermal form. *Europ. Heart J.* 1986;7:673-678.
58. Ryden L, Schaffrath R. Buccal versus sublingual nitroglycerin administration in the treatment of angina pectoris: a multi centre study. *Europ. Heart J.* 1987;8:994-1001.
59. Anderson E, Haymaker W, Henderson E. Successful sublingual therapy in Addison's disease. *J. Am. Med. Assoc.* 1940;115:216-217.
60. Miescher K, Gasche P. Zur lingualen Applikation von männlichem sexualhormon; Beitrag zur Therapie mit "Perandren-Linguetten". *Schweiz. Med. Wochenschr.* 1942;72:279-281.
61. Escamilla RF, Bennett LL. Pituitary infantilism treated with purified growth hormone, thyroid and sublingual methyltestosterone. Case report. *J. Clin. Endocrinol.* 1951;11:221.-228.
62. Thorburn DN, Ferguson MM. Topical corticosteroids and lesions of the oral mucosa. *Adv. Drug Deliv. Rev.* 1994;13:135-149.
63. Bardgett D, Howard C, Murray GR, Calvey TN, Williams NE. Plasma concentration and bioavailability of buccal preparation of morphine sulphate. *Br. J. Clin. Pharmacol.* 1984;17:198P-199P.
64. Bell MDD, Murray GR, Mishra P, Calvey TN, Weldon BD, Williams NE. Buccal morphine - a new route for analgesia? *Lancet* 1985;i:71-73.
65. Fisher AP, Vine P, Whitlock J, Hanna M. Buccal morphine premedication. *Anaesthesia* 1986;41:1104-1111.
66. Fisher AP, Fung C, Hanna M. Serum morphine concentrations after buccal and intramuscular morphine administration. *Br. J. Clin. Pharmacol.* 1987;24:685-687.
67. Samaranayake LP. Oral mycoses in HIV infection. *Oral Surg. Oral Med. Oral Pathol.* 1990;73:171-180.
68. Samaranayake LP, Ferguson MM. Delivery of antifungal agents to the oral cavity. *Adv. Drug Deliv. Rev.* 1994;13:161-179.
69. Nair MK, Chien YW. Development of anticandidal delivery systems: (II) Mucoadhesive devices for prolonged drug delivery in the oral cavity. *Drug Dev. Indust. Pharm.* 1996;22:243-253.
70. Fujioka N, Akazawa R, Sakamoto K, Ohashi K, Kurimoto M. Potential application of human interferon-alpha in microbial infections of the oral cavity. *J. Interferon Cytokine Res.* 1995;15:1047-1051.
71. Asthana OP, Woodcock BG, Wenchel M, Frömming KH, Schwabe L, Rietbrock N. Verapamil disposition and effects on PQ intervals after buccal, oral and intravenous administration. *Drug Res.* 1984;34:498-502.
72. Robinson BF, Dobbs RJ, Kelsey CR. Effects of nifedipine on resistance of vessels, arteries and veins in man. *Br. J. Clin. Pharmacol.* 1980;10:433-438.
73. Miller GW. Induction of labour by buccal administration of oxytocin. *J. Am. Osteopath. Assoc.* 1974;72:1110-1113.
74. Merkle HP, Wolany G. Buccal delivery for peptide drugs. *J. Cont. Rel.* 1992;21:155-164.

Chapter Four

Oesophageal Transit

INTRODUCTION

The oesophagus serves to move boluses of food, drink or drug formulations from the buccal cavity, through the lower oesophageal sphincter and into the stomach. In normal healthy people, ingested materials have a very short contact time with oesophageal tissue, but this is slightly lengthened when individuals are supine due to the loss of the effect of gravity.

The appreciation that oesophageal transit of formulations could be the first stumbling block that orally administered solid drug formulations could encounter appears to stem from the introduction of wax-based matrix tablets of potassium chloride produced in the 1960s[1]. Since this time there have been numerous reports in the literature of drugs that have the potential to cause damage to the mucosa. Although most of the injuries were self-limiting, with symptoms such as retrosternal pain and dysphagia, there were occasional instances of serious complications such as perforation and haemorrhage leading to death. Another significant consequence of retention of a formulation in the oesophagus is that it can reduce or delay absorption of the drug.

ANATOMY AND PHYSIOLOGY

Oesophagus

The oesophagus is a 25 cm long, 2 cm diameter muscular tube which joins the pharynx to the cardiac orifice of the stomach. The stratified squamous epithelium lining the buccal cavity continues through the pharynx and down the oesophagus. The lowest 2 cm or so of the oesophagus which lies within the abdominal cavity is normally lined with gastric mucosa and covered by peritoneum. The stratified squamous epithelium provides a tough impermeable lining resisting the abrasive nature of food boluses, whilst the gastric mucosal lining resists damage by gastric acid. The lumen of the oesophagus is highly folded in the relaxed state. The pH of the normal oesophageal lumen is usually between 6 and 7.

The oesophagus has four coats, a fibrous external layer, a muscular layer, a submucous or areolar layer and an internal or mucous layer (Figure 4.1).

a) The fibrous coat consists of elastic fibres embedded in a layer of areolar tissue.

b) The muscular layer is composed of circular muscle surrounded by longitudinal muscle. Smooth muscle is found in the lower third of the oesophagus, striated muscle in the upper part and both types are found in the middle section.

c) The areolar or submucous coat contains the larger blood vessels, nerves and mucous glands. It loosely connects the mucous and muscular coats.

d) The mucosal layer consists of a layer of stratified squamous epithelium, one of connective tissue, and a layer of longitudinal muscle fibres, the muscularis mucosae. It forms longitudinal folds in its resting state which disappear when distended.

Two types of secretory glands are found in the oesophagus. The majority of oesophageal glands are simple glands located in the lamina propria, but in the lower 5 cm of the oesophagus the glands are compound and identical to the cardiac glands of the stomach (Chapter 5) which secrete mucus rather than acid.

The oesophageal glands are distributed throughout the length of the oesophagus and are located in the submucosa. These are small racemose glands of the mucous type and each opens into the lumen by a long duct which pierces the muscularis mucosae. There are probably no more than 300 in total, of which the majority lie in the proximal half of the oesophagus. The relatively few glands present make the oesophagus a moist rather than a wet environment with the majority of fluid coming from swallowed saliva (approximately 1 litre per day). The principal reason for secretion is to lubricate food and protect the lower part of the oesophagus from gastric acid damage.

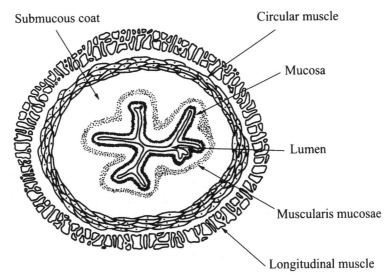

Submucous coat   Circular muscle

Mucosa

Lumen

Muscularis mucosae

Longitudinal muscle

Figure 4.1 Cross section through the oesophagus

The oesophagus possesses both sympathetic and parasympathetic innervation. Extrinsic innervation consists of a supply from the vagus nerves and sympathetic fibres derived from the cervical and thoracic ganglia. The intrinsic supply is derived from the Auerbach and Meissner plexuses. Neurites are found in the circular muscle of the oesophagus. They also run over the surfaces of interstitial cells which are not present in the longitudinal layer. These cells are called interstitial cells of Cajal and they possess a round or oval nucleus and a long, flat broad process which extends between the muscle fibres. The precise function of these cells has not yet been discovered, but it is thought that they co-ordinate muscle contraction.

Gastro-oesophageal junction or cardia

The distal or lower oesophageal sphincter, also called the cardia, represents the transition between the oesophagus and the stomach. As no definite anatomical sphincter exists, there are several definitions of the lower oesophageal sphincter:

a) the junction of squamous and columnar epithelium,

b) the point at which the oesophagus enters the stomach,

c) the junction between the oesophageal inner muscle layer and the inner layer of oblique muscle of the stomach (Figure 4.2).

These features all occur in the human stomach within 1 cm of each other. The definition by manometry is a high pressure zone, 2 to 6 cm in length, with an intraluminal pressure of 15 to 40 mm Hg above intragastric pressure. This "sphincter" prevents gastro-oesophageal reflux, i.e. acidic gastric contents from reaching stratified epithelia of the oesophagus, where it can cause inflammation and irritation.

MOTILITY OF THE OESOPHAGUS

Swallowing is a highly complex set of events controlled by a swallowing centre in the medulla. A normal adult swallows between 100 and 600 times per day, one-third of these accompany eating and drinking and the remaining events occur when breathing out. Relatively few swallows occur during sleep (< 10%). The primary stimulus for swallowing food is provided by sensory stimuli originating from receptors located within the sensory fields of the mouth and pharynx. Non-prandial swallowing is driven by salivation and occurs without apparent cerebral participation.

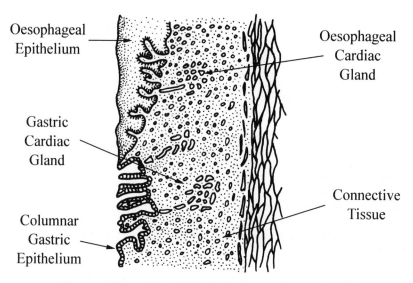

Oesophageal Epithelium

Oesophageal Cardiac Gland

Gastric Cardiac Gland

Columnar Gastric Epithelium

Connective Tissue

Figure 4.2 Transverse section through the cardia

The resting pressure in the oesophagus reflects the changes due to breathing which cause cycles of positive and negative intrathoracic pressure between -5 to -10 mm Hg (Torr) during inspiration, to 0 to +5 mm Hg during expiration. On swallowing, the upper oesophageal sphincter relaxes for a period of about 1 second and then constricts. The swallow is associated with a transient decrease in pressure followed by a primary peristaltic wave of high pressure which travels towards the stomach at a speed of 2 to 6 cm s^{-1} in the proximal oesophagus, gradually becoming faster by the time it reaches the distal oesophagus (Figure 4.3). The lower oesophageal sphincter relaxes usually about 2 seconds after the initiation of swallowing for a period of 5 to 10 seconds allowing entry of the swallowed bolus.

The peak of the peristaltic wave is usually above 40 mm Hg, but there is considerable intra-subject variation. If a second swallow is taken before the peristaltic wave from the first swallow has reached the base of the oesophagus, then the initial peristaltic wave is

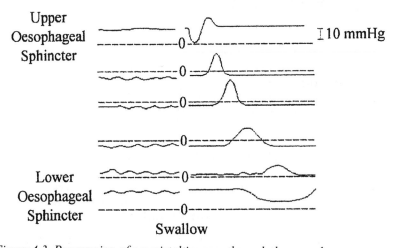

Upper Oesophageal Sphincter

$\mathbb{I}$10 mmHg

Lower Oesophageal Sphincter

Swallow

Figure 4.3 Progression of a peristaltic wave through the oesophagus

interrupted by the second peristaltic wave. When swallows are repeated in quick succession, then the contraction of the oesophagus is inhibited until the last swallow occurs; only the final peristaltic wave proceeds uninterrupted to the cardia carrying any food bolus or drug formulation with it.

If the subject is upright, gravity assists the movement of the swallowed material which may arrive at the lower oesophageal sphincter before relaxation has begun. This is especially true for non-viscous liquids whose entry in stomach may be slightly delayed until the lower oesophageal sphincter relaxes. Secondary peristaltic waves arise from distension of the oesophagus and serve to move sticky lumps of food or refluxed materials into the stomach. Initiation of secondary peristalsis is involuntary and is not normally sensed. Variation in the size of the bolus being swallowed leads to a variation in the amplitude of oesophageal contraction.

The pH of the oesophagus is between 6 and 7. After a meal, reflux of gastric acid is seen as sharp drops in pH which rapidly return to baseline. This is a normal physiological occurrence. Gastro-oesophageal reflux disease (heartburn) occurs when gastric acid damages the oesophageal mucosa either through prolonged contact or reduced resistance of the mucosa to damage.

OESOPHAGEAL TRANSIT OF DOSAGE FORMS
Measurement
Oesophageal transit is usually assessed clinically by x-ray study of a swallowed bolus of barium sulphate suspension. Very early studies also used barium to assess oesophageal transit of variety of substances such as gelatin cylinders[2], marshmallows[3 4], cotton pledgets, tablets[5 6] and capsules[7]. However, later studies demonstrated that dense materials such as barium have faster transit than more physiological substances. In addition, X-ray contrast techniques are difficult to quantify and are associated with a significant radiation burden on the subjects. Consequently, gamma scintigraphy has become the method of choice to assess oesophageal transit. It has the advantages that any suitably labelled test material, food or dosage forms can be followed and radiation dosimetry is very small allowing repeat studies in individuals. It is a quantifiable technique since transit can be expressed as position of radioactivity against time (Figure 4.4).

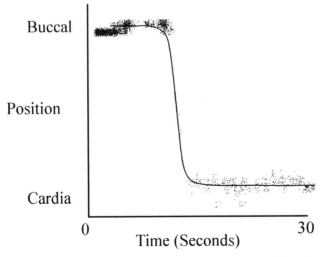

Figure 4.4 Plot of position of activity versus time for a swallow of technetium-99m - DTPA labelled water

Table 4.1 Typical transit times for various pharmaceutical dosage forms
*ODT – Orally dissolving tablet

Formulation	Weight & dimensions	Transit time Seconds	Posture
Tablet Round	100mg 6mm diameter	13	Supine[8]
Tablet Oval	14mm x 9mm Film-coated	3	Erect[9]
Tablet Oval	14mm x 9mm, Film-coated	>300	Supine[9]
Tablet Oval	14mm x 9mm	>300	Supine[9]
Tablets	Various sizes & shapes	8	Supine[10]
Tablets	Various	4	Erect[11]
Capsule	Hard gelatin, Size 2	10	Supine[12]
Capsule	Hard gelatin, Size 2 (0.59g)	10	Supine[11]
Capsule	Hard gelatin, Size 2 (1.2g)	80	Supine[9]
Capsule	Hard gelatin, Size 2 (0.59g)	9	Erect[9]
Capsule	Hard gelatin, Size 2 (1.2g)	3	Erect[9]
Capsule	Hard gelatin, Size 0 (1.2g)	3	Erect[9]
Capsule	Hard gelatin, Size 0 (1.2g)	45	Supine[9]
Capsule	Hard gelatin, Size 0 (0.67g)	9	Erect[9]
Capsule	Hard gelatin, Size 0 (1.2g)	9	Supine[9]
Liquid	10 ml	9	Supine[12]
Zydis™	12 mm diameter, 0.25 ml	14	Supine[12]
Suspension	90 – 125 µm (5 mg)	9	Seated[14]
Suspension	20 – 40 µm (5 mg)	7	Seated[14]
ODT*	90 – 125 µm (5 mg resin)	35	Seated[14]
ODT*	20 – 40 µm (5 mg resin)	39	Seated[14]
Water	1.5 ml	8	Seated[14]

Typical transit times

Normally, the oesophageal transit of dose forms is extremely rapid, usually of the order of 10 to 14 seconds. Typical transit times for various pharmaceutical dosage forms are shown in Table 4.1.

These data suggest that large oval tablets have a shorter oesophageal transit than large round tablets, but the influence of size and shape of formulations on oesophageal transit is insignificant when compared to the influence of the posture of the subject. Oesophageal transit is slower in supine patients than upright ones. Although studies are often carried out in supine patients to eliminate the effects of gravity, the differences in oesophageal transit produced with varying size and shape of a tablet are only observed in upright subjects and not supine ones. Interestingly, the transit of a heavy capsule is significantly faster than a light capsule in erect subjects, but the order is reversed in supine subjects[15]. The transit of large but not small capsules is significantly faster than plain oval tablets in both erect and supine volunteers [15].

Bolus composition can markedly affect transit. Liquids clear rapidly, with one swallow regardless of whether the subjects were supine or seated, but capsules or liver cubes when ingested without water, frequently remained in the oesophagus up to 2 hours after administration, without the subject being aware of their presence[13].

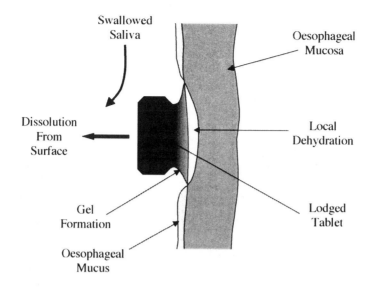

Figure 4.5 Mechanism of adhesion of a dosage form

OESOPHAGEAL ADHESION OF DOSAGE FORMS

There are normal anatomic narrowings of the oesophagus located at the cricopharyngeus, aortic arch and left main stem bronchus which increase the contact time of a bolus and hence are potential sites for adhesion in healthy subjects. It is well recognised that there is approximately a 20% incidence of adhesion of dosage forms to the oesophagus, particularly for tablets or capsules. Only 3% of patients are aware that the tablet/capsule has stuck in the oesophagus[16]. The risk of adhesion of dosage forms to the oesophagus is increased to about 50% for people who take their medication whilst recumbent or semi-recumbent and/or who take formulations with little or no water. If patients sleep whilst the dose form is lodged in the oesophagus, disintegration will be very slow since saliva production is greatly reduced compared to waking levels.

The recommended method of taking tablets and capsules to avoid oesophageal retention is upright, with a sip of water before the dose form and then at least 100 ml of water with the medication. Hospital dosing cups in particular should be marked with a minimum fill line for water to assist staff to give the correct amount when dosing patients, particularly since they are likely to be recumbent or semi-recumbent.

Although the outer surface of many dosage forms will rapidly disintegrate when placed in fluid under sink conditions, the small amount of fluid available in the oesophagus will only moisten the surface. If this quickly becomes sticky, then the dosage form has the potential to adhere, a problem that is exacerbated by the highly folded nature of the oesophageal lumen in the resting state which will press the sticky dosage form against the mucosa. The mucosa will partly dehydrate at the site of contact as the unit hydrates, resulting in formation of a gel between the formulation and the mucosa (Figure 4.5). The unit then disintegrates from its non-contact side. Disintegration of the lodged formulation is slow, firstly because the amount of dissolution fluid available is low, being dependent on the volume of swallowed saliva and secondly due to the reduced surface area available for dissolution.

In some patients, solid dosage forms will still adhere to the oesophagus even when reasonable volumes of water are taken, these patients may have reduced peristaltic pressures or have cardiac pathologies in which the left side of the heart is enlarged. In these patients liquid preparations should be used or alternative routes of drug administration should be explored to avoid oesophageal damage by delivery of high concentration of drug to a small area of mucosa.

Factors predisposing formulations to adhere

There have been many studies carried out examining the potential for various dosage forms to adhere in the oesophagus. The main discrepancies in the literature arise from whether the data is derived from *in vitro* preparations of animal oesophagus or human studies. *In vitro* studies often use isolated porcine mucosa. Here the formulations are moistened, placed in contact with the mucosa and the force required to detach them is measured. *In vivo* studies generally measure transit in humans using fluoroscopy or gamma scintigraphy. In the transit studies all the factors which influence the tendency of a formulation to adhere e.g. shape, size, density etc are measured, whereas the *in vitro* experiments only study the tendency of the surface layer to adhere.

Tablets are often coated to render them more acceptable to the patient or to protect the drug from gastric acid etc., but the coatings themselves may affect the tendency for formulations to adhere. *In vitro* studies using isolated oesophageal preparations have concluded that that hard gelatin capsules had the greatest tendency to adhere, followed by film coated tablets, uncoated tablets, with sugar coated tablets demonstrating the least adhesion[17 18]. It was estimated that hard gelatin capsules have 6 times the tendency to adhere than that of sugar coated tablets and 1.5 times that of soft gelatin capsules when calculated per unit area. The difference between hard and soft gelatin capsules in their tendency to adhere is not borne out in human studies[16]. Although coated tablets have significantly shorter oesophageal transit times than plain tablets, if they do lodge, they take longer to disintegrate. Coatings made from cellulose acetate phthalate, shellac, methacrylate copolymer and a copolymer composed from of vinyl acetate and crotonic acid all have a low tendency to adhere. The tendency of hydroxypropylmethylcellulose to adhere can be altered by incorporation of sucrose which reduces surface stickiness; conversely addition of lactose or titanium oxide and talc increases the tendency to adhere. In contrast, polyethylene glycol 6000 coating demonstrated the greatest tendency to adhere.

A variety of studies in humans have demonstrated that capsules lodge in the oesophagus with a much higher incidence than tablets[10-12 19]. If the passage through the oesophagus of a hard gelatin capsule is delayed for more than two minutes, it can absorb sufficient water to become adherent to the mucosa. Apart from gelatin, other materials which become sticky as they hydrate are cellulose derivatives and guar gum. Recently it was reported that guar gum, formulated into a slimming product, hydrated and formed a large viscous mass which was sufficient to cause oesophageal obstruction[20]. A further report of an anhydrous protein health food tablet, which adhered to the oesophagus so firmly that it had to be removed at endoscopy, shows that it is not only pharmaceutical dosage forms which have potential to stick, but now nutriceuticals also have to be evaluated for this possible hazard[21].

Dosage forms are being developed which can be swallowed with little or no water. There has been some concern that material from these dose forms is retained in the mouth and oesophagus since they rely on saliva for clearance. The Zydis® formulation (Scherer DDS Ltd) is an example of a rapidly disintegrating solid dosage form which can be taken without water. The general pattern of buccal clearance of the fast dissolving dosage form was either to dissolve rapidly in the mouth and hence clear with several swallows, or to pass intact through the oesophagus (Figure 4.6)[12].

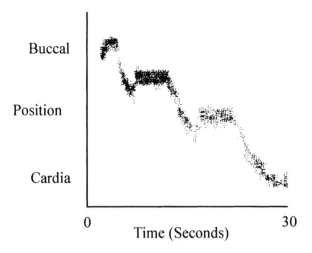

Figure 4.6 Clearance of a fast-dissolving dosage form from the oesophagus

CONSEQUENCES OF ADHESION OF DOSAGE FORMS
Delay in drug absorption

Retention of the dosage form in the oesophagus can delay drug absorption and consequently the onset of action (Figure 4.7)[22]. Drugs cannot easily pass through the stratified squamous epithelium of the oesophageal mucosa. Passage of the drug into the stomach and through to the small intestine where it is absorbed will be dependent upon the disintegration time of the unit in the oesophagus.

Oesophageal damage

If a dosage form adheres to the oesophagus, a very concentrated solution of drug is presented to an extremely small area of the mucosa and it is not surprising that oesophageal injury can occur. Repeated insult to the mucosa can result in dysphagia and even stricture formation, both of which exacerbate the original problem. Drugs which are irritant to the gastric mucosa are often given as enteric coated formulations; however, failure of these coatings may result if units lodge in the oesophagus where the pH is near 7.

Medication induced oesophageal injury was first reported in 1970[1], and was reviewed in 1983[23]. During the period between 1960 and 1983, 221 cases were reported due to 26 different medications, and since then there have been numerous reports in the literature[24][25]. Antibiotics account for half the reported cases regardless of brand, although it has been reported for numerous other drugs including emepronium bromide, theophylline, doxycycline monohydrate and bisphosphonates[26]. This may reflect the various proportions of drugs which are prescribed, but this has not been studied. Endoscopic surveillance in healthy volunteer studies has shown that oesophagitis is detectable in 20% of subjects taking non-steroidal anti-inflammatories (NSAIDs)[27]. NSAIDs are also believed to have a causative role in oesophageal stricture in patients with gastro-oesophageal reflux[28].

Drugs can cause local injury by a range of mechanisms including caustic or acidic effects, hyperosmotic effect, heat production, gastro-oesophageal reflux, impaired oesophageal clearance of acid and accumulation within the basal layer of the epithelium, in addition to any specific toxic effects caused by the drug.

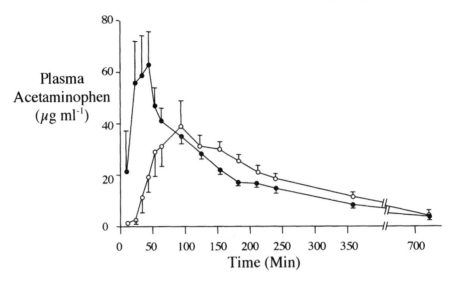

Figure 4.7 Plasma concentrations of 400 mg acetaminophen in patients with delayed oesophageal transit (○) and normal transit (•)[23]

Endoscopy demonstrates a redness and friability of the mucosa, an erosion about the size of a coin, or a deep ulcer[29]. Occasionally particles of drug may be seen to be adhered to the mucosa. The majority of lesions are located at the level of the aortic arch or slightly above it (Figure 4.8). Less commonly lesions can be seen higher in the oesophagus, particularly in bedridden patients. Lesions have also been reported in the lower third of the oesophagus, just above the gastro-oesophageal junction. In severe cases, stricture may result. Most patients are apparently healthy people who are suddenly hit by symptoms of oesophageal injury. Men and women alike are affected and patients between 9 and 98 years of age have been reported in the literature. A single dosage form can cause problems, particularly if the patient takes the tablets/capsules immediately before retiring to bed and without water. The patient wakes up a few hours later, or in the morning with severe retrosternal pain which is not relieved by drinking or eating. The patient avoids swallowing as it is painful. If medical attention is sought, a doctor will rule out heart disease and prescribe an analgesic or antacid. The pain can persist for days and will only resolve when the patients alters his method of taking medication.

EFFECT OF AGEING

Impairment of the ability to swallow with advancing age has been identified as a major healthcare problem in an ageing population. Radiological studies of an asymptomatic group of 56 patients with a mean age of 83 years showed that a normal pattern of deglutition was present in only 16% of individuals[30]. Oral abnormalities, which included difficulty in controlling and delivering a bolus to the oesophagus following ingestion, were noted in 63% of cases. Structural abnormalities capable of causing oesophageal dysphagia include neoplasms, strictures and diverticula although only minor changes of structure and function are associated directly with ageing. The difficulty appears therefore to relate to neurological mechanisms associated with the coordination of tongue, oropharynx and upper oesophagus during a swallow.

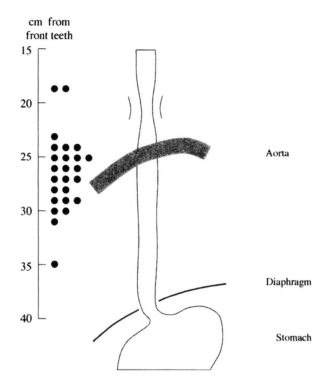

Figure 4.8 Location of twenty five drug induced ulcers.
(scale on the left hand side indicates distance of the lesions from the teeth[29])

Impaired swallowing in the elderly will result in even small tablets (4 mm) adhering to the oesophagus[31]. Low dose tablets, including the aminobisphosphonates used to inhibit bone resorption, have been reported to cause ulceration[32]. This has led to an FDA recommendation that these medications be consumed with 240 ml water, the subject to remain erect for 30 minutes after administration. Dosage forms which float on the co-administered water may also present problems to the elderly by sticking to the roof of the oropharynx.

PATIENT PREFERENCE AND EASE OF SWALLOWING

Patients prefer taking capsules to large oval or round tablets, partly due to the smooth surface and the shape which assists swallowing. The difficulty in swallowing large round tablets increases over the age of 60 years when up to 60% of healthy subjects may report a problem. There is a tendency amongst these patients to chew the tablets and capsules or to open the capsule and disperse the pellets in food or a drink. This can lead to an unknown loss of a proportion of the dose. Chewing formulations will destroy the integrity of any surface coating and it is a particular problem for sustained or controlled release formulations that are designed to be swallowed intact. Chewing will destroy matrix structures and increase the surface area available for drug dissolution.

EFFECT OF DISEASED STATES ON TRANSIT

Oesophageal transit may be influenced by diseased states such as oropharyngeal dysphagia or achalasia. Oral pharyngeal dysphagia is a common problem particularly in the elderly which carries a significant morbidity and mortality[33]. Oral-pharyngeal dysphagia

Table 4.2 Potential risk factors for stricture development in subjects with pill-induced oesophageal damage[38]

Risk factor	Pill-induced oesophageal damage without stricture	Pill-induced oesophageal stricture
Age (years, mean ±s.d)	36 ± 19	60 ± 16
Sex (M:F)	43:95	18:17
Number taking sustained release formulations	14/155 (9%)	17/33 (52%)
Number in reclining position	60/121 (50%)	18/25 (72%)
Number with left atrial engorgement	11/119 (9%)	15/25 (63%)
Number with pre-existing oesophageal disease	1/120 (1%)	5/32 (16%)

copuld be caused by neurogenic dysfunction, with stroke being the commonest cause, but could also be due to local structural lesions[34]. Achalasia is caused by local structural lesions in which transit is impaired by an oesophageal stricture or inability of the lower oesophageal sphincter to relax. Oesophageal retention of food results. Additionally, abnormalities in oesophageal function can occur as a result of a variety of diseased states such as diabetes mellitus, chronic alcoholism and scleroderma, although an abnormality of the oesophagus is not a prerequisite for adhesion of dosage forms. Oesophageal dysfunction has been shown to be more common in asthmatics than normal subjects[35], so drugs such as theophylline may show an increased incidence of adhesion[36].

Reflux of gastric contents can cause injury to the oesophageal mucosa and the oesophagitis produced can lead to stricture. The acid reflux may actually exacerbate the oesophageal damage produced by some drugs such as doxycycline monohydrate which are poorly water soluble and should produce little damage under normal conditions. If gastro-oesophageal reflux of acid occurs, the monohydrate may be converted to the highly ulcerogenic hydrochloride. In humans, this problem would be compounded since delayed transit is associated with hiatus hernia and gastro-oesophageal reflux with typical clearance times of 50 s compared to 9.5 s in normals[37].

Where there is an existing stricture due to reflux or previous 'pill-induced' damage, the likelihood of further damage is increased. Risk factors associated with age, posture and formulation for stricture and non-stricture groups are illustrated in Table 4.2[38].

TARGETING THE OESOPHAGUS

In the past attention has been focused on reproducible smooth and rapid oesophageal transit. In some instances, for example in the treatment of oesophageal damage from gastro-oesophageal reflux or oesophageal cancer, delivery of drugs to the oesophageal mucosa would be desirable. In 1990, the use of ultrafine ferrite (γ-Fe_2O_3), utilising a dye and polymer as an adhesion/release controlling delivery system was reported for the delivery of drugs to treat oesophageal cancer[39]. More recently, poly(oxyethylene-b-oxypropylene-b-oxyethylene)-g-poly(acrylic acid) which is composed of polyacrylic acid and a block co-polymer of ethylene oxide and propylene oxide has been explored for this use. The material shows strong mucoadhesive properties and undergoes reverse thermal gelation at body temperature[40]. Approximately ten percent of the formulation was observed to remain in the oesophagus 10 minutes after administration (Figure 4.9).

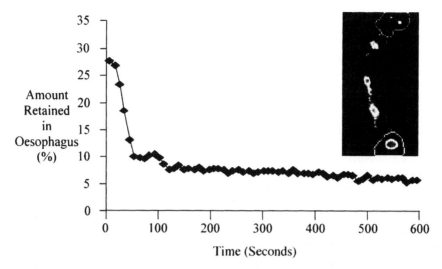

Figure 4.9 Distribution of smart hydrogel

CONCLUSIONS

Oesophageal adhesion of dosage forms is surprisingly common and can cause problems of local ulceration or delayed drug absorption. In general, there are several factors which predispose a formulation to adhere: a) shape of dosage form, b) size of dosage form, c) position of subject, d) volume of water with which the dosage form is administered, e) surface characteristic of the dosage form. It is important to emphasise the correct method of swallowing tablets, particularly in high risk groups. New technologies are emerging which can locally deliver drugs to treat disorders of the oesophagus.

REFERENCES

1. Pemberton J. Oesophageal obstruction and ulceration caused by oral potassium therapy. *Br. Heart. J.* 1970;32:267-268.
2. Mickey PM. Method for measuring lumen of the oesophagus. *Radiology* 1929;13:469-471.
3. McNally EE, Del Gaudio W. The radiopaque esophageal marshmallow bolus. *Am. J. Roentgenol. Rad. Therap. Nucl. Med.* 1967;101:485-489.
4. Kelly JE. The marshmallow as an aid to radiologic examination of the esophagus. *New Eng. J. Med.* 1961;265:1306-1307.
5. Wolf BS. Use of half-inch barium tablet to detect minimal esophageal strictures. *J. Mt. Sinai Hosp.* 1961;28:80-82.
6. Evans KT, Roberts GM. Where do all the tablets go? *Lancet* 1976;2:1237-1239.
7. Schatzki R, Gary JE. Dysphagia due to diaphragm-like localised narrowing in the lower esophagus (lower esophageal ring). *Am. J. Roentgenol. Rad. Therapy and Nuclear Med.* 1953;70:911-922.
8. Wilson CG, Washington N, Peach J, Murray GR, Kennerley J. The behaviour of a fast-dissolving dosage form (Expidet) followed by gamma scintigraphy. *Int. J. Pharmaceut.* 1987;40:119-123.
9. Channer KS, Virjee JP. The effect of formulation on oesophageal transit. *J. Pharm. Pharmacol.* 1985;37:126-129.
10. Hey H, Jorgensen F, Sorensen K, Hasselbalch H, Wamberg T. Oesophageal transit of six commonly used tablets and capsules. *Br. Med. J.* 1982;285:1717-1719.
11. Channer KS, Virjee JP. The effect of size and shape of tablets on their esophageal transit. *J. Clin. Pharmacol.* 1986;26:141-146.

12. Wilson CG, Washington N, Norman S, Peach J, Pugh K. A gamma scintigraphic study to compare the oesophageal clearance of an "Expidet" formulation, tablets and capsules in supine volunteers. *Int. J. Pharmaceut.* 1998;46:241-46.

13. Kjellén G, Svedberg JB, Tibbling L. Computerised scintigraphy of oesophageal bolus transit in asthmatics. *Int. J. Nucl. Med. Biol.* 1981;8:153-158.

14. Burton S, Washington N, Steele RJC, Musson R, Feely L. Intragastric distribution of ion-exchange resins: A drug delivery system for the topical treatment of the gastric mucosa. *J. Pharm. Pharmacol.* 1995;47:901-906.

15. Channer KS, Virjee JP. The effect of formulation on oesophageal transit. *J. Pharm. Pharmacol.* 1985;37:126-129.

16. Evans KT, Roberts GM. The ability of patients to swallow capsules. *J. Clin. Hosp. Pharm.* 1981;6:207-208.

17. Marvola M, Vahervuo K, Sothmann A, Marttila E, Rajaniemi M. Development of a method for study of the tendency of drug products to adhere to the esophagus. *J. Pharmaceut. Sci.* 1982;71:975-977.

18. Swisher DA, Sendelbeck SL, Fara JW. Adherence of various oral dosage forms to the oesophagus. *Int. J. Pharmaceut.* 1984;22:219-228.

19. Perkins AC, Wilson CG, Blackshaw PE, Vincent RM, Dansereau RJ, Juhlin KD, et al. Impaired oesophageal transit of capsule versus tablet formulations in the elderly. *Gut* 1994;35:1363-1367.

20. Opper FH, Isaacs KL, Warshauer DM. Esophageal obstruction with a dietary fibre product designed for weight reduction. *J. Clin. Gastroenterol.* 1990;12:667-669.

21. Roach J, Martyak T, Benjamin G. Anhydrous pill ingestion: a new cause of esophageal obstruction. *Ann. Emerg. Med.* 1987;16:913-914.

22. Channer KS, Roberts CJC. Effect of delayed esophageal transit on acetaminophen absorption. *Clin. Pharmacol. Ther.* 1985;37:72-76.

23. Kikendall JW, Friedman AC, Oyewole MA, Fleischer D, Johnson LF. Pill-induced esophageal injury: case reports and a review of the medical literature. *Dig. Dis. Sci.* 1983;28:174-182.

24. Collins FJ, Matthews HR, Baker SE, Strakova JM. Drug induced oesophageal injury. *Br. Med. J.* 1979;1:1673-1676.

25. Ovartlarnporn B, Kulwichit W, Hiranniramol S. Medication-induced esophageal injury: report of 17 cases with endoscopic documentation. *Am. J. Gastroenterol.* 1991;86:748-750.

26. Enzenauer RW, Bass JW, McDonnell JT. Esophageal ulceration associated with oral theophylline (letter). *N. Engl. J. Med.* 1984;310:261.

27. Santucci L, Patoia L, Fiorucci S, Farroni F, Favero D, Morelli A. Oesophageal lesions during treatment with piroxicam. *Br. Med. J.* 1990;300:1018.

28. Heller SR, Fellows IW, Ogilvie AL, Atkinson M. Non-steroidal anti-inflammatory drugs and benign oesophageal stricture. *Br. Med. J.* 1982;285:167-168.

29. Weinbeck M, Berges W, Lübke HJ. Drug-induced oesophageal lesions. *Baillière's Clin. Gastroenterol.* 1988;2:263-274.

30. Ekeberg O, Feinberg MJ. Altered swallowing function in eldely patients without dysphagia: radiological findings in 56 cases. *Am. J. Roentgenol.* 1991;156:1181-1184.

31. Robertson CS, Hardy J.G. Oesophageal transit of small tablets. *J. Pharm. Pharmacol.* 1988;40:595-596.

32. De Groen PC, Lubbe DF, Hirsch LJ, Daifotis A, Stephenson W, Freedholm D, et al. Esophagitis associated with the use of alendronate. *New Engl. J. Med.* 1996;335:1016-1021.

33. Lindgren M, Janzon L. Prevalence of swallowing complaints and clinical findings among 50-79 year old men and women in an urban population. *Dysphagia* 1991;6:187-192.

34. Cook IJ. Investigative techniques in the assessment of oral-pharyngeal dysphagia. *Dig. Dis.* 1998;16:125-133.

35. Kjellén G, Brundin A, Tibbling L, Wranne B. Oesophageal function in asthmatics. *Eur. J. Resp. Dis.* 1981;62:87-94.

36. D'Arcy PF. Oesophageal problems with tablets and capsules. *Pharm. Int.* 1984; 5:109.

37. Eriksen CA, Sadek SA, Cranford C, Sutton D, Kennedy N, Cuschieri A. Reflux oesophagitis and oesophageal transit: evidence for a primary oesophageal motor disorder. *Gut* 1988;29:448-452.

38. McCord GS, Clouse RE. Pill-induced esophageal strictures: clinical features and risk factors for development. *Am. J. Med.* 1990;88:512-518.

39. Ito R, Machida Y, Sannan T, Nagai T. Magnetic granules: A novel system for specific drug delivery to esophageal mucosa in oral administration. *Int. J. Pharmaceut.* 1990;61:109-117.

40. Potts AM, Jackson SJ, Washington N, Gilchrist P, Ron ES, Schiller M, Wilson CG. The oesophageal retention of a thermally sensitive hydrogel. *Proc. 24th Int. Symp Cont. Rel. Soc.* 1997:335-336.

Chapter Five

The Stomach

ANATOMY AND PHYSIOLOGY

The stomach has several functions:

1. it acts as a reservoir for food,
2. it processes it into fluid chyme which facilitates the absorption of nutrients from the small intestine,
3. it regulates the delivery of food to the small intestine where the nutrients are absorbed,
4. it produces acid which is bacteriostatic, since ingested food is not sterile, and it also produces the correct pH for pepsin to function.

The stomach is located in the left upper part of the abdomen immediately below the diaphragm. In front of the stomach are the liver, part of the diaphragm, and the anterior abdominal wall. The pancreas, the left kidney, the left adrenal, the spleen and the colon are located behind it. When the stomach is empty, it contracts, and the transverse colon ascends to occupy the vacated space. The size, shape, and position of the stomach can vary quite considerably depending upon the extent of its contents as well as upon the tension in the muscles of its walls. The opening from the oesophagus into the stomach is the gastro-oesophageal sphincter or junction. It is also known as the *cardia*. The pylorus is the outlet from the stomach into the duodenum.

Organisation of the stomach

The stomach can also be divided into three anatomical regions (Figure 5.1). The uppermost part is the *fundus*, which after a meal is often seen to contain gas. It also produces slow sustained contractions which exert a steady pressure on the gastric contents gradually pressing them in an aboral direction. The largest part of the stomach is the *body* which acts as a reservoir for ingested food and liquids. The *antrum* is the lowest part of the stomach. It is almost funnel-shaped, with its wide end joining the lower part of the body of the stomach and its narrow end connecting with the pyloric canal. The pyloric portion (the antrum plus the pyloric canal) of the stomach tends to curve to the right and slightly upward and backward and thus gives the stomach its J-shaped appearance.

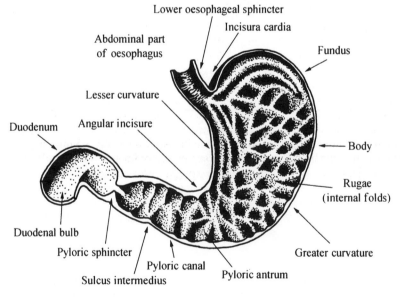

Figure 5.1 Structure of the stomach

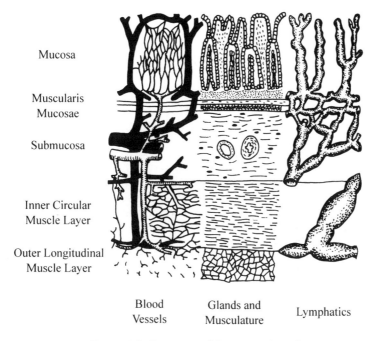

Mucosa

Muscularis Mucosae

Submucosa

Inner Circular Muscle Layer

Outer Longitudinal Muscle Layer

Blood Vessels

Glands and Musculature

Lymphatics

Figure 5.2 Structure of the stomach wall

The stomach adapts to increasing volumes of food by receptive relaxation, which allows the stomach to expand with little variation in intragastric pressure. The distal or antral portion of the stomach has a wall composed of thicker muscle and is concerned with regulation of emptying of solids by contraction, and by acting as a gastric homogenizer and grinder. It is co-ordinated with the body in the propulsion of gastric contents towards the pylorus. The pyloric sphincter has two functions. It sieves the chyme and prevents large particles of food from being emptied from the stomach before solid masses have been sufficiently reduced in size. It also prevents reflux of duodenal material containing bile and pancreatic enzymes which may damage the gastric mucosa.

Mucosa

The mucosa of the stomach (Figure 5.2) is thick, vascular and glandular and is thrown into numerous folds or rugae, which for the most part run in the longitudinal direction, and flatten out when distended. The mucosal surface of the stomach is lined by a single layer of simple columnar epithelium, 20 to 40 μm in height. Approximately 3.5 million gastric pits (foveolae) puncture the lining, each of which serves approximately 4 gastric glands (Figure 5.3). The distribution of gastric glands varies throughout the stomach. The first region, 1.5 to 3 cm in length, around the gastric cardia or gastro-oesophageal junction, contains the cardiac glands. The second region, the fundus and body, contains the acid-secreting glands. The third region, which contains the pyloric or antral glands, includes the pylorus and extends past the antrum to the lesser and greater curvatures.

Gastric mucus

The surface of the mucosa is always covered by a layer of thick tenacious mucus that is secreted by the columnar cells of the epithelium. Gastric mucus is a glycoprotein which lubricates food masses, facilitating movement within the stomach, and forms a protective

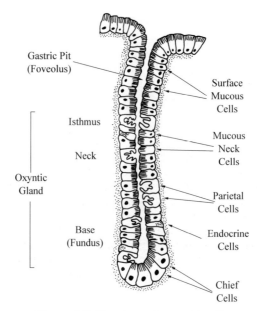

Figure 5.3 Structure of a gastric pit

layer over the lining epithelium of the stomach cavity. This protective layer is approximately 140 µm thick in humans and is a defence mechanism to prevent the stomach from being digested by its own proteolytic enzymes (Figure 5.4). The barrier is enhanced by the secretion of bicarbonate into the surface layer from the underlying mucosa. As the hydrogen ions diffuse across the mucus layer from the lumen, they meet bicarbonate secreted from the underlying mucosa, thus setting up a pH gradient. The mucus is continually digested from the luminal surface and is continually being replaced from beneath. It has been estimated that the turnover time of the mucus layer, i.e. from production to digestion, is in the order of 4 to 5 hours. However, it may be slower since any interaction with the mucosa causes it to secrete copious amounts of mucus, making accurate measurements problematic.

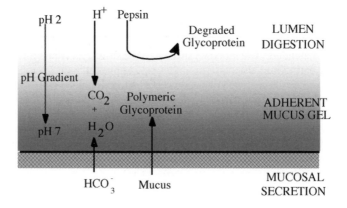

Figure 5.4 Mucus degradation in the stomach

Gastric glands

The gastric glands are located beneath the surface epithelium and open into small pits or foveolae gastricae. There are approximately 100 gastric pits per square millimetre of surface epithelium. Between three and seven glands open into each pit.

The gastric mucosa contains five different types of cells. In addition to the tall columnar surface epithelial cells mentioned above, the other common cell types found in the various gastric glands are:

(1) Mucoid cells which secrete mucus and are found in all the gastric glands. They predominate in the gastric glands in the cardiac and pyloric areas of the stomach. The necks of the glands in the body and fundus are also lined with mucoid cells.

(2) The chief or zymogen cells are located predominantly in the gastric glands in the body and fundus. These cells secrete pepsinogen, the precursor for the enzyme pepsin.

(3) Hydrochloric acid is secreted by the parietal or oxyntic cells which are mainly located in the body and fundus of the stomach (Figure 5.5). They are also responsible for secreting most of the water which is found in the gastric juice and a protein called intrinsic factor. Parietal cells are almost completely absent from the antrum.

(4) Endocrine cells or endocrine-like cells. The endocrine cells throughout the antrum secrete the acid-stimulating hormone gastrin. The endocrine cells are scattered, usually singly, between the parietal and chief cells.

Blood and nerve supply

Arterial blood is brought to the stomach via many branches of the celiac trunk. The celiac trunk is a short, wide artery that branches from the abdominal portion of the aorta, the main vessel conveying arterial blood from the heart to the systemic circulation. Blood from the stomach is returned to the venous system via the portal vein, which carries the blood to the liver.

Both parasympathetic and sympathetic divisions of the autonomic nervous system supply the stomach. The parasympathetic nerve fibres are carried in the vagus (10th cranial) nerves. As the vagus nerves pass through the opening in the diaphragm together with the oesophagus, branches of the right vagus nerve spread over the posterior part of the

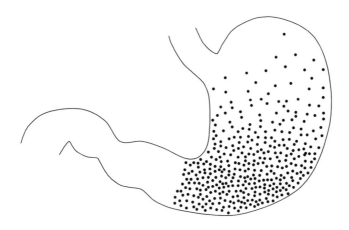

Figure 5.5 Distribution of parietal cells in the stomach. Note their absence in the antrum

stomach, while the left vagus supplies the anterior part. Sympathetic branches from a nerve network called the celiac, or solar plexus accompany the arteries of the stomach into the muscular wall.

Gastric secretion

The human stomach secretes between 1.0 and 1.5 litres of gastric juice per day. This juice is highly acidic because of its hydrochloric acid content, and it is rich in enzymes. Gastric juice provides a medium for soluble food particles to dissolve and it initiates digestion, particularly for proteins.

Acid secretion

The composition of the gastric juice varies according to the stimulus and the secretion rate (Figure 5.6). It is a mixture of water, hydrochloric acid, electrolytes (sodium, potassium, calcium, phosphate, sulphate, and bicarbonate) and organic substances (mucus, pepsins, and protein). Parietal cells can secrete hydrogen ions at a concentration of 150 mmolar. In comparison, the hydrogen ion concentration in the blood is 40 nmolar. Pure parietal cell secretion is diluted to between 20 and 60 mmolar by non-parietal cell secretion. Normal adults produce a basal secretion of up to 60 ml per hour containing approximately 4 mmoles of H^+. This can rise to more than 200 ml, and between 15 and 50 mmoles per hour, when maximally stimulated.

Hydrogen ions are produced by metabolic activity in the parietal cells (Figure 5.7). The key reaction between water and carbon dioxide is catalysed by carbonic anhydrase. The bicarbonate produced diffuses back into the bloodstream and after a meal, its concentration is sufficient to produce a marked alkalinity in the urine called the "alkaline tide". The hydrogen ions are actively pumped into the stomach lumen in exchange for potassium ions. Potassium also diffuses passively out of the cell, hence pure parietal secretion is a mixture of hydrochloric acid and potassium chloride.

Hydrochloric acid is produced by the parietal cells in response to histamine, gastrin or acetylcholine stimulation. Histamine is released from gastric mast cells in response to food ingestion, and acts on the H_2 receptors in the parietal cells, directly causing acid secretion. Gastrin is released in response to reduced acidity of the gastric contents when food enters the stomach, and in particular by the presence of peptides. Acetylcholine is released

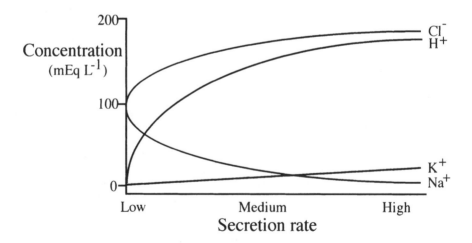

Figure 5.6 Variation in composition of gastric juice with secretion rate

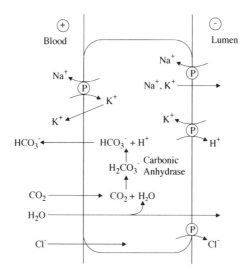

Figure 5.7 Mechanism of acid production by the parietal cell

when stimuli descend the vagus nerve in response to the sight, smell and taste of food and to the physical effects of chewing and swallowing. It is likely that acetylcholine and gastrin may operate by activating the mast cells which then release histamine, so that histamine is the final common pathway by which the parietal cell is activated.

The process of gastric secretion has been divided into three phases: cephalic, gastric and intestinal, which have different primary mechanisms. The phases of gastric secretion overlap, and there is an interrelation and some interdependence between the neural and humoral pathways.

The cephalic phase of gastric secretion occurs in response to stimuli received by the senses; that is, taste, smell, sight, and sound. This phase is entirely reflex in origin and is mediated by the vagus nerves. The gastric juice that is secreted in response to vagal stimulation is rich in enzymes and is highly acidic.

The gastric phase is mediated both by the vagus nerves and by the release of gastrin. Acid continues to be secreted during the gastric phase in response to distension, and to the peptides and amino acids liberated from food as protein digestion proceeds. The free amino acids and peptides liberate gastrin from the antrum into the circulation. When the pH of the antral contents falls below 2.5, a feedback mechanism inhibits the release of gastrin, thus the system is self-limiting. The gastric phase continues until the food leaves the stomach.

During the intestinal phase the chyme in the small intestine continues to elicit acid secretion for many hours, although the amount of acid released diminishes progressively during the digestion and absorption processes in the small intestine. Some of the actions of the intestinal phase are due to gastrin released from the duodenum, but there is evidence that another hormone-like substance not yet characterised may be responsible. Finally, as certain amino acids and small peptides are infused into the circulation during this phase, they also promote gastric acid secretion. It is possible, therefore, that the absorption of the products of protein digestion also may have a role in the intestinal phase.

Once food reaches the small intestine, it stimulates the pancreas to release fluid containing a high concentration of bicarbonate. This neutralizes the highly acidic gastric juice, which would otherwise destroy the intestinal epithelium, resulting in a duodenal ulcer. Other secretions from the pancreas, gallbladder, liver, and glands in the intestinal wall add to the total volume of chyme.

Pepsin

Pepsinogen is converted to the active enzyme, pepsin, by hydrolysis of the precursor by hydrochloric acid. The hydrochloric acid present in the stomach provides the correct pH for the pepsins to act, i.e. between 1.8 and 3.5; above pH 5 they are denatured. Human pepsins are endopeptidases which hydrolyse several peptide bonds within the interior of ingested protein molecules to form polypeptides, but little free amino acid. The susceptible bonds involve the aromatic amino acids tyrosine or phenylalanine. The polypeptides produced have N-terminal amino acids with lipophilic side chains which facilitate absorption.

Other enzymes

Some other enzymes, including gastric lipase and gastric amylase and gelatinase can be found in gastric juice. Gastric lipase is highly specific tributyrase acting solely on butterfat which is largely tributyrin. It is not capable of digesting medium- and long-chain fatty acids, but since there is only a small proportion of short-chain fatty acids in food, little fat digestion proceeds in the stomach. Gastric amylase plays a minor role in the digestion of starches and the enzyme gelatinase helps liquefy some of the proteoglycans in meats.

Intrinsic factor of Castle

Parietal cells also secrete a glycoprotein known as intrinsic factor of Castle (m. w. 1350 Dalton) which is required for the absorption of vitamin B_{12}. It is continuously secreted, even in the absence of any gastric secretory stimulus in man. Its basal secretion greatly exceeds the minimum amount required for normal vitamin B_{12} absorption.

Prostaglandins

Prostaglandins are hormone-like substances which are derived from dietary lipids. They are present in virtually all animal tissues and body fluids, and are involved in the contraction and dilatation of blood vessels, the aggregation of platelets (clotting), and the contraction and relaxation of the smooth muscle of the gastrointestinal tract. Prostaglandins also inhibit the secretion of hydrochloric acid by the stomach in response to food, histamine, and gastrin. They also protect the mucosa from damage by various chemical agents. This protection is not related to their ability to influence acid secretion. Prostaglandins increase the secretion of mucus and bicarbonate from the mucosa, and they stimulate the migration of cells to the surface for repair and replacement of the mucosal lining.

Digestion and absorption

Salivary amylase acts on food starch while the acidity of the mixture is low, around pH 6, but ceases when the acidity of the mixture increases with greater acid secretion. Gastric pepsins account for only about 10 to 15 percent of the digestion of protein and are most active in the first hour of digestion. The stomach is primarily a processing organ and not an absorptive one and is not essential to life. It is possible, for example, after total gastrectomy (the complete removal of the stomach) for a person to remain, or to become, obese because most of the digestion and absorption of food takes place in the intestine. The stomach can absorb some substances, including glucose and other simple sugars, amino acids, and some fat-soluble substances. A number of alcohols, including ethanol, are readily absorbed from the stomach. The pH of the gastric contents controls the absorption of certain ionizable materials such as aspirin, which is readily absorbed in its unionized form when the stomach is acidic, but more slowly when the gastric contents are neutral. The absorption of water and alcohol can be slowed if the stomach contains food, especially fat, probably because gastric emptying is delayed and most water in any situation is absorbed from the jejunum.

Water moves freely from the gastric contents across the gastric mucosa into the blood. The net absorption of water from the stomach is small, however, because water moves just as easily from the blood across the gastric mucosa to the lumen of the stomach. In tracer experiments using deuterium oxide, about 60 percent of the (isotopic) water placed in the stomach is absorbed into the blood in 30 minutes.

GASTRIC pH

Gastric pH is primarily influenced by two factors; acid secretion and gastric content. In a 24 hour period, the median daytime pH for eight subjects was 2.7 (range 1.8 to 4.5) in the body and 1.9 (range 1.6 to 2.6) in the antrum of the stomach[1]. Food buffers and neutralizes gastric acid, producing an increase in pH. The pH is not uniform in the stomach, due to the differences in the distribution of parietal cells, and the different patterns of motility in various regions of the stomach. These effects are illustrated by the experiment shown in Figure 5.8, in which pH electrodes were placed 5 cm, 10 cm and 15 cm below the gastro-oesophageal junction prior to administering a test meal. Initially all electrodes showed a low basal pH. The meal raised the pH in the fundus to approximately 4.5, but this rapidly began to decline, returning to baseline after 2.5 h. The pH in the body of the stomach was slower to respond, again increasing to about 4.5, 15 minutes later than the fundus. This region returned to basal pH 3.5 h after meal ingestion. The magnitude of the change in pH in the antrum was much smaller, indicating that in this region the food is acidic for the majority of the time. In the body of the stomach, the large concentration of parietal cells

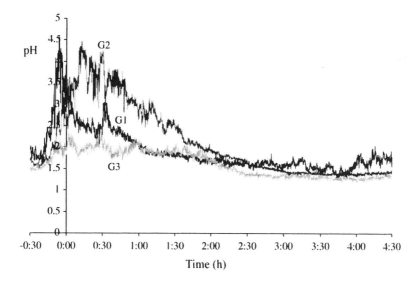

Figure 5.8 Gastric pH after a meal. Electrode positions are G1 = 5 cm, G2 = 10 cm and G3 = 15 cm below the gastro-oesophageal sphincter

causes rapid acid production, but mixing in this region is poor, so that the extended buffer-ing effect of the food is observed. As the food moves into the antrum, the vigorous mixing not only reduces particle size of the food, but mixes it with the gastric acid which was produced higher in the stomach. The pH in the antrum remains low, despite the fact that there are no parietal cells in this region, since much of the food has been neutralized while stored in the body of the stomach (note: the small peak seen after 30 minutes was due to the administration of 50 ml of water for a separate phase of the experiment, and should be ignored).

Acid secretion is increased after hot or cold meals even though temperature of the meal per se does not alter gastric emptying. It takes significantly longer for cold meals to be brought to body temperature than hot meals[2]. Content of the meal also affects gastric pH; for example, a pure carbohydrate meal given as a pancake has no detectable effect on acid-ity[3], while a protein meal of similar calorific value has a significant buffering effect[4]. A liquid meal, rather than a mixed phase meal, with a balance of carbohydrate and protein has a strong buffering effect but the pH rapidly returns to basal levels as the liquid is emptied. The situation is complicated by feedback effects; for example pepsin normally hydrolyses proteins to peptides and amino acids, which are potent secretagogues, and increase the acidification of gastric contents. However pepsin is inactivated above pH 5, so a large meal which raises the pH above this value will prevent the production of these substances, and peak gastric acid secretion will be reduced.

Circadian rhythm of acidity

A circadian rhythm of basal gastric acidity is known to occur with acid output being highest in the evening and lowest in the morning (Figure 5.9)[5]. The daytime patterns of gastric pH vary greatly between individuals, in part due to the differences in the composi-tion of meals and the variable responses of acid secretion and gastric emptying. However, nocturnal patterns of gastric acidity are very similar with very low pHs between midnight and early morning[3]. The later in the day the evening meal is taken, the later the nocturnal peak of acidity occurs[6]; it is therefore important to standardise the time for the evening meal when comparing the nocturnal effects of anti-secretory drugs.

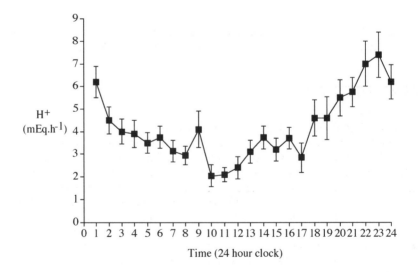

Figure 5.9 Circadian variation in gastric acidity

Night-time transient increases in pH can be detected by electrodes placed in the antrum and body of the stomach. They have been interpreted as evidence of duodeno-gastric reflux flowing from the antrum into the body[7] since the increase often occurs in the fundus before that in the body. The same phenomenon may explain the observation that if a group of subjects are kept awake at night, the pH of the gastric juice is observed to rise compared to sleeping levels, which may be due to increased duodeno-gastric reflux in subjects who are denied sleep.

pH and gender

Healthy women secrete significantly less basal and pentagastrin-stimulated acid than men, with a median 24 h integrated acidity of 485 mmol.h^{-1} versus 842 mmol.h^{-1}. In a sample of 365 healthy subjects, the average basal pH was 2.16 ± 0.09 for men and 2.79 ± 0.18 in women[8].

pH and age

It has always been assumed that gastric acid secretion decreases with age, however this has been shown not to be true. A group of healthy subjects with a mean age of 51 years (range 44 - 71 years) had a higher basal acid production than a group with a mean age of 33 years (range 23 - 42 years)[9]. The age related increase in secretion was greater in men than women and was not correlated with height, weight, body surface area or fat-free body mass, or by the increased incidence of *Helicobacter pylori* infection.

Occasionally, babies are intubated for the purposes of investigating oesophageal reflux, but results are sparse in older children. In twelve healthy children aged 8-14 years, the mean fasting gastric pH was 1.5 and the duodenal pH was 6.4. The pH gradually rises down the small intestine reaching a peak value of 7.4 in the distal ileum[10]. The pH dropped to 5.9 in the caecum but increased to 6.5 in the rectum. In 11 healthy adults, the median pH was 7.0 in duodenum, dropped to pH 6.3 in the proximal part, but rose to 7.3 in the distal part of the small intestine[11]. These values are quite similar and allay fears that, for example, sustained-release or enteric coated dose forms evaluated in adults may not work correctly in children.

pH and smoking

Daytime intragastric acidity is higher in smokers (median pH 1.56) compared to non-smokers (median pH 1.70); however, there is no significant difference in 24 hour or night time pH[12].

GASTRIC MOTILITY

The fasted state

The stomach will revert to the fasted pattern of motility in the absence of digestible food, or when it is empty (Figure 5.10). After a meal, the digestible food will have been processed to chyme and passed to the small intestine leaving a residue of mucus and undigested solids. These remain in the stomach until the small intestine has finished absorbing nutrients from the chyme i.e. approximately 2 h after the last of the digestible food has left the stomach. At this point the digestive phase of activity ceases and is replaced by the interdigestive phase, which is also the normal resting condition of the stomach and small intestine. All gastric residues which the stomach has failed to process to chyme are removed in this phase, the migrating myoelectric complex (MMC) or so-called 'housekeeper contractions'. The MMC removes debris from the stomach by strong contractions against an open pylorus.

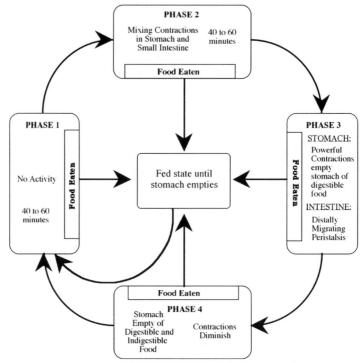

Figure 5.10 The migrating myoelectric complex

Starting from a state in which the stomach and small intestine show no motor activity (Phase I), the activity front begins simultaneously in the antrum and duodenum producing a series of mixing contractions which build up over a period of 60-90 minutes (Phase II). These end in a series of powerful circular peristaltic waves which sweep from the site of origin down the entire small bowel to the caecum emptying all the large solid particles from the stomach and small intestine (Phase III). The waves then subside to the resting phase. The whole cycle repeats every two hours until a meal is eaten, when they are immediately interrupted to initiate the digestive phase of motility. The peristaltic waves can also be halted by an intravenous infusion of a hormone, motilin.

Gastric emptying of the basal gastric secretion occurs even during fasting to prevent accumulation of fluid, as there is very little net absorption by the gastric mucosa.

The fed state

The adult capacity of the stomach is about 1500 ml. The average (western) daily intake of food and drink is 3 to 4 kg, and it is estimated that another 5 litres of fluids such as saliva, gastric juice, pancreatic juice and other body liquids are added to this. The greatest secretory activity occurs in the stomach within the first hour of eating and the volume of gastric juices produced may be up to twice that of the meal.

The uppermost third of the stomach, or fundus, adapts to the varying volume of ingested food by relaxing its muscular wall, holding the food while it undergoes the first stages of digestion. The adaptive process allows it to accommodate the ingested food without increasing intragastric pressure.

The stomach not only elicits a fed pattern of motility in response to the presence of food with calorific value, but it will also respond to the presence of a large quantity of small particle size indigestible material, suggesting that gastric distention is also a contributory factor[13]. Indigestible material of small diameter (1-3 mm) will elicit the fed pattern of motor activity in dogs, and the duration of postprandial antroduodenal motility patterns can be influenced solely by the size of a meal which comprises only indigestible material.

The mixing, grinding and emptying of food all occur together. The dispersion of food is more a mechanical process than an enzymatic one. Mixing and grinding are carried out by a series of peristaltic waves which originate in mid-body as a shallow indentation and gradually deepen as they progress toward the duodenum. The velocity of the wave increases until the final 3 to 4 cm of the antrum is reached, at which stage the antrum and pylorus appear to contract simultaneously. This is often called antral systole. Liquids and solids within the distal antrum are compressed as the antral wave deepens. The wave does not occlude the lumen and hence liquid and suspended particles are retropelled through the wave, but larger and denser solids are trapped ahead of the constriction. Once the pylorus has closed, the antral systole grinds and then retropels the solids into the proximal antrum (Figure 5.11). The grinding action, combined with the shear forces produced during retro-pulsion, reduces the particle size and mixes the particles with gastric juice. The motion and acid-pepsin digestion account for the physical breakdown of solid food in this region. The rate of emptying from the human stomach decreases if the ingested solid food is composed of larger masses. Solids are only emptied after they are ground to particles smaller than approximately 1 mm, and the larger, harder particles will take longer to reach this size.

Tonic or sustained motor activity decreases the size of the lumen of the stomach, as all parts of the gastric wall seem to contract simultaneously. It is this type of activity that accounts for the stomach's ability to accommodate itself to varying volumes of gastric content. Mixing contractions and peristaltic contractions are superimposed upon the tonic contraction, which is independent of the other contractions. Both the mixing and the peristaltic contractions occur at a constant rate of three per minute when recorded from the gastric antrum. This rate is now recognised as the basic rhythm, although some drugs are capable of abolishing both types of contractions or of stimulating the strength of contractions. The distension of the body of the stomach by food activates a neural reflex that initiates the activity of the muscle of the antrum.

About twice per minute between 1 and 5 ml of antral contents escape into the duodenum, and decrease the duodenal pH. Emptying from the pylorus occurs in discrete episodes of 2 to 5 seconds only, and the majority of these occur as the terminal antrum, pylorus and duodenum relax at the start and end of each peristaltic cycle[14]. Transpyloric flow ceases

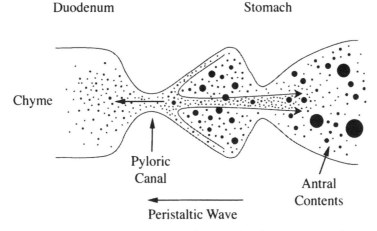

Duodenum   Stomach

Chyme

Pyloric Canal

Antral Contents

Peristaltic Wave

Figure 5.11 Grinding and mixing action of the antral mill. Note retropulsion of large particles i.e. sieving

approximately 2 seconds before the antral systole occurs[14 15]. It was assumed that the particle size cut-off was produced by the narrow pyloric diameter, but neither pyloroplasty nor
pylorectomy alters the size distribution of food passed into the duodenum[16] and the antrum
alone can selectively retain solids in the absence of the pylorus. The pylorus appears to be
wide open, having an aperture larger than 5 mm, for approximately 15 to 20% of the time[17].
The length of time for which the pylorus is wide open does not completely determine the
emptying rate of liquids because the duodenum also seems to apply a braking mechanism.
The periodic opening of the pylorus during the fed phase of motility can explain how some
large particles, including intact large fragments of tablets, can be emptied during this cycle.

Solids and liquids do not empty from the stomach together as a homogeneous mass.
Liquids empty according to the pressure gradient between the stomach and duodenum, with
isotonic liquid meals emptying more rapidly than hypotonic or hypertonic mixtures. The
liquid component of a meal empties exponentially, but the emptying of solids is linear after
a variable lag time (Figure 5.12). The lag phase is dependent upon the size of the food
particles in the stomach. Larger particles require a longer period of digestion to break them
down into a size suitable to exit through the pylorus. Small indigestible solids of between 1
to 5 mm in diameter are progressively emptied during the whole postprandial period even
before liquid emptying is completed. Certain liquids and solids can be clearly seen as two
separate layers on magnetic resonance images (Figure 5.13). Interestingly, during episodes
of heartburn or gastro-oesophageal reflux, food and acid are refluxed into the oesophagus
independently of each other[18]. It is likely that this occurs because the food forms a central
core in the body of the stomach. As gastric acid is secreted around the outside of the food
mass, it is only mixed effectively with the food in the antrum. Refluxed material originates
largely from the upper part of the stomach where mixing is irregular.

Receptors in the duodenal bulb detect the calorific value and hydrogen ion concentration of the chyme causing relaxation of the lower part of the duodenum, and allowing
gastric emptying to start. During a duodenal contraction, the pressure in the duodenal bulb
rises above than that in the antrum, and the pylorus prevents reflux by closing. The vagus

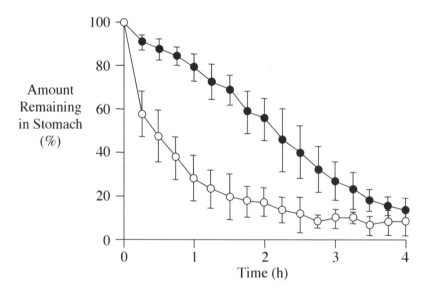

Figure 5.12 Gastric emptying of liquid (O) and solid (●) components of a meal

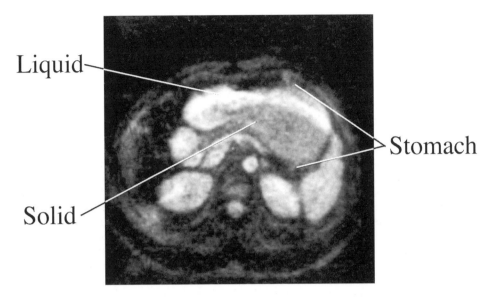

Figure 5.13 MRI cross section through the body. The large organ at the top is the stomach, which clearly shows the liquid layer(white) floating on the solid (grey) matter

nerve has an important role in the control of emptying, but studies on paraplegia caused by injury to the spinal cord indicate that the sympathetic division of the autonomic nervous system is also involved.

Effect of meal size and composition on gastric emptying

The empty stomach has a volume of approximately 50 ml which increases to over 1 litre when full. The stomach empties the three different components of the meal, liquid, digestible solid and indigestible solid, at different rates. For example, in a study of the emptying of a mixed meal consisting of soft drink, scrambled egg and radioopaque markers, the separate components had T_{50}'s (the time for half the component to be emptied) of 30 ± 7 minutes, 154 ± 11 minutes and 3 to 4 hours respectively[19].

In general, the larger the amount of food ingested, the longer the period of fed activity; large meals tend to empty more slowly in the first hour and then more quickly compared to a small meal. Gastric emptying rates correlate with the nutritive density of the meal; foodstuffs slow gastric emptying equally when their concentration is expressed as kilocalories per millilitre. It is now believed that two types of receptors exist which control the rate at which the energy density is delivered to the duodenum. Two sets of duodenal receptors are involved, one stimulated by the osmotic properties of the digestion products of carbohydrate and protein, and one by the digestion products of fat. Energy is not actually sensed, but the two sets of receptors behave in tandem to control the delivery of the chyme to the duodenum by energy density.

The emptying of amino acids appears to be solely dependent upon their osmolarity, except for L-tryptophan which delays gastric emptying in concentrations which can be obtained from normal protein digestion[20]. Fatty acids, monoglycerides and diglycerides all delay gastric emptying, but the greatest delay is produced by fatty acids of chain lengths of 10-14 carbon atoms[21]. The slowing of gastric emptying produced by triglycerides depends upon their rate of hydrolysis to long-chain fatty acids.

Manometric and scintigraphic studies indicate that bland liquids such as water and saline empty from the stomach in gushes associated with co-ordinated contractions of the antrum and duodenum[22]. For example, during the emptying of 600 ml of a bland liquid, 1-3% passed into the duodenum very quickly, followed by a lag phase of 4-6 minutes, with the overall emptying having a T_{50} of only 15 minutes [23].

Food was believed to form layers in the body of the stomach in the order in which it was swallowed, since for the first hour after ingestion of a meal peristalsis is weak, allowing the food to remain relatively undisturbed[24], with the food ingested first being closest to the stomach wall. This data was generated from a study in which rats were fed successive portions of bread, each coloured with a different dye. The animals were killed, the stomachs removed, frozen and sectioned. The portions were found to be separate[25]. This is a simplified case which bears little resemblance to a typical human meal, which consists of a mixture of components of varying density. The human stomach is of course much larger than the rat stomach, so that the effects of sedimentation and stratification are likely to be very different. Pellets with a density of 1.2 g cm[3] sink through food to the base of the greater curvature and are emptied after the majority of food (Figure 5.14). Increasing the viscosity of the gastric contents increases the rate at which dense spheres will empty from the stomach[26]. This suggests that the high viscosity of the medium prevents the spheres from settling into the base of the greater curvature, away from the mixing, grinding and emptying function of the antrum. Materials which have been demonstrated to float *in vivo* can be refloated from the antrum of the stomach to the fundus by the subsequent intake of food[27] thus casting doubt on the theory of stratification.

The effects of fats and oils on gastric emptying

Although it is widely recognised that the fat content of food is the most important factor controlling gastric emptying, the majority of studies over the past 15 years have been carried out in animals such as rats, mice and dogs. The fundamental difference between

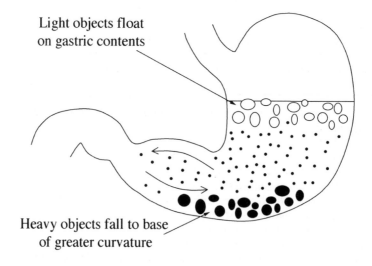

Light objects float
on gastric contents

Heavy objects fall to base
of greater curvature

Figure 5.14 The effect of density on gastric distribution

these species and man is posture, and since certain types of fat will layer in the stomach, their presentation to the pylorus and duodenum naturally will be different in relation to other components of the meal. This is due to the effect of gravity. This effect can be demonstrated in man since olive oil empties more slowly than an aqueous component of a meal when subjects are seated whereas, in the decubitus position (lying), it empties faster[28][29].

The delayed emptying of fat is not just due to the fact that it floats on the meal, and hence empties last when subjects are upright, but the presence of fat in the intestine causes the fundus to relax. This lowers the intragastric pressure, increasing the reservoir function of the stomach. It also inhibits antral contractile activity, increases pyloric contraction and narrows the pyloric lumen[15]. This has the effect of significantly increasing the lag phase of the meal after an initial amount has entered the small intestine[23]. The movement of food from the proximal to the distal stomach still occurs; however, it is followed by a retrograde movement of food back to the proximal stomach, and this may also contribute to the increased lag phase. This redistribution of food in the stomach is also seen after intraduodenal infusion of lipid[30]. Interestingly, the emptying of the oil follows a linear pattern rather than the expected monoexponential emptying typical of liquids.

Dietary fat is ingested in three forms: 1) in solid food, 2) as aqueous emulsions, and 3) as unemulsified, liquid oil. To complicate matters, the gastric residence of a meal with identical composition will be prolonged if the fat content is used to fry the food rather than ingested as the cold oil[31]. Ingestion of a high fat meal increases satiety and a feeling of epigastric fullness for a longer period than an energy-matched low fat meal. It will influence the amount of food taken at the next meal even though the amount of food remaining in the stomach from the first meal is approximately the same[32]. The addition of fat to a meal will also prolong the time for which the meal elevates gastric pH[33].

The behaviour of oils within the stomach is also affected by the other constituents of the meal. When 60 ml of ^{99m}Tc labelled oil was given to subjects with 290 ml of ^{113m}In-labelled soup, gastric emptying of the oil was significantly slower than the soup (time to 50% emptying 139 versus 48 min)[34]. Oil was retained in the proximal stomach and retrograde movement of oil from distal into proximal stomach was noted. The second arm of this study investigated the relative gastric residence time of ^{113m}In-labelled minced beef, ^{99m}Tc-labelled oil and non-labelled soup. In this case, there was no difference in emptying of oil and beef from the stomach, but again more oil was retained in the proximal stomach whereas more beef was retained in the distal stomach. In another study[35] the effect of adding 60 g of margarine into either the soup or mashed potato component of a meal was investigated. The addition of margarine to either component significantly delayed the gastric emptying of the mashed potato, but the pattern of emptying of the potato varied depending which component was fat-enriched. Incorporation of fat into the soup increased the lag phase but did not influence the slope of emptying of the mashed potato, while incorporation of fat into the mashed potato reduced the slope of emptying of the mashed potato but did not influence its lag phase.

When ingested as part of a mixed meal, water invariably leaves the stomach faster than fat[36]. Solid fat, extracellular fat, and intracellular fat phases of a meal empty together, in parallel, after an initial lag[26]. The way in which fat is emptied from the stomach is species dependent. In humans, significantly less extracellular fat than intracellular fat empties from the stomach on or in solid food particles (22% versus 51%). In dogs, 81% of the extracellular fat empties as an oil, 13% empties on the solid particles, and only 6% empties as a stable, aqueous emulsion. Sixty-six percent of the intracellular fat emptied in the solid food particles, 20% as a stable, aqueous emulsion, and 14% as an oil. The conclusion from this study was that the majority of the intracellular fat empties within the solid food phase, whereas most of the extracellular fat empties as an oil phase[26].

Dietary fats leave the stomach faster, but are absorbed less efficiently, after homogenised meals, compared to being given as a mixed phase meal[37]. Co-ingestion of fat with carbohydrate results in a significant flattening of the postprandial glucose curves, the effect being more pronounced for carbohydrates such as mashed potatoes which are more rapidly absorbed than carbohydrates such as lentils[38].

In humans, duodenogastric reflux occurs both after meals and under fasting conditions. The reflux rate is on the average 13 times smaller than the emptying rate, but is higher with a lipid than with a protein meal, and is independent of the rate of gastric emptying. The concentration and total amount of duodenal contents refluxed back to the stomach were higher after lipid than after protein meals. The increased gastric concentration and accumulation of duodenal contents after lipid meals is due to slowed gastric clearing and increased reflux of duodenal contents. Under fasting conditions, the reflux rate was lower and the gastric concentration of duodenal contents was higher than after either type of meal[39].

The distribution of the fat within the stomach can be changed with disease. Patients with non-ulcer dyspepsia demonstrate an abnormal intragastric distribution of dietary fat. In control subjects, approximately three-quarters of the fatty test meal was located in the proximal stomach during the lag period and during emptying. In the group of patients with non-ulcer dyspepsia, significantly less of the fatty test meal was found in the proximal stomach during emptying, and the time taken for half the meal to empty was significantly delayed[40].

It is often believed that a high fat meal produces nausea in conjunction with motion. However, the nausea produced does not appear to be related to the fat being present in the stomach, but rather the small intestine[41]. Nausea is at its greatest when motion of the body occurs when half of a fatty meal has emptied into the small intestine, but is interesting that gastric residence of the fat is not correlated with the symptoms.

There is a positive correlation between lipid intake and reflux in morbidly obese people[42]. This is likely to be due to a combination of an increase in gastric residence of the meal due to the high calorific density of the fat, and a decrease in lower oesophageal sphincter pressure produced by fatty meals. Interestingly, intravenous lipid emulsions do not affect lower oesophageal sphincter pressure or increase pathological reflux episodes[43].

Physiological factors which influence gastric emptying

Gastric emptying follows a circadian rhythm, with slower emptying occurring in the afternoon compared to the morning (Figure 5.15)[44]. This effect can be very marked; in the study illustrated there was over a 50% decrease in emptying rate in the solid phase of the meal when it was eaten in the evening compared to the morning.

In women, pregnancy and the menstrual cycle can drastically alter the transit of materials in various regions of the gastrointestinal tract. Often pregnant women suffer from heartburn and constipation which is attributed to decreased oesophageal pressure and impaired colonic motility. During the normal menstrual cycle mouth to caecum transit is significantly longer in the luteal phase than in the follicular phase[45].

There are conflicting reports as to the effect of obesity on gastrointestinal transit. Some studies show no effect, whilst others report delayed emptying of solids particularly in men, a phenomenon which is not reversed after significant weight loss[46][47]. Other studies show an inverse association between body mass index and mean gastric emptying time of test meals such as radiolabelled cellulose fibre. Body mass index had no influence on other transit variables[48].

Heavy exercise was found to increase the gastric emptying rate of digestible solids in healthy men[49].

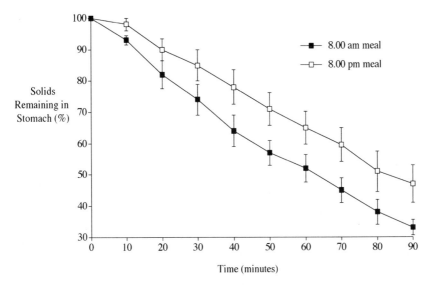

Figure 5.15 The effect of time of day on the rate of gastric emptying

Effect of disease on gastric emptying

Diseases which affect gastric motility and emptying are predominantly diseases of the gastrointestinal tract itself, disorders involving smooth muscle and extraintestinal diseases. Some diseases only affect one of the phases of gastric emptying. Generally duodenal ulcer produces accelerated emptying, while gastric ulcer reduces antral motility, producing normal emptying of liquids but delayed emptying of solids[50]. Emptying of a solid meal is slowed in patients with pernicious anaemia[51] and atrophic gastritis[52], but in achlorhydric patients liquids empty rapidly[53].

Gastro-oesophageal reflux is a common disease affecting between 10 and 20% of the general population[54], although the true magnitude of the condition is not known since a large proportion of sufferers self-medicate[55]. It is therefore likely that within a given patient group a significant proportion will be suffering from this disease to some extent. The effect of this disease on gastric emptying is unclear since some studies report no effect on the emptying of liquids[56] or mixed meals[57], whilst others demonstrate a delay[58-60]. It is possible that the emptying of solids in a mixed meal is selectively delayed[61] suggesting impaired antral motility. This would lead to a greater difference in emptying between liquids, pellets and tablets than in normal subjects.

Migraine is frequently associated with nausea (95%) and vomiting (20%) and there is some evidence that gastric emptying is delayed during migraine attacks.

The eating disorders bulimia nervosa and anorexia nervosa are believed to affect between 5 and 10% of adolescent females and young women in the western world. Bulimia does not affect gastric emptying, but anorexia produces both delayed solid and liquid emptying[62].

DISPERSION OF DOSAGE FORMS IN THE STOMACH

The most commonly used type of dosage form is the conventional compressed tablet. Despite the use of scintigraphy to evaluate more sophisticated dose forms [63], there has been surprisingly little study of the behaviour of ordinary tablets. Most workers assume that tablets will disintegrate rapidly *in vivo* due to the use of superdisintegrants and the evidence of *in vitro* dissolution tests; however this is often not the case. Endoscopy has demonstrated that when multiple tablets are administered, all lie in the same place in the stomach, at the base of the greater curvature. This is a particular problem with formulations which cause gastric irritation or damage, for example non-steroidal anti-inflammatory drugs which can produce focal erosions due to repeated insult to a small area of the mucosa. Iatrogenically-produced ulcers can often be differentiated from those of natural origin, since drug-induced erosions usually occur at the base of the greater curvature, whereas peptic ulcers form on the lesser curvature. Multiple unit dose forms can also cause mucosal damage; for example microencapsulated potassium chloride showed similar gastric mucosal irritation to single units. This was attributed to poor dispersion of the potassium chloride, with clumps of the drug held together with gastric mucus[64].

Hard gelatin capsules

Hard gelatin capsules have found a variety of applications in drug formulation. The capsule can be used as a container for powdered drug, multiparticulate systems, a liquid-fill matrix or oily vehicle. The nature of the interior of the fill of the capsule is known to affect the rate of disintegration within the stomach. A hydrophobic interior reduces the rate of disintegration of the capsule compared to that of a water soluble material, and in addition it reduces the dispersion of the released material. When capsules contain components which are insoluble in gastric juice, then their disintegration time is of the order of 30 minutes in fasted volunteers and 100 minutes in fed volunteers[65]. Changing the fill to a water soluble material decreases the break-up time to 6 minutes.

The dispersion of the capsule fill is limited in fasted subjects, and the material empties from the stomach as a bolus[66-68]. Dispersion is increased if the capsule is taken with a meal, particularly if the meal has a high liquid content. This is of importance since patients are often instructed to take medications with a meal, but it is unclear whether this means before, during or after food. If capsules are given with 100 ml of water, they will initially float above the gastric folds. Rapidly the ends of the capsule become sticky and can become attached to the gastric wall, which may be another explanation for the poor dispersion of the capsule contents[64].

The dispersion of milled resin administered in a hard gelatin capsule in fasted volunteers was greatly reduced when it was milled from 25 μm to 9 μm[66 68]. It was proposed that this was due to changes in the hydrophobicity of the surfaces, arising from chemical and physical variations in the resin through the bulk of the particle. It is equally likely that milling changes the wettability of the material due to variations in particle surface roughness.

Soft gelatin capsules

There have been relatively fewer studies of the behaviour of soft gelatin capsules in man. Pilot studies indicate that the time of disintegration of soft gelatin capsule formulations is highly variable, particularly if the formulations are given without food. The capsules were predominantly broken up as they entered the pylorus immediately prior to leaving the stomach (unpublished data). Armstrong and co-workers [69] have compared the dispersion of oils from soft gelatin capsules in man and rabbits using x-ray techniques and gamma scintigraphy. Soft gelatin capsules were filled with iodinated cotton seed oil (Lipiodol) for x-ray studies, or iodine-123 labelled ethyl oleate for gamma camera studies in humans. In x-ray studies of rabbits, disintegration of the capsule began after 2 to 3 minutes, swelling into a more isometric shape. This behaviour was observable *in vitro* and was associated with the breakdown of the capsule at the sealing line. Subsequently it was difficult to assess whether the shell had dissolved with the oil as one discrete globule, or whether the oil had emerged from the shell before it had completely dissolved. When a surfactant (1% polysorbate 80) was added to the formulation, the mean disintegration time of the soft gelatin capsule decreased markedly.

GASTRIC EMPTYING OF DOSAGE FORMS

For the majority of cases, oral drug delivery is the cheapest and most convenient method of dosing. Unfortunately it is difficult to achieve a precise control of the plasma concentration-time profile, which shows marked intra- and inter-subject variation even under the rigidly controlled conditions of the clinical trial. In the unrestricted patient this is exaggerated by poor compliance and anything more complicated than a b.d. schedule is impractical. Daily patterns such as food intake, activity and posture are large contributors to inter- and intra-subject variation. The nature of food intake is not only specific to race and geographic location but unique for each person, and varies on a day-to-day basis. This factor probably produces the largest physiological variation in the behaviour of oral dose forms. The rate of gastric emptying, the presence of food or other drugs, the particular formulation of the drug (size, shape and rate of disintegration), and the vehicle carrying it all influence the absorption of the drug.

Once the dosage form has reached the stomach, it meets a highly variable environment in terms of food content and pH. The gastric emptying of tablets, pellets and liquids is highly dependent on the presence and amount of food in the stomach. Large tablets can either disintegrate in the stomach and empty with the digestible phase of the meal, or if they are designed to remain intact will be treated as indigestible material since they do not possess a significant calorific value. Large non-disintegrating capsules will empty with phase III of the MMC, and since ingestion is not synchronised to any particular part of the cycle, the emptying will appear erratic, occurring any time between a few minutes and 3 hours after administration.

When a large unit is given after a light meal (1500 kJ) the emptying becomes more predictable at around 2 to 3 hours. The meal serves to put the motility cycle into phase by initiating the fed pattern until the small calorific load has been passed to the duodenum. The next MMC then removes the tablet approximately 2 hours after the stomach has been cleared of the digestible components of the meal. Dosage forms are often administered to fasting subjects during pharmacokinetic studies in an attempt to reduce variability, but the effect of erratic emptying can affect the time of appearance of the drug in the plasma. However if the formulation is given with food to synchronise motility, the absorption of the drug can be influenced by the food. A possible solution is to give the drug with apple juice, which is a clear liquid, but has sufficient calories to synchronise gastric motility.

If a large single unit is given with a heavy meal (3600 kJ) and the subject is fed at regular intervals, the unit can remain in the stomach for longer than 8 hours due to prolonged suppression of the MMC. The only time at which the stomach can revert to the fasted pattern of motility is during the night when there is a sufficient interval between dinner and breakfast[70]. The length of the retention is proportional to the meal size. Thus when given with a meal of 650kJ, the mean residence time of a controlled release ibuprofen formulation was 2.0 ± 0.9 h; when the size of the meal was increased to 3330 kJ, the mean residence time was in excess of 9 ± 3 h. In the fasted state, the mean residence time was 1.0 ± 0.4 h[70].

The effect of administering a large non-disintegrating tablet (11 x 6 mm, density 1.4 g ml^{-1}) with several different feeding regimens is shown in Figure 5.16[71]. It can clearly be seen that the continual intake of small meals throughout the day, such as is common in the Western world, can delay the emptying of the tablets for more than 10 hours. Increasing the calorific value of a liquid meal by nearly 4-fold did not produce a proportionate increase in gastric residence time, but a mixed meal with similar calorific value to the liquid meal

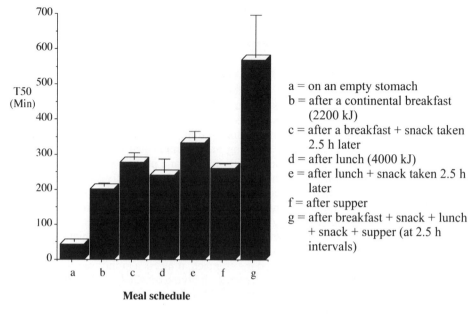

a = on an empty stomach
b = after a continental breakfast
    (2200 kJ)
c = after a breakfast + snack taken
    2.5 h later
d = after lunch (4000 kJ)
e = after lunch + snack taken 2.5 h
    later
f = after supper
g = after breakfast + snack + lunch
    + snack + supper (at 2.5 h
    intervals)

*Figure 5.16 Gastric residence time of a large non-disintegrating unit (11 x 6
mm, density 1.4 g ml^{-1}) with different feeding regimens.*

nearly doubled the residence time of the tablet. The ingestion of snacks increased the gas-tric residence time of the tablet by about 1.5 hours, but as the original meal size increased the difference became less significant due to the greater variation in emptying.

The effect of meal size on the gastric emptying times of single units is extremely important, especially for enteric coated preparations since this is the main factor influenc-ing the onset of drug release from enteric coated tablets[72]. The definition of a "large" tablet is still not known for humans. Tablets of between 3 and 7 mm empty similarly from the stomach after light, medium and heavy meals, and it is the calorific value of the meal and not the size which influences the emptying significantly[73].

The gastric emptying rates of multiparticulate dosage forms are not as severely af-fected by the presence or absence of food as are large single units. The gastric emptying of encapsulated pellets from the fasted stomach depends upon the nature of the capsule, the speed at which it disintegrates and the degree of dispersion of the pellets in the low volume of gastric contents available[74]. It has been proposed that dispersion of the capsule contents occurs into the mucus, followed by clearance at the normal mucus turnover rate, so that the emptying of pellets from the fasted stomach was a random event with the pellets emptying as a series of boluses. When pellets are administered with a meal, they tend to empty in a similar fashion to the digestible component of the meal (Figure 5.17).

The discrimination of the emptying of dosage forms produced by the presence of food can clearly be seen in a study in which a large non-disintegrating single unit (an os-motic pump device) and a pellet formulation were administered together (Figure 5.18). When administered with the light breakfast, in the majority of subjects, the single unit had emptied by 2 hours amidst the pellets; however the heavy breakfast greatly delayed the gastric emptying of the single unit to more than 9 hours. The emptying of the pellets was also prolonged by the heavier meal, but not to the same extent as the single unit[75].

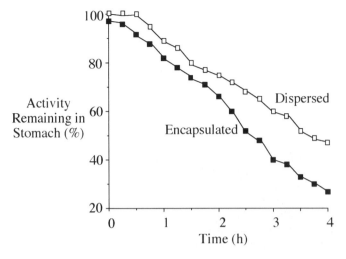

Figure 5.17 The gastric emptying of multiparticulates in a hard gelatin capsule taken either with a meal or dispersed within a meal

Time of dosing relative to a meal

Often patients are instructed to take their medication "with a meal", but instructions are never precise and this can be interpreted by the patient as taking the medication immediately before, midway through or just after the food. After dosing with a capsule containing pellets during or 10 minutes after a meal, pellets tend to remain in the upper half of the stomach. In these cases, the gastric emptying pattern is approximately linear with time. If the capsule is taken 10 minutes prior to a meal, the pellets empty faster following an exponential pattern (Figure 5.19)[76].

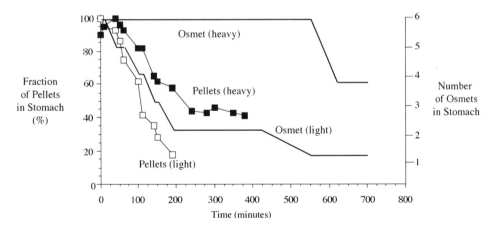

Figure 5.18 The effect of meal size on the emptying of single units (Osmets®) and multiparticulates. Note that at 12 h four of the large units were still in the stomach, however, the released drug had emptied from the stomach

Anti-reflux agents provide an example of how certain medications, particularly those which float on the gastric contents, are affected by time of dosing relative to a meal. Ingestion of an anti-reflux agent prior to meal causes it to empty before the food, and in addition it does not form the floating raft which is required for its action[77]. However, the anti-reflux agent does float when administered 30 minutes after a meal and hence its emptying is delayed with respect to the food. The gastric residence of floating formulations can be prolonged by frequent intake of meals[27] since ingestion of subsequent meals will delay the emptying of both the original meal and the formulation[78].

Retention of formulations in the stomach

There are several advantages in the use of formulations which remain in the stomach. For example, improvement in local delivery of drug to treat infections such as *Helicobacter pylori,* or prolonging the exposure of the upper small intestine to high concentrations of drug. This also may be advantageous for drugs which are acid soluble. Gastroretentive dosage forms will significantly extend the period of time over which drugs may be released, and thus prolong dosing intervals and increase patient compliance.

Many systems have been reported in the literature and the majority rely on flotation mechanisms to produce gastric retention. The prolonged gastric emptying of these formulations relies entirely on the presence of food in the stomach and they are generally emptied either at the end of the digestive phase, or with the MMC if they are large.

A hydrodynamically balanced system (HBS) was the first low-density formulation to be described. It is simply a capsule containing a mixture of drug, gel-forming hydrophilic polymer and excipients such as hydrophobic fatty materials. Upon contact with gastric fluid the capsule shell dissolves and the drug-hydrocolloid mixture absorbs water and swells to form a soft-gelatinous barrier. As the outer layer is eroded, a new layer is continually formed and the drug is released by diffusion through the hydrated layer[79]. To improve buoyancy and drug release the formulation was modified by the addition of a second layer of HPMC. Flotation of the HBS was visualised in volunteers using endoscopy[80].

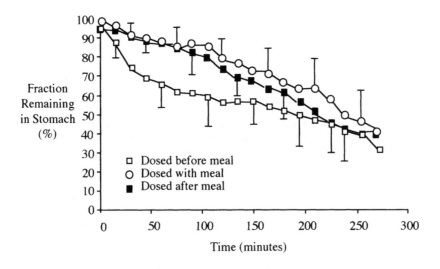

Figure 5.19 The effect on emptying of dosing time of a multiparticulate with respect to a meal

In order to improve buoyancy, an important strategy has been to incorporate gas producing agents such as sodium bicarbonate within the formulation. The systems may be composed of single or multiple layers and the gas-generation agent can be incorporated into any of the layers. Alternatively, ion-exchange resin can be loaded with bicarbonate and coated with a semipermeable membrane. Another approach has been to start with a buoyant core e.g. an empty hard gelatin capsule, polystyrene foam or concave tablet shell[81].

In vivo studies have shown that gastrically retained dose forms can produce up to 25% increase in bioavailability for agents such as riboflavin[82], but others report no effect for drugs such as acetaminophen in fasted or fed states[83]. Floating formulations can be a disadvantage for some drugs such as amoxycillin trihydrate, which show a reduction in bioavailability compared to conventional systems[84].

In contrast to floating systems, high density systems also have been investigated as a method for retaining dose forms in the stomach. The rationale behind this approach is that a dense object will fall through food and sit at the bottom of the greater curvature away from antral mixing. These devices have been used to great effect in animals, particularly ruminants, and early work in humans appeared promising at first. The studies reported that increasing the density of a multi-particulate dose form from 1 to 1.6 gcm^{-3} significantly increased the transit time in ileostomy subjects[85]. Unfortunately the results were later found not to be reproducible[86]. No differences in transit were found for pellets of 0.94 and 1.96 g cm^3 [87] or for single units with densities of 1.03 and 1.61 g cm^3 [88]. A number of subsequent studies have also failed to find an effect of formulation density until very high densities are reached e.g. 2.8 g cm^{-3} [89]. In this case gastric emptying can be significantly prolonged in both fasted and fed subjects, but small intestinal transit time is unaffected.

Studies conducted in dogs have demonstrated that spheres empty from the fed stomach as a function of their diameter, their density and the viscosity of the gastric contents[90]. The smaller the diameter (between 1 and 5 mm), the faster the spheres emptied; however spheres smaller than 1 mm did not empty any faster than 1 mm spheres. Spheres which were more or less dense than water emptied more slowly than the same size spheres with unit density. The explanation given for this is that the lighter spheres floated and the heavier spheres sank and so moved out of the central aqueous stream. Increasing the viscosity of the gastric contents caused even large dense spheres to empty more quickly, possibly because it retarded the layering of the spheres to the base of the stomach. This phenomenon has been observed in human subjects dosed with different density pellets. Pellets which floated on or sank to the base of the stomach emptied more slowly then pellets of a similar density to food. When the light and heavy pellets were administered with a small meal, their emptying was similar to that seen with pellets of a similar density to food when administered with a large meal (Figure 5.20). This suggests that the light and heavy pellets are not caught up in the antral flow.

The gastric retention of solid dosage forms may also be achieved by mucoadhesion, in which case the dosage form will adhere to the mucosal surface of the stomach wall. Once attached, it will remain there until mucus turnover sloughs it off. The mucoadhesives which have been tried are polycarbophil and Carbopol®. Studies in animals and humans have produced rather disappointing results and the main problem appears to be that these polymers are such good adhesives that they stick to anything they come into contact with. Hence they will stick to the gelatin released from the capsules in which they were dosed, or to water-soluble proteins present in the stomach, and also sloughed mucus. This non-specific adhesion severely reduces the amount of bioadhesive available to stick to the epithelial mucus.

Earlier studies conducted in dogs used slurries of polycarbophil particulates (1 - 3 mm in diameter) at doses of 30 and 90 g[13]. The meal containing the 90 g polycarbophil slurry demonstrated a decreased rate of gastric emptying. At autopsy, the particles were

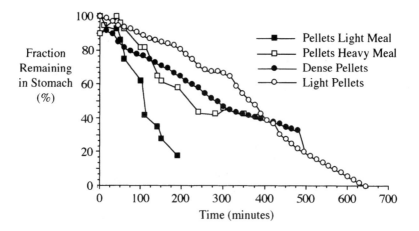

Figure 5.20 The effect of pellet density and size of a meal on the gastric emptying of multiparticulates

shown not to have adhered to the mucosa, but to have formed large intragastric boluses. Apparently that the slow rate of emptying of the polycarbophil was due to the action of the stomach squeezing the particles together, causing a loss of surface-bound water and forming a large bolus; occasional retropulsion mixed the bolus with the gastric secretions causing some re-dispersion of particles. The gastric distension produced by the large indigestible mass elicited the fed pattern of activity and the fasting peristaltic waves were suppressed.

Another gastroretentive system is the magnetic dose form. This usually contains a magnet, or a mass of magnetic material such as a ferrite, in its centre and an externally placed magnet serves to anchor the dose form within the body. Drugs which have been delivered by this method include cinnarizine, acetominophen and riboflavin, all of which showed improved bioavailability. The major drawback with this method is that placing the external magnet to hold the tablet in the stomach is technically quite difficult. To make magnetic tablets commercially viable a better method for applying the magnetic field needs to be produced than that currently available.

Dose forms that unfurl or expand in the stomach, becoming too large to exit through the pylorus, have also been proposed to achieve prolonged gastric residence. Geometric shapes which have been studied include a continuous solid stick, a ring and a planar membrane. In fasted beagle dogs retention times of over 24 h were reported[91], but in humans the time was reduced to 6.5 h in the fed state and 3 h in the fasted state. The main problem with this type of system is that they have to exit the stomach eventually, and hence have to be biodegradable as well as having expanding properties. This can pose severe design restrictions. In addition, like all sustained release devices, the systems would have to have a high reliability since they would be designed to administer a large dose of drug over an extended period. Adhesion of dosage form to the oesophagus is common, and the possibility of a device sticking and expanding in the oesophagus is unpleasant to say the least. Swellable systems would also have to be able to withstand the 80 to 100 mmHg pressures generated in the human pylorus[22 92]. These combined difficulties have outweighed any potential advantages for manufacturers to date.

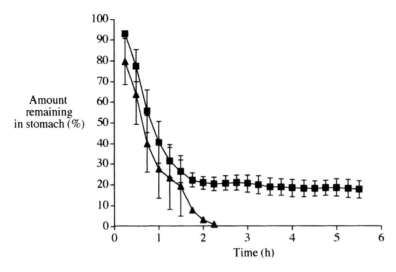

Figure 5.21 - Gastric retention of a suspension of 20-40 μm ion exchange resin (■) compared to 99mTc-DTPA (▲) which is a water soluble marker

One promising method of achieving gastric retention is by the use of micronised ion exchange resins[93]. Ionic resins are already in use as drug delivery vehicles[94], in which release from the resin occurs through the replacement of the drug by another ion of the same charge. Recent studies[95] have shown that if micronized resins are administered in a small volume of water, they coat the stomach uniformly, and approximately 20% of the resin is retained for 5-6 hours and is not dislodged by subsequent meals (Figure 5.21). Anionic resins such as cholestyramine have been shown to display better mucoadhesive properties *in vitro* than cationic polymers[96]. This was thought to be due to ionic interactions between the highly charged surface of the polymers and the mucus.

Posture effects

Moving from the upright to the supine position markedly affects the emptying of formulations and hence the rate and extent of drug absorption. Bland, unbuffered liquids and pellet formulations empty more slowly from the stomach when the subject is lying down compared to when upright or sitting erect[67 97]. For floating formulations, such as raft-forming alginates, the buoyant raft empties faster than food in subjects lying on their left side or their backs, and slower in subjects lying on their right side with the raft positioned in the greater curvature[98]. When the subjects lay on their left side the raft was presented to the pylorus ahead of the meal and so emptied first. Oily materials float and hence also empty more slowly than the aqueous phase of the meal when subjects are in the sitting position[28]. Posture also affects the emptying of large non-disintegrating capsules from the fasted stomach. Capsules are only passed into the duodenum during phase III of the first MMC initiated when the subjects are lying in the right lateral position[99]. The gastric residence of floating and non-floating capsules is similar in supine subjects[100].

Posture can also affect drug absorption. The time to maximum plasma concentration of coadministered soluble paracetamol, nifedipine, and its metabolite produced at first pass, was significantly decreased when subjects are standing or lying on their right side compared to when they lay on their left side[101]. These postures also resulted in a significantly higher peak plasma concentration and area under the plasma concentration-time curve of the nifedipine, but not its metabolite. The increased absorption of these drugs also produced a significantly higher heart rate. Lying down decreased the rate of gastric emptying when compared to sitting, and a combination of sitting and standing produced the most rapid gastric emptying[102].

Drug-induced effects on gastric emptying

Drugs contained within the formulations may also alter gastric motility. For example adrenergic agonists, particularly β_2-agonists such as salbutamol, delay gastric emptying. In asthmatic subjects an variable quantity of the inhaled drug may be swallowed, and hence even though the drug is not taken by the oral route, it may still have an effect on the gastric emptying of other drugs. Tricyclic antidepressants and some anti-Parkinsonian drugs depress gastrointestinal motility. Dopaminergic antagonists e.g. domperidone, and cholinergic agonists e.g. bethanechol, enhance gastric motor activity.

GASTRIC pH AND ENTERIC COATINGS

In the past, the pH chosen by most formularies to represent the conditions in the stomach is 1.0 (100 mM HCl). However, there is some evidence that the basal gastric pH can be surprisingly high. It has been reported that 35% of humans have a resting gastric pH of 6 or above[103]. Less than 2% of the human subjects had a resting pH below 1.5. Basal gastric pH in normal healthy students is around 1.8, but occasional cases of achlorhydria are seen. Meals markedly alter the pH, which can increase to 3 - 5 after eating, particularly if the meal contains large amounts of easily digested protein.

These variations in pH will be especially important when developing products designed to be gastro-resistant, e.g. enteric coatings for acid-labile or potentially irritant drugs. In these cases gamma scintigraphy may be combined with *in vivo* pH measurement to investigate the efficiency and operation of the enteric coating. In a study which administered both radiolabelled pH radiotelemetry capsules and radiolabelled enteric coated naproxen tablets to fed subjects[72], it was found that the pH remained below 2 within the stomach, except for a transient rise after food. Five tablets disintegrated in the small intestine approximately 1.2 h after gastric emptying, one disintegrated in the stomach at pH 1.1 and one tablet remained intact in the stomach for 9 h.

DRUG/FORMULATION INDUCED ULCERATION

Acute and/or chronic lesions on the gastric mucosa may result from the ingestion of alcohol, and some drugs such as anti-inflammatory drugs, reserpine, histamine and caffeine. Salicylates are often reported to produce dyspepsia and gastric ulcers due to their widespread use. A single dose of two aspirin tablets produced haemorrhaging in the stomach of normal volunteers within 1 hour of ingestion, continued intake (two tablets every 6 hours) resulted in gastric erosions in all subjects and duodenal erosions in 50% of the subjects[104]. Patients who require aspirin on a regular basis should take enteric coated or adequately buffered preparations.

ANIMAL MODELS FOR GASTRIC EMPTYING

Dogs are widely used to assess the absorption of drugs. However, the drug absorption profiles differ quite considerably from those in humans, and this is a particular problem when attempting to obtain useful data for either sparingly water-soluble drugs or sustained release preparations.

The anatomy and dimensions of the upper gastrointestinal tract of dogs and humans are essentially similar. The volume of the stomach is 1 – 1.6 L in man and about 1 L in dogs. The length of the duodenum is 25 cm in both species and the jejunum is 185-250 cm in dogs and 300 cm in man. The diameter of the small intestine is 2 – 2.5 cm in dogs and 3-4 cm in man. The ileum and colon are substantially shorter in dogs than man.

During fasting, intragastric pH in man varies between 1.3-1.8, but the corresponding pH in the dog is between 0.8 and 8. Kuna [103] reported that 77% of 403 dogs had a fasting pH of 6 or above. Sometimes the resting gastric pH is indistinguishable from the duodenal pH. The rate of acid secretion is much lower in dogs, being 0.1 mEqh^{-1} compared to 2-5 mEqh^{-1} in man.

It is also thought that dogs have a faster total gastrointestinal transit time than man, and hence bioavailability is generally underestimated. However, in dogs, a normal meal can induce a fed pattern for approximately 12 to 14 hours, but in humans this usually only lasts for between 3 and 4 hours. Rigidity is an important factor in the retention of dosage forms. In dogs, rigid rings with a diameter of 3.6 cm are well retained in the stomach for 24 hours, whilst pellets and strings demonstrated rapid emptying[105]. In dogs pellets tend to empty from the stomach entrapped in plugs of mucus[106]. Dogs have a delayed onset of MMC compared to man[107 108].

Pigs are also not a good model for the gastrointestinal transit of large non-disintegrating capsules. One study demonstrated a gastric residence time of 5 days for an enteric coated non-disintegrating magnesium hydroxide caplet (1.5 g ml density, 19.6 x 9.5 mm, 1.2 g weight)[109]. As a result of these differences, studies of oral dose forms in animals must be interpreted with caution, particularly if the operation of the formulation depends on its detailed behaviour in the gastrointestinal tract.

REFERENCES

1. McLaughlan G, Fullarton GM, Crean GP, McColl KEL. Comparison of gastric body and antral pH: a 24 hour ambulatory study in healthy volunteers. *Gut* 1989;30:573-578.
2. McArthur K, Hogan D, Isenberg JI. Relative stimulatory effects of commonly ingested beverages on acid secretion in humans. *Gastroenterol.* 1982;83:199-204.
3. Bumm R, Blum AL. Lessons from prolonged gastric pH monitoring. *Aliment. Pharmacol. Therap.* 1987;1:518S-526S.
4. Richardson CT, Walsh JH, Hicks MI, Fordtran JS. Studies on the mechanisms of food-stimulated gastric acid secretion in normal human subjects. *J. Clin. Invest.* 1976;58:623-681.
5. Moore JG. Circadian dynamics of gastric acid secretion and pharmacodynamics of H$_2$ receptor blockade. *Ann. New York Acad. Sci.* 1991;618:150-158.
6. Lanzon-Miller S, Pounder RE, McIsaac RI, Wood JR. Does the timing of the evening meal affect the pattern of 24 hour intragastric acidity. *Gut* 1988;29:A1472.
7. Bauerfriend P, Cilluffo T, Fimmel CJ, Gasser T, Kohler W, Merki H, et al. Die intragastrale Langzeit-pH-Metrie (Continuous intragastric pH-metry). *Scweitz. Med. Wochenschr.* 1985;115:1630-1641.
8. Feldman M, Barnett C. Fasting gastric pH and its relationship to true hypochlorhydria in humans. *Dig. Dis. Sci.* 1991;36:866-869.
9. Goldschmiedt M, Barnett CC, Schwarz BE. Effect of age on gastric acid secretion and serum gastric concentrations in healthy men and women. *Gastroenterol.* 1991;101:977-990.
10. Dantas RO, Dodds WJ. Measurement of gastrointestinal pH and regional transit times in normal children. *J. Ped. Gastroenterol. Nutr.* 1990;11:211-214.
11. Ke MY, Li RQ, Pan GZ. Gastrointestinal pH and transit times in healthy subjects with ileostomy. *Aliment. Pharmacol. Therapeut.* 1990;4:247-253.
12. Kaufmann D, Wilder-Smith CH, Kempf M. Cigarette smoking, gastric acidity and peptic ulceration. What are the relationships? *Dig. Dis. Sci.* 1990;35:1482-1487.

13. Russell J, Bass P. Canine gastric emptying of fiber meals: Influence of meal viscosity and antroduodenal motility. *Am. J. of Physiol. - Gastrointest. Liver Physiol.* 1985;12:G662-G667.
14. King PM, Adam RD, Pryde A, McDicken WN, Heading RC. Relationships of human antroduodenal motility and transpyloric fluid movement: non-invasive observations with real-time ultrasound. *Gut* 1984;25:1384-1391.
15. Kumar D, Ritman EL, Malagelada JR. Three-dimensional imaging of the stomach: Role of pylorus in the emptying of liquids. *Am. J. of Physiol. - Gastrointest. Liver Physiol.* 1987;253:G79-G85.
16. Meyer JH, Thomson JB, Cohen MB, Shadcher A, Madola SA. Sieving of solid food by the canine stomach and sieving after gastric surgery. *Gastroenterol.* 1979;76:804-813.
17. Hausken T, Ødegaard S, Berstad A. Antroduodenal motility studied by real time ultrasonography. *Gastroenterol.* 1991;100:59-63.
18. Washington N, Steele RJC, Jackson SJ, Washington C, Bush D. Patterns of food and acid reflux in patients with low grade oesophagitis: the role of an anti-reflux agent. *Alim. Pharmacol. Therap.* 1998;12:53-58.
19. Feldman M, Smith HJ, Simon TR. Gastric emptying of solid radiopaque markers: Studies in healthy subjects and diabetic patients. *Gastroenterol.* 1984;87:895-902.
20. Stephens JR, Woolson RF, Cooke AR. Effects of essential and non-essential amino acids on gastric emptying in the dog. *Gastroenterol.* 1975;69:920-927.
21. Hunt JN, Knox MT. A relation between the chain length of fatty acids and the slowing of gastric emptying. *J. Physiol.* 1968;194:327-336.
22. Houghton LA, Read NW, Heddle R, Maddern GJ, Downton J, Toouli J, Motor activity of the gastric antrum, pylorus and duodenum under fasted conditions and after a liquid meal. *Gastroenterol.* 1988;94:1276-1284.
23. Houghton LA, Mangnall YF, Read NW. Effect of incorporating fat into a liquid test meal on the relation between intragastric distribution and gastric emptying in human volunteers. *Gut* 1990;31:1226-1229.
24. Hunt JN, Knox MT. Regulation of gastric emptying. In: Code CF, Heidel W, editors. *Handbook of Physiol.*. Washington D. C. Am. Physiol. Soc., 1968:1917-1935.
25. Sanford PA. The stomach. *Dig. System Physiol.,*. London: Edward Arnold, 1982:36, Chapter 3.
26. Meyer JH, Mayer EA, Jehn D, Gu Y, Fink AS, Fried M. Gastric processing and emptying of fat. *Gastroenterol.* 1986;90:1176-1187.
27. Moss HA, Washington N, Greaves JL, Wilson CG. Anti-reflux agents: Stratification of floatation? *Europ. J. Gastroenterol. Hepatol.* 1990;2:45-51.
28. Horowitz M, Jones K, Edelbroek MAL, Smout AJPM, Read NW. The effect of posture on gastric emptying and intragastric distribution of oil and aqueous meal components and appetite. *Gastroenterol.* 1993;105:382-390.
29. Carney BI, Jones KL, Horowitz M, Sun WM, Penagini R, Meyer JH. Gastric-emptying of oil and aqueous meal components in pancreatic insufficiency - Effects of posture and on appetite. *Am. J. of Physiol.-Gastrointest. Liver Physiol.* 1995;31:G 925-G 932.
30. Heddle R, Collins PJ, Dent J, Horowitz M, Read NW, Chatterton B, Houghton LA. Motor mechanisms associated with slowing of the gastric emptying of a solid meal by an intraduodenal lipid infusion. *J. Gastroenterol. Hepatol.* 1989;4:437-447.
31. Benini L, Brighenti F, Castellani G, Brentegani MT, Casiraghi MC, Ruzzenente O, et al. Gastric-emptying of solids is markedly delayed when meals are fried. *Dig. Dis. Sci.* 1994;39:2288-2294.
32. Sepple CP, Read NW. Effect of prefeeding lipid on food intake and satiety in man. *Gut* 1990;31:158-l61.
33. Konturek JW, Thor P, Domschke W, Konturek SJ. Role of CCK in the control of gastric emptying and gastric secretory response to fatty meal in humans. *Biomed.Res.* 1995;16(Suppl. 2):141-146.

34. Edelbroek M, Horowitz M, Maddox A, Bellen J. Gastric-emptying and intragastric distribution of oil in the presence of a liquid or a solid meal. *J. Nucl. Med.* 1992;33:1283-1290.

35. Cunningham KM, Read NW. The effect of incorporating fat into different components of a meal on gastric emptying and postprandial blood glucose and insulin responses. *Br. J. Nutr.* 1989;61:285-290.

36. Cortot A, Phillips SF, Malagelada JR. Gastric emptying of lipids after ingestion of a solid-liquid meal in humans. *Gastroenterol.* 1981;80:922-927.

37. Cortot A, Phillips SF, Malagelada JR. Parallel gastric emptying of nonhydrolyzable fat and water after a solid-liquid meal in humans. *Gastroenterol.* 1982;82:877-881.

38. Collier G, McLean A, Odea K. Effect of co-ingestion of fat on the metabolic responses to slowly and rapidly absorbed carbohydrates. *Diabetologia* 1984;26:50-54.

39. Sonnenberg A, MuellerLissner SA, Weiser HF, Effect of liquid meals on duodenogastric reflux in humans. *Am. J. Physiol. - Gastrointest. Liver Physiol.* 1982;6:G42-G47.

40. Mangnall YF, Houghton LA, Johnson AG, Read NW. Abnormal distribution of a fatty liquid test meal within the stomach of patients with non-ulcer dyspepsia. *Europ. J. Gastroenterol. and Hepatol.* 1994;6:323-327.

41. Feinle C, Grundy D, Read NW. Fat increases vection-induced nausea independent of changes in gastric emptying. *Physiol. Behav.* 1995;58:1159-1165.

42. Rigaud D, Merrouche M, Le Moel G, Vatier J, Paycha F, Cadiot G, Facteurs de reflux gastro-oesophagien acide dans l'obesite severe (Gastro-oesophageal reflux in morbid obesity). *Gastroenterol. Cliniq. Biologiq.* 1995;19:818-825.

43. Casaubon PR, Dahlstrom KA, Vargas J, Hawkins R, Mogard M, Ament ME. Intravenous fat emulsion (intralipid) delays gastric emptying, but does not cause gastroesophageal reflux in healthy volunteers. *J. Parenter. Enter. Nutr.* 1989;13:246-248.

44. Goo RH, Moore JG, Greenberg E, Alazaki NP. Circadian variation in gastric emptying of meals in man. *Gastroenterol.* 1987;93:515-518.

45. Wald A, Van Thiel DH, Hoechstetter L, Gavaler JS, Egler KM, Verm R, et al. Gastrointestinal transit: the effect iof the menstrual cycle. *Gastroenterol.* 1980;80:1497-1500.

46. Wright RA, Krinsky S, Fleeman C, Trujillo J, Teague E. Gastric emptying and obesity. *Gastroenterol.* 1983;84:747-751.

47. Hutson WR, Wald A. Obesity and weight-reduction do not influence gastric-emptying and antral motility. *Am. J. Gastroenterol.* 1993;88:1405-1409.

48. Madsen JL. Effects of gender, age, and body mass index on gastrointestinal transit times. *Dig. Dis. Sci.* 1992;37:1548-1553.

49. Moore JG, Datz FL, Christian E. Exercise increases solid meal gastric-emptying rates in men. *Dig. Dis. Sci.* 1990;35:428-432.

50. Miller LJ, Malagelada JR, Longstreth GF, Go VLW. Dysfunctions of the stomach with gastric ulceration. *Dig. Dis. Sci.* 1980;25:857-846.

51. Bromster D. Gastric emptying rate in gastric and duodenal ulceration. *Scand. J. Gastroenterol.* 1969;4:193-201.

52. Davies WT, Kirkpatrick JR, Owen GM, Shields R. Gastric emptying in atrophic gastritis and carcinoma of the stomach. *Scand. J. Gastroenterol.* 1971;6:297-301.

53. Halvorsen L, Dotevall G, Walan A. Gastric emptying in patients with achlorhydria or hyposecretion of hydrochloric acid. *Scand. J. Gastroenterol.* 1973;8:395-399.

54. Castell DO, Holtz A. Gastroesophageal reflux. Don't forget to ask about heartburn. *Postgrad. Med.* 1989;86:141-144.

55. Graham DY, Smith JL, Patterson DJ. Why do apparently healthy people use antacid tablets? *Am. J. Gastroenterol.* 1983;78:257-260.

56. Behar J, Ramsey G. Gastric emptying and antral motility in reflux esophagitis. *Gastroenterol.* 1978;74:253-256.

57. Coleman SC, Rees WDW, Malagelada J-R. Normal gastric function in esophageal reflux (abstract). *Gastroenterol.* 1979;76:1115.

58. Baldi F, Corinaldesi R, Ferrarini F, Stanghellini V, Miglioli M, Barbara L. Gastric secretion and emptying of liquids in reflux esophagitis. *Dig. Dis. Sci.* 1981;26:886-889.

59. Hillemeier AC, Grill BB, McCallum R, Gryboski J. Esophageal and gastric motor abnormalities in gastroesophageal reflux during pregnancy. *Gastroenterol.* 1983;84:741-746.

60. Donovan IA, Harding LK, Keighley MRB, Griffin DW, Collis JL. Abnormalities of gastric emptying and pyloric reflux in uncomplicated hiatus hernia. *Br. J. Surg.* 1977;64:847-848.

61. McCallum RW, Berkowitz DM, Lerner E. Gastric emptying in patients with gastrooesophageal reflux. *Gastroenterol.* 1981;80:285-291.

62. Hutson WR, Wald A. Gastric-emptying in patients with bulimia nervosa and anorexia-nervosa. *Am. J. Gastroenterol.* 1990;85:41-46.

63. Wilson CG, Washington N. Assessment of disintegration and dissolution of dosage forms *in vivo* using gamma scintigraphy. *Drug Dev. Ind. Pharm.* 1988;14:211-281.

64. Graham DY, Smith JL, Bouvet AA. What happens to tablets and capsules in the stomach - endoscopic comparison of disintegration and dispersion characteristics of two microencapsulated potassium formulations. *J. Pharmaceut. Sci.* 1990;79:420-424.

65. Casey DL, Beihn RM, Digenis GA, Shambhu MB. Method for monitoring hard gelatin disintegration times in humans using external scintigraphy. *J. Pharmaceut. Sci.* 1976;65:1412-1413.

66. Hunter E, Fell JT, Calvert RT, Sharma H. *In vivo* investigation of hard gelatin capsules in fasting and non-fasting subjects. *Int. J. Pharmaceut.* 1980;4:175-183.

67. Hunter E, Fell JT, Sharma H. The gastric emptying of pellets contained in hard gelatin capsules. *Drug Dev. Ind. Pharm.* 1982;8:751-757.

68. Hunter E, Fell JT, Sharma H. The gastric emptying of hard gelatin capsules. *Int. J. Pharmaceut.* 1983;17:59-64.

69. Armstrong NA, James KC. Drug release from lipid-based dosage forms *Int. J. Pharmaceut.* 1980;6:185-193.

70. Wilson CG, Washington N, Greaves JL, Kamali F, Rees JA, Sempik AK, Bimodal release of ibuprofen in a sustained-release formulation: a scintigraphic and pharmacokinetic open study in healthy volunteers under different conditions of food intake. *Int. J. Pharmaceut.* 1989;50:155-161.

71. Ewe K, Press AG, Bollen S, Scuhn I. Gastric emptying of indigestible tablets in relation to composition and time of ingestion of meals studied by metal detector. *Dig. Dis. Sci.* 1991;36:146-152.

72. Hardy JG, Evans DF, Zaki I, Clark AG, Tønnesen HH, Gamst ON. Evaluation of an enteric coated naproxen tablet using gamma scintigraphy and pH monitoring. *Int. J. Pharmaceut.* 1987;37:245-250.

73. Khosla R, Feely LC, Davis SS. Gastrointestinal transit of non-disintegrating tablets in fed subjects. *Int. J. Pharmaceut.* 1989; 53:107-117.

74. Hunter E, Fell JT, Sharma H, McNeilly AM. The *in vivo* behaviour of hard gelatin capsules filled with thixotropic liquids. Part 2: Quantitative aspects. *Pharmazeutische Industrie* 1983;45:433-434.

75. Davis SS, Hardy JG, Taylor MJ, Whalley DR, Wilson CG. The effect of food on the gastrointestinal transit of pellets and an osmotic device (Osmet). *Int. J. Pharmaceut.* 1984;21:331-340.

76. O'Reilly S, Hardy JG, Wilson CG. The influence of food on the gastric emptying of multiparticulate dosage forms. *Int. J. Pharmaceut.* 1987;34:213-216.

77. Washington N, Greaves JL, Wilson CG. Effect of time of dosing relative to a meal on the raft formation of an anti-reflux agent. *J. Pharm. Pharmacol.* 1990;42:50-53.

78. Horowitz M, Maddox A, Bochner M, Wishart J, Bratasiuk R, Collins P, Relationships between gastric-emptying of solid and caloric liquid meals and alcohol absorption. *Am. J. Physiol.* 1989;257:G291-G298.

79. Sheth PR, Tossounian J. The hydrodynamically balanced system (HBS™): A novel drug delivery system for oral use. *Drug Dev. Ind. Pharm.* 1984;10:313-339.

80. Khattar D, Ahuja A, Khar RK. Hydrodynamically balanced systems as sustained release dosage forms for propranolol hydrochloride. *Pharmazie* 1990;45:356-358.

81. Watanabe S, Kayano M, Ishino Y, Miyao K. Solid therapeutic preparations remaining in the stomach. *US Patent* 1976;3,976,764.

82. Ingani HM, Timmermans J, Moes AJ. Conception and *in vivo* investigation of peroral sustained release floating dosage forms with enhanced gastrointestinal transit. *Int. J. Pharmaceut.* 1987;35:157-164.

83. Phuapradit W, Bolton S. The influence of tablet density on the human oral absorption of sustained release acetominophen matrix tablets. *Drug Dev. Ind. Pharm.* 1991;17:1097-1107.

84. Hilton AK, Deasy PB. *In vitro* and *in vivo* evaluation of an oral sustained-release floating dosage form of amoxicillin trihydate. *Int. J. Pharmaceut.* 1992;86:79-88.

85. Bechgaard H, Ladefoged K. Distribution of pellets in the gastrointestinal tract. The influence on transit time exerted by density or diameter of pellets. *J. Pharm. Pharmacol.* 1978;30:690-692.

86. Bogentoft C, Appelgren C, Jonnson WE, Sjögren J, Alpsten M. Intestinal transit time of 51Cr-labelled pellets of different densities. In *Radionuclide Imaging in Drug Research.* Wilson, CG, Hardy, JG, Frier, M. and Davies, SS (eds) 1982;Croom Helm, London:294-296.

87. Bechgaard H, Christensen FN, Davis SS, Hardy JG, Wilson CG,Taylor MJ, Whalley DR, Gastrointestinal transit of pellet systems in ileostomy subjects and the effect of density. *J. Pharm. Pharmacol.* 1985;37:718-721.

88. Kaus LC, Fell JT, Sharma H, Taylor DC. The intestinal transit of of a single non-disintegrating unit. *Int. J. Pharmaceut.* 1984;20:315-323.

89. Devereux JE, Newton JM, Short MB. The influence of density on the gastrointestinal transit of pellets. *J. Pharm. Pharmacol.* 1990;42:500-501.

90. Meyer JH, Dressman J, Fink AS, Amidon G. Effect of size and density on gastric emptying of indigestible solids (abstract). *Gastroenterol.* 1985;88:1502.

91. Curatoto WJ, Lo J. Gastric retention systems for controlled drug release. *U.S. Patent* 1995;5,443,843.

92. Houghton LA, Read NW, Heddle R, Horowitz M, Collins PJ, Chatterton B, Dent J. Relationship of the motor activity antrum, pylorus and duodenum to gastric emptying of a solid-liquid mixed meal. *Gastroenterol.* 1988;94:1285-1291.

93. Burton S, Washington N, Steele RJC, Musson R, Feely L. Intragastric distribution of ion-exchange resins: A drug delivery system for the topical treatment of the gastric mucosa. *J. Pharm. Pharmacol.* 1995;47:901-906.

94. Borodkin S. Ion-exchange resin delivery systems. In: *Polymers for Controlled Drug Delivery.* Tarcha P, (ed.) Florida: CRC Press, Boca Raton, 1991:215-230.

95. Thairs S, Ruck S, Jackson SJ, Steele RJC, Feely L, Washington C, Washington N. Effect of dose size, food and surface coating on the gastric residence and distribution on an ion exchange resin. *Int. J. Pharmaceut.* 1998;176:47-53.

96. Park H, Robinson JR. Physico-chemical properties of water insoluble polymers important to mucin/epithelial adhesion. *J. Cont. Rel.* 1985;2:47-57.

97. Hunt JN, Knox MT, O'Ginskey A. The effect of gravity on gastric emptying of various meals. *J. Physiol. (London)* 1965;178:92-97.

98. Bennett CE, Hardy JG, Wilson CG. The influence of posture on gastric emptying of antacids. *Int. J. Pharmaceut.* 1984;21:341-347.

99. Mojaverian P, Chan K, Desai A, John V. Gastrointestinal transit of a solid indigestible capsule as measured by radiotelemetry and dual gamma scintigraphy. *Pharmaceut. Res.* 1989;6:719-724.

100. Sangekar S, Vadino WA, Chaundry I, Parr A, Beihn R, Digenis G. Evaluation of the effect of food and specific gravity of tablets on gastric retention time. *Int J. Pharmaceut.* 1987;35:187-191.

101. Renwick AG, Ahsan CH, Challenor VF, Daniels R, Macklin BS, Waller DG, et al. The influence of posture on the pharmacokinetics of orally-administered nifedipine. *Br. J. Clin. Pharmacol.* 1992;34:332-336.
102. Moore JG, Datz FL, Christian PE, Greenberg E, Alazraki N. Effect of body posture on radionuclide measurements of gastric-emptying. *Dig. Dis. Sci.* 1988;33:1592-1595.
103. Kuna S. The pH of gastric juice in the normal resting stomach. *Arch Int Pharmacodyn.* 1964;151:79-97.
104. O'Laughlin JC, Hoftiezer JW, Ivey KJ. Effect of aspirin on the human stomach in normals: endoscopic comparison of damage produced one hour, 24 hours and 2 weeks after administration. *Scand. J. Gastroenterol.* 1981;16 Suppl. 67:211-214.
105. Cargill R, Caldwell LJ, Engle K, Fix JA, Porter PA, Gardner CR. Controlled gastric emptying. 1. Effects of physical properties on gastric residence times of nondisintegrating geometric shapes in beagle dogs. *Pharmaceut. Res.* 1988;5:533-536.
106. Gruber P, Rubinstein A, Hon Kin Li V, Bass P, Robinson JR. Gastric emptying of nondigestible solids in the fasted dog. *J. Pharmaceut. Sci.* 1987;76:117-122.
107. Kaniwa N, Aoyagi N, Ogata H, Ejima A. Gastric emptying rates of drug preparations. I Effects of size of dosage forms, food and species on gastric emptying rates. *J. Pharmacobiol. Dyn.* 1988;11:563-570.
108. Kaniwa N, Aoyagi N, Ogata H, Ejima A, Motoyama H, Yasumi H. Gastric emptying rates of drug preparations. II. Effects of size and density of enteric-coated drug preparations and food on gastric emptying rates in humans. *J. Pharmacobiol. Dyn.* 1988;11:571-575.
109. Hossain M, Abramowitz W, Watrous BJ, Szpunar GJ, Ayres JW. Gastrointestinal transit of nondisintegrating, nonerodible oral dosage forms in pigs. *Pharmaceut. Res.* 1990;7:1163-1166.

Chapter Six

Drug Absorption from the Small Intestine

ANATOMY AND PHYSIOLOGY OF THE SMALL INTESTINE

The small intestine is between 5 and 6 metres in length and its main functions are to mix food with enzymes to facilitate digestion, to mix the intestinal contents with the intestinal secretions to enable absorption to occur, and to propel the unabsorbed materials in an aboral direction. The small intestinal epithelium has the highest capacity for nutrient and drug absorption within the gastrointestinal tract, due to the large surface area provided by epithelial folding and the villous structures of the absorptive cells.

Gross morphology

The small intestine is the longest section of the digestive tube and it is arbitrarily divided into three parts. The first 20 to 30 cm is termed the duodenum, the second 2.5 metres the jejunum and the final 3.5 metres the ileum. These regions are not anatomically distinct, although there are differences in absorptive capability and secretion. There is no definite sphincter between the stomach and duodenum although in some studies a zone of elevated pressure between the two regions has been reported to exist. The duodenum has a thick wall with a deeply folded mucous membrane and contains duodenal digestive glands and Brunner's glands. Brunner's glands are found only in the submucosa of the duodenum and produce a protective alkaline secretion which does not contain any enzymes, but serves to neutralize gastric acid. The jejunum is thicker walled and more vascular than the duodenum and has larger and more numerous villi than the ileum. In the ileum, the lymphatic follicles (Peyer's patches) are larger and more numerous than elsewhere in the intestine.

Most of the small intestine is suspended from the body wall by an extension of the peritoneum called the mesentery. The blood vessels which supply the small intestine lie between the two sheets of the mesentery.

Mucosa

The small intestine consists of the serosa, the muscularis, the submucosa and the mucosa (Figure 6.1). The serosa is an extension of the peritoneum, and consists of a single layer of flattened mesothelial cells overlying some loose connective tissue. The muscularis has an outer longitudinal layer and an inner circular layer of muscle. The submucosa consists largely of dense connective tissue sparsely infiltrated by lymphocytes, fibroblasts, macrophages, eosinophils, mast and plasma cells. The submucosa contains an extensive lymphatic network.

The intestinal mucosa itself can be divided into three layers:

a) the muscularis mucosa, which is the deepest layer consisting of a sheet of muscle 3 to 10 cells thick that separates the mucosa from the submucosa.

b) the lamina propria, the middle layer, is mainly connective tissue and forms the core of the numerous villi and surrounds the crypts. The lamina propria usually contains many types of cells, e.g. plasma cells, lymphocytes, mast cells, macrophages, smooth muscle cells and non-cellular elements such as collagen and elastin fibres. The lamina propria provides structural support, and there is increasing evidence that it has an important role in preventing the entry of microorganisms and foreign substances.

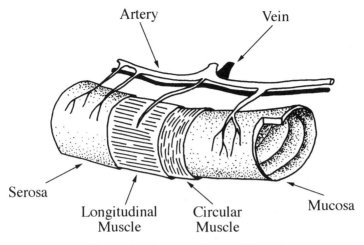

Figure 6.1 Section of the small intestine

c) the epithelium, which is the innermost layer of the mucosa and consists of a single layer of columnar epithelial cells or enterocytes, which lines both the crypts and the villi.

Organisation of the mucosa

The surface area of the small intestinal mucosa is greatly increased by the folds of Kerckring, villi and microvilli (brush border) and is about 200 m² (or roughly the size of a tennis court!) in an adult (Figure 6.2).

Folds of Kerckring

A particularly prominent feature in the small intestine is the folding of the epithelium, known as the folds of Kerckring. The folds increase the surface area by a factor of 3. These folds extend circularly most of the way around the intestine and are especially well developed in the duodenum and jejunum, where they protrude by up to 8 mm into the lumen. They also act as baffles which aid mixing of the chyme in the small intestine.

Villi

The surface of the mucous membrane of the small intestine possesses about 5 million villi, each about 0.5 to 1 mm long. Although the villi are often described as "finger-like", their shape changes along the gut and duodenal villi are shorter and broader than those found in the jejunum. Further down the gut the villus height decreases. Diet and environment markedly affect mucosal morphology and intestinal biopsies demonstrate differences between human populations. There is also a species difference, for example, the villi of the chick are pointed and leaf-like.

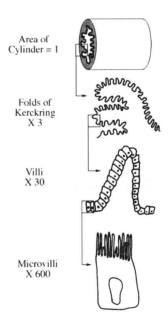

Figure 6.2 Increases in surface area in the small intestine due to folding

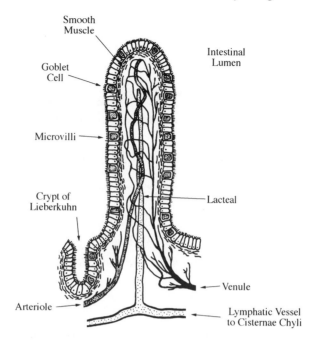

Figure 6.3 Structure of a villus. Note blood and lymph flow

The major features of a villus are illustrated in Figure 6.3. Each villus contains an arteriole and a venule, and also a blind-ending lymphatic vessel called a lacteal. The arteriole and venule do not anastomose in the small intestine as they do in the gastric mucosa. Small molecules absorbed through the villus pass into the descending loop of the villus capillary and diffuse into the ascending vessel. This creates a counter-current exchange system in each villus, which is relatively inefficient since it decreases the concentration gradient for passive diffusion. The efficiency of this process has been estimated to be around 15% and has the net effect of slowing the rate of absorption.

Microvilli

Each enterocyte has about 1000 minute processes or microvilli which project into the intestinal lumen. Multiple actin filaments extending into the interior of each microvillus are believed to be responsible for contraction of the microvilli and thus the movement of the fluid immediately in contact with the surface.

The membrane which forms the microvilli on the outer surface of the absorptive cells is rich in protein, cholesterol and glycolipids and contains enzymes, disaccharidases and peptidases which are localised within the surface membrane. Specific receptor proteins are located on the microvillus membrane-surface coat complex which selectively bind substances prior to their absorption, including the intrinsic factor-vitamin B_{12} complex in the ileum and conjugated bile salts in the distal intestine.

Epithelium

The epithelium which covers the intestinal villi is composed of absorptive cells, goblet cells, a few endocrine cells and tuft or calveolated cells. The goblet and endocrine cells closely resemble those found in the crypts. The tuft or calveolated cells are characterized by long, broad apical microvilli and an intra-cytoplasmic system of tubules and vesicles.

These cells are uncommon and their function is not known. The absorptive cells or enterocytes are tall, columnar cells, with their nuclei located close to their base.

Crypts of Lieberkühn

The cells between the villi form the germinal area known as the crypts of Lieberkühn. The main functions of the crypts are cell renewal and water, ion, exocrine and endocrine secretion. The crypt epithelium consists of at least 4 different cell types:

a) the Paneth cells which secrete large amounts of protein-rich materials, and in the rat are known to phagocytose selected protozoa and bacteria. Human Paneth cells contain lysozyme, IgA and IgG.

b) goblet cells which secrete mucus. These cells are able to tolerate a higher osmotic stress than the enterocytes and are more firmly attached to the basement membrane. Exposure to toxins or hypertonic vehicles leads to accumulation of goblet cells at the apex of the villus, goblet cell capping, and a hypersecretion of mucus presumably as a protective response[1].

c) undifferentiated cells, the most common type, whose major function is in the renewal process of the epithelium. Cells in the enterocyte lineage divide several more times as they migrate up the crypts. As they migrate onto the villi, they will differentiate further into the mature absorptive cells that express all the transport proteins and enzymes characteristic of those cells.

d) endocrine cells which produce hormones and peptides such as gastrin, secretin, cholecystokinin, somatostatin, enteroglucagon, motilin, neurotensin, gastric inhibitory peptide, vasoactive peptide and serotonin.

Stem cells in the crypts divide to form daughter cells. One daughter cell from each stem cell division is retained as a stem cell. The other becomes committed to differentiate along one of the four pathways mentioned above.

The volume of intestinal secretions formed by the cells in the crypts is around 1800 ml per day and is almost pure extracellular fluid, with a pH of between 7.5 and 8.0. The fluid is rapidly absorbed by the villi and provides the watery vehicle required for the absorption of substances from chyme.

The gastrointestinal circulation

The gastrointestinal circulation is the largest systemic regional vasculature and nearly one third of the cardiac output flows through the gastrointestinal viscera, with 10% (500 ml min^{-1}) supplying the small intestine. Each anatomical region (salivary glands, pharynx, oesophagus, stomach, liver and intestine) possesses separate blood vessels. The blood vessels of the jejunum and ileum are derived from the superior mesenteric artery. Arterioles branch off and supply the muscular coat and form plexuses in the submucosal layer. From each plexus, tiny vessels direct blood to the villi and the glands in the mucosa.

The distribution of the blood flow varies according to the metabolic demands of the cells within each region. The highly metabolic villi receive 60% of the blood flow to the mucous layer, while the muscle layer with its lower demand for oxygen receives only 20% of the blood flow. During periods of enhanced absorption or electrolyte secretion, the blood flow is preferentially distributed to the mucosa, whilst increased intestinal motility causes diversion of the blood flow to the muscle layers. After a meal, blood flow increases by 30 to 130% of basal flow and the hyperaemia is confined to the segment of the intestine exposed to the chyme. Long chain fatty acids and glucose are the major stimuli for hyperaemia, which is probably mediated by hormones such as cholecystokinin released from mucosal endocrine cells[2].

The blood from the small intestine flows into the large hepatic portal vein which takes the blood directly to the liver. The liver has the highest drug metabolising capacity in the body and, in a single pass, can remove a large proportion of the absorbed drug before it reaches the systemic circulation. This process, termed first-pass metabolism, may have a significant effect on drug bioavailability when formulations are given by the oral route. The blood supply from the buccal cavity and the anal sphincter do not drain to the portal vein, and a greater proportion of a drug with a high hepatic extraction may be absorbed from these regions.

The lymphatic system

The lymphatic system is important in the absorption of nutrients, especially fat, from the gastrointestinal tract and provides a route by which electrolytes, protein and fluids can be returned from the interstitial spaces to the blood. It is also responsible for removal of red blood cells lost into tissues as a result of haemorrhage or bacteria which may have invaded tissues.

Structure of the lymphatics

The gastrointestinal tract is richly supplied with lymphatic vessels. Lymphatic vessels are lined by flattened endothelium with an incomplete basement membrane. Smooth muscle and connective tissue also surround the larger lymph vessels. The contractile activity of lymphatic vessels is most likely to be related to the amount of associated smooth muscle. The valves found in the larger vessels assist with the propulsion of lymph.

In the oesophagus, stomach and intestine, there is a plexus of lymph vessels present in the mucosal, submucosal and muscular layers with short vessels linking the networks together, and passing through lymph nodes which act as filters for lymph directed into larger vessels. The major lymphatic trunks are found on the left side of the body with the bulk of the lymph entering the circulation at the left jugulo-sub-clavian tap which is located at the base of the neck.

The lymphatic vessels of the small intestine are called the lacteals. The central lymphatic vessel is a blind-ending tube. The walls consist of a single layer of thin endothelium and resemble blood capillaries, however the small fenestrations seen in the blood vessel walls are not found in the lymphatics. The intestinal villi rhythmically contract and relax which probably serves to pump lymph into the lacteals of the submucosa. The flow of lymph in the thoracic duct is about 1-2 ml min^{-1} between meals but this can increase by 5 to 10 fold during absorption and digestion of a meal.

In addition to its main function of absorption, the gastrointestinal tract is a lymphoid organ. The lymphoid tissue is referred to as the gut-associated lymphoid tissue or GALT. The number of lymphocytes in the GALT is roughly equivalent to those in the spleen.

Lymphatic tissue can be seen in certain areas of the gastrointestinal tract close to epithelial surfaces, or as large aggregates e.g. pharyngeal tonsils and Peyer's patches in the ileum. Peyer's patches are lymphoid follicles located in the mucosa and extending into the submucosa of the small intestine, especially the ileum. Peyer's patches are usually situated on the ante-mesenteric border. Each patch typically comprises 40 to 50 nodules which are separated from the gut lumen by a layer of epithelial cells, the M-cells or microfold cells. There is a thin layer of vascularised connective tissue between the nodules and the serosa. The patches have their own blood supply. M-cells lack fully developed microvilli, are pinocytic and contain numerous vesicles. These cells may play an essential role in the intestinal immune response since they transport macromolecules and therefore have a specific role in antigen uptake. At this point in the intestine the mucosal barrier may be breached by pathogens. M cells do not digest proteins, but transport them into the underlying tissue, where they are taken up by macrophages. The macrophages which receive antigens from M cells present them to T cells in the GALT, leading ultimately to appearance of immunoglobulin A-secreting plasma cells in the mucosa. The secretory immunoglobulin A is transported through the epithelial cells into the lumen, where, for example, it interferes with adhesion and invasion of bacteria.

In adults, B lymphocytes predominate in Peyer's patches. Smaller lymphoid nodules can be found throughout the intestinal tract. Lamina propria lymphocytes are lymphocytes scattered in the lamina propria of the mucosa. A majority of these cells are IgA-secreting B cells. Intraepithelial lymphocytes are lymphocytes positioned in the basolateral spaces between luminal epithelial cells, beneath the tight junctions. These are inside the epithelium, not inside epithelial cells as the name may suggest.

Formation of lymph

Lymph is a component of the extracellular fluid of the body and is largely derived from fluid and solute filtered from the blood circulation across the capillary wall. A mixture of hydrostatic forces and osmotic pressure controls the fluid content of the blood. The high pressure within the arteriolar capillaries forces plasma into the intercellular spaces, the majority of which is returned to the bloodstream at the venous end of the capillary. The volume and solute concentration of the filtrate is modified by passage through the tissues and the lymphatic vessel endothelium before becoming lymph. About 10% of the fluid flowing from the arterial capillaries is absorbed by the lymphatic capillaries and returns to the bloodstream through the lymphatic system.

The sparse and incomplete basement membrane of the endothelium of small lymphatics is a weak barrier to the passage of solutes, fluids and large particles. In addition, the intercellular adhesion is poor and hence large particulates and even cells can occasionally pass between them. Specific vesicular transport may also be an important route of entry.

Composition of lymph

All plasma proteins are found in lymph. The protein concentration of lymph from all parts of the alimentary tract tends to be high; e.g. thoracic duct lymph has a protein concentration of 66% of that of serum. Lymph contains relatively less of the larger proteins compared to plasma, suggesting that molecular size is important in lymph filtration. Materials with a molecular weight of less than 10,000 are found in similar concentrations in both lymph and plasma. Additional proteins, mainly immunoglobulins, are added to the lymph on passage through the lymph nodes. Finally, lymph also contains reticulo-endothelial cells (lymphocytes) to destroy bacteria.

Lymph contains all the coagulation factors found in the blood, but it clots less readily. The electrolyte composition is very similar. Cholesterol and phospholipids in lymph are mainly associated with protein as lipoprotein, and together with triglycerides synthesised in the enterocytes form submicrometre droplets known as chylomicrons. This renders the triglycerides water-miscible. The concentration of chylomicrons varies with the amount of protein present in the lymph. The amount of neutral fat in the chylomicrons depends upon the degree of absorption from the gastrointestinal tract. Immediately after meals there are large quantities of lipoproteins and fats in the lymph which have been taken up from the gastrointestinal tract, but this drops to a low level between meals.

Stimulation of lymphatic transport

Many substances given by mouth increase the flow of lymph e.g. olive oil and corn oil[3-5]. In rats, lymph flow is enhanced after intragastric administration of substances such as water, 0.9% sodium chloride, 10% serum albumin or 10% glucose[6]. Of these, sodium chloride is a particularly potent lymphagogue, and some workers use an intragastric infusion of this solution to maintain a good mesenteric lymph flow in a period immediately after creating a lymph fistula.

Secretions into the small intestine

Glands

Two types of glands are found in the small intestine.

1. Brunner's glands which are confined to the duodenum and secrete bicarbonate and mucus.

2. The intestinal cells which are present throughout the small intestine and secrete mucus and a few enzymes.

The intestinal juice or succus entericus produced by the intestinal glands has an electrolyte composition similar to that of extracellular fluid. It has a pH of 7.5 to 8.0. The only enzyme of importance in the succus entericus is enteropeptidase (enterokinase) derived from the microvillous membrane, which converts trypsinogen to trypsin.

Pancreatic secretion

The human pancreas is a large gland, often more than 20 cm long, which secretes approximately 1 litre of pancreatic juice per day. The pancreatic juice has two major components: (i) alkaline fluid and (ii) enzymes. At all rates of secretion pancreatic juice is isotonic with extracellular fluid. The pancreatic acinar cells synthesize and secrete the majority of the enzymes which digest food. All the pancreatic proteases are secreted as inactive enzyme precursors and are converted to the active form in the lumen, whereas pancreatic amylase and lipase are secreted in active forms. The secretion of the aqueous phase and the bicarbonate component is largely regulated by the pH of the chyme delivered into the small intestine from the stomach. The secretion of pancreatic enzymes is primarily regulated by the amount of fat and protein entering the duodenum.

Biliary secretion

The liver secretes bile which is necessary for the digestion and absorption of lipids. All hepatic cells continually form a small amount of bile which is secreted into bile canaliculi. It is stored and concentrated in the gall bladder in man. Approximately 600 ml of hepatic bile is produced per day, but within 4 hours, up to 90% of the water present in the hepatic bile can be removed by the gall bladder. Concentration takes place by removal of sodium ions, and chloride and water then follow passively.

Bile is a variable and complex mixture of water, organic and inorganic solutes. The major organic solutes are bile acids, phospholipids (particularly lecithin), cholesterol and bilirubin. Sodium and potassium ions are found in proportions similar to that found in plasma whilst the concentrations of Cl^- and HCO_3^- are often lower and the bile acids make up the remainder of the ion balance. The bile acids are derivatives of cholesterol in which hydroxyl and carboxylic acid groups are attached to the steroid nucleus, converting it into a powerful natural surfactant. The major pigment of bile is bilirubin. Its formation is of considerable biological significance as it is the most important means by which haem, produced by the breakdown of haemoglobin, is eliminated. Up to 20% of the bilirubin present in bile is produced from other resources such as myoglobin and cytochromes.

Bile salts have two important actions:

(i) emulsification of the fat content of food, producing small droplets of fat in aqueous suspension.

(ii) assisting in the absorption of fatty acids, monoglycerides, cholesterol and other lipids from the intestinal tract by forming submicron clusters of fat and surfactant called mixed micelles.

Brief periodic bursts of bile flow occur under fasting conditions, coincident with the passage of phase 3 of the migrating motor complex (MMC) through the duodenum. When a meal is ingested, the gall bladder contracts and the bile salts are secreted into the duodenum where they can emulsify dietary fat. Bile acids are poorly absorbed in the proximal small intestine, unlike the majority of nutrients, but are absorbed by an active process in the terminal ileum. After absorption, bile acids have a high hepatic clearance and are also re-secreted in the bile. This process is known as enterohepatic recirculation.

Secretion and absorption of water

An adult human takes in roughly 1 to 2 litres of dietary fluid every day. In addition, another 6 to 7 litres of fluid is received by the small intestine as secretions from salivary glands, stomach, pancreas, liver and the small intestine itself. By the time the ingesta enters the large intestine, approximately 80% of this fluid has been absorbed. The absorption of water is absolutely dependent on absorption of solutes, particularly sodium.

Within the intestine, there is a proximal to distal gradient in osmotic permeability. Further down the small intestine, the effective pore size through the epithelium decreases, hence the duodenum is much more "leaky" to water than the ileum and the ileum more leaky than the colon. However, the ability to absorb water does not decrease, but water flows across the epithelium more freely in the proximal compared to distal gut because the effective pore size is larger. The distal intestine actually can absorb water better than the proximal gut. The observed difference in permeability to water across the epithelium is due almost entirely to differences in conductivity across the paracellular path as the tight junctions vary considerably in "tightness" along the length of the gut.

Regardless of whether water is being secreted or absorbed, it flows across the mucosa in response to osmotic gradients. In the case of secretion, two distinct processes establish an osmotic gradient that pulls water into the lumen of the intestine. Firstly, the increases in luminal osmotic pressure resulting from influx and digestion of food cause water to be drawn into the lumen. Chyme when passed into the small intestine from the stomach is slightly hyperosmotic, but as its macromolecular components are digested, osmolarity of that solution increases dramatically. For example, starch which is a large molecule, will only contribute a small amount to osmotic pressure when intact. As it is digested, thousands of molecules of maltose are generated, each of which is as osmotically active as the parent molecule. Thus, as digestion proceeds the osmolarity of the chyme increases dramatically and water is pulled into the lumen. Then, as the osmotically active molecules are absorbed, osmolarity of the intestinal contents decreases and water is then reabsorbed.

Secondly, crypt cells actively secrete electrolytes, which leads to water secretion. The apical or luminal membrane of crypt epithelial cells contain a cyclic AMP-dependent chloride channel known also as the cystic fibrosis transmembrane conductance regulator or CFTR because mutations in the gene for this ion channel result in the disease cystic fibrosis. This channel is responsible for secretion of water. Elevated intracellular concentrations of cAMP in crypt cells activate the channel which results in secretion of chloride ions into the lumen. The increase in concentration of negatively-charged chloride anions in the crypt creates an electrical potential which attracts sodium, pulling it into the lumen across the tight junctions. The net result is secretion of sodium chloride into the crypt which creates an osmotic gradient across the tight junction, hence water is drawn into the lumen. Abnormal activation of the cAMP-dependent chloride channel in crypt cells has resulted in the deaths of millions of people. Several types of bacteria produce toxins, the best known of which is the cholera toxin, that strongly and often permanently activate the adenylate cyclase in crypt enterocytes. This leads to elevated levels of cAMP, causing the chloride channels to essentially become stuck in the "open" position. The result is massive secretion of water which produces the classic symptom of severe watery diarrhoea.

The most important process which occurs in the small intestine which makes absorption possible is maintenance of an electrochemical gradient of sodium across the epithelial cell boundary of the lumen. To remain viable, all cells are required to maintain a low intracellular concentration of sodium. In polarized epithelial cells like enterocytes, a low intracellular sodium concentration is maintained by a large number of sodium pumps or Na^+/K^+ ATPases embedded in the basolateral membrane. These pumps export 3 sodium ions from the cell in exchange for 2 potassium ions, thus establishing a gradient of both charge and sodium concentration across the basolateral membrane. In rats, there are about 150,000 sodium pumps per small intestinal enterocyte, which allows each cell to transport about 4.5 billion sodium ions out of each cell per minute[7]. This flow and accumulation of sodium is ultimately responsible for absorption of water, amino acids and carbohydrates. The transport of water from lumen to blood often occurs against an osmotic gradient, allowing the intestine to absorb water into blood even when the osmolarity in the lumen is higher than osmolarity of blood. The proximal small intestine functions as a highly permeable mixing segment, and absorption of water is basically isotonic. That is, water is not absorbed until the ingesta has been diluted to just above the osmolarity of blood. The ileum and especially the colon are able to absorb water against an osmotic gradient of several hundred milliosmoles.

Digestion and absorption of nutrients

Food assimilation takes place primarily in the small intestine and it is optimized by the increased surface area produced by Kerckring's folds, villi and microvilli. The chyme presented to the duodenum from the stomach consists of a mixture of coarsely emulsified fat, protein and some metabolites produced by the action of pepsin, and carbohydrates including starch, the majority of which would have escaped the action of the salivary amylase.

The chyme is acidic and this is buffered by bile and the bicarbonate present in the pancreatic juice to between pH 6.5 and 7.6. The digestive enzymes are located in the brush border of the glycocalyx and they can be altered by changes in diet, especially by the proportion of ingested disaccharides. The protein content of the diet does not affect the proteases, but a diet deficient in protein leads to a reduction in all enzymes.

It is important to recognize that the epithelium of the gut is not a monotonous sheet of functionally identical cells. As chyme travels through the intestine, it is sequentially exposed to regions having epithelia with very different characteristics. This diversity in function results from differences in the number and type of transporter molecules expressed in the epithelial plasma membrane, and the structure of the tight junctions. Even within a given segment there are major differences in the type of transport that occurs, for example, cells in the crypts have different transporter systems than cells on the tips of villi.

Blood passing through the minute veins of the capillaries is brought into close proximity with the intestinal contents in an area estimated to be about 10 m^2. The capillaries are fenestrated, hence allowing a very rapid exchange of absorbed materials. During digestion and absorption the villi contract fairly quickly at regular intervals and relax slowly. The contraction probably serves to pump lymph into the lacteals of the submucosa and stir the intestinal contents. The veins in the villi ultimately open into the portal vein, which leads directly to the liver and hence all materials carried from the small intestine undergo "first-pass" metabolism.

The site of absorption of the small intestine depends upon the relationship between the rate of transit and that of absorption. This is more apparent for drugs than for food, since excipients may control the rate of drug release. For example the duodenum can be demonstrated to have a high rate of absorption, however the passage through this region is extremely rapid and so the net absorption in this region is probably quite low. The function of the duodenum is to sample the chyme which is delivered from the stomach and thus regulate the delivery of the food according to its calorific value by a feedback process. Virtually all nutrients from the diet are absorbed into blood across the mucosa of the small intestine. The absorption of water and electrolytes plays a critical role in maintenance of body water and acid-base balance.

Carbohydrates

The principal dietary carbohydrates are starches, sucrose and lactose. Starch is a glucose-containing polysaccharide with a molecular weight which varies from 100,000 to more than 1 million. The two major polysaccharides of starch are amylose and amylopectin. Indigestible carbohydrates e.g. cellulose are the main constituents of dietary fibre.

Salivary and pancreatic amylases initiate the hydrolysis of starch and exhibit their optimal activity near a neutral pH. The salivary amylase is inactivated once it reaches the acid in the stomach. The intraluminal digestion of carbohydrates occurs rapidly in the duodenum due to the large amount of amylase secreted by the pancreas. The final oligosaccharide products of luminal digestion are formed before the chyme reaches the jejunum. The major products of starch digestion are maltose and maltotriose. Carbohydrates are absorbed in the proximal part of the small intestine and they have completely disappeared from the lumen by the time the meal reaches the ileum.

The disaccharides are further digested to monosaccharides by the brush border enzymes lactase, sucrase, maltase and isomaltase during their transfer across the epithelium. It is likely that the enzymes and carriers are so orientated spatially that hydrolysis and subsequent absorption are sequential events. Both passive diffusion and active transport absorb glucose rapidly and completely. The brush border possesses a sodium-dependent carrier which transports sugars across the membrane in either direction.

Proteins

Most protein digestion occurs principally in the small intestine under the influence of the proteolytic enzymes of the pancreatic secretion. When the proteins leave the stomach they are mainly in the form of large polypeptides. Immediately upon entering the small intestine, the partial breakdown products are attacked by the pancreatic enzymes. Trypsin and chymotrypsin split protein molecules into small polypeptides, carboxypolypeptidase then cleaves individual amino acids from the carboxyl ends of the polypeptides. The brush border of the small intestine contains several different enzymes for hydrolysing the remaining small peptides. The constituent amino acids are then absorbed. Most naturally occurring amino acids are L-isomers which are transported against concentration gradients by sodium-dependent carrier mechanisms. There are four carrier systems for amino acids: for neutral amino acids (histidine), for basic amino acids (lysine), for dicarboxylic acids (glutamic acid) and a fourth transports the amino acids proline, hydroxyproline and glycine.

Enterocytes do not have transporters to carry proteins across the plasma membrane and proteins cannot permeate tight junctions. However, studies suggest that very small amounts of proteins may be absorbed intact. In most instances, the extent of this absorption is small and nutritionally not significant, however it can result in immune reactions, hormonal or toxic effects. This is most clearly seen in neonates. This enhanced ability, which is rapidly lost, is of immense importance because it allows the newborn babies to acquire passive immunity by absorbing immunoglobulins from colostral milk.

Fats

Dietary intake of lipid is mainly in the form of triglycerides which are composed of a glycerol chain and three fatty acids. There are also small quantities of cholesterol,

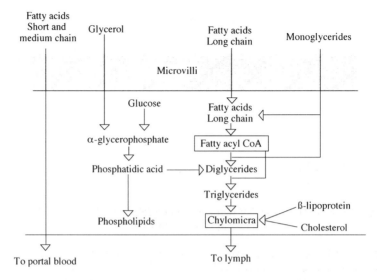

Figure 6.4 Metabolism and transport of fat into the lymphatic and systemic circulation

phospholipids and cholesterol esters in chyme. Fat is emulsified by the bile salts into small droplets which disperse in water allowing access of digestive enzymes.

Lipase in the pancreatic juice and enteric lipase from the epithelial cells of the small intestine both hydrolyse emulsified triglycerides to monoglycerides and fatty acids. The short and medium chain fatty acids are absorbed passively through the epithelium into the blood. The long chain fatty acids and monoglycerides remain as mixed micelles with the bile salts and are internalized by the epithelium. They are reassembled into triglycerides within the cell and excreted into the lymph as small (0.1 μm) droplets called chylomicra (or chylomicrons) (Figure 6.4).

Iron

Heme iron is absorbed from meat more efficiently than dietary inorganic iron and in a different manner[8]. Thus, iron deficiency is less frequent in countries where meat constitutes a significant part of the diet. Proteolytic digestion of myoglobin and hemoglobin results in the release of heme, which is maintained in a soluble form by globin degradation products so that it remains available for absorption. Heme enters the small intestinal absorptive cell as an intact metalloporphyrin. This may be facilitated by a vesicular transport system[9]. In the absorptive cell the porphyrin ring is split by heme oxygenase. The released inorganic iron becomes associated with mobilferrin and paraferritin, which acts as a ferrireductase to make iron available for production of iron-containing end products such as heme proteins. Mucosal transfer of iron into the body occurs competitively with dietary iron that enters the absorptive cell as inorganic iron, because they both share a common pathway within the intestinal cell. Dietary inorganic iron as the ferric iron is solubilized at the acid pH level of the stomach where it chelates mucins and certain dietary constituents to keep them soluble and available for absorption in the more alkaline duodenum.

PATTERNS OF MOTILITY IN THE SMALL INTESTINE

The small intestine, like the stomach, displays two distinct patterns of motility. The fed pattern is characterized by random motor activity, in groups of 1 to 3 sequential contractions, separated by 5 to 40 seconds of inactivity. The physical and chemical nature of the

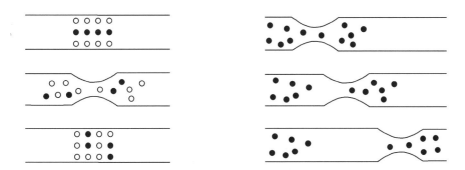

*Figure 6.5 Segmental contractions (left) and propulsive contractions (right)
of the small intestine*

food determines the number of contractions; for example, twice as many contractions occur when solid food is ingested than when an equicalorific liquid is consumed[2]. Carbohydrates stimulate the largest number of contractions, followed by proteins and lipids. The fed pattern of motility consists of segmental and peristaltic contractions, the segmental contractions being the most frequent (Figure 6.5). Initially a segment of the bowel, less than 2 cm in length, contracts while the adjacent segments are relaxed; the procedure is then reversed, as the contracted segment relaxes and vice versa. This type of motility mixes chyme by continually moving it in the lumen and increasing contact with the absorbing surface, but since there are less frequent contractions aborally than orally, there is a net movement of chyme towards the large bowel. This movement is enhanced by peristaltic contractions which occur less frequently than segmental contractions, and each move the chyme a few centimetres. The continuous movement shears the chyme resulting in effective mixing (Figure 6.6).

The interdigestive migrating myoelectric complex (Chapter 5) continues from the stomach to the small intestine. Phase I is a period of no activity, Phase II is characterized by random activity and Phase III is a period of intense activity which is associated with the aboral movement of the intestinal contents. The migrating myoelectric complex occurs every 140 to 150 minutes, and as one complex reaches the ileum, another starts at the duodenum. The velocity of the contractile wave decreases as it approaches the ileum and only rarely does it reach the terminal ileum[10].

Motility in the small intestine, as in all parts of the digestive tube, is controlled predominantly by excitatory and inhibitory signals from the enteric nervous system. These local nervous signals are modulated by inputs from the central nervous system, and to some degree by a number of gastrointestinal hormones.

Stagnation at the ileocaecal junction

The ileocaecal junction divides the terminal small intestine from the caecum. The junction or sphincter appears to formed by papillary protrusions into the lumen of the caecum, rather than two flat lips of a valve[11]. Its function seems to be to retain chyme in the small intestine until digestion is largely complete and then to empty its contents into the large bowel. The ileocaecal junction also serves to prevent the spread of the colonic bacteria into the small intestine[12]. Contraction of the ileocolonic sphincter is produced by a-adrenergic agonists including phenylephrine, adrenaline and noradrenaline, and by cholin-

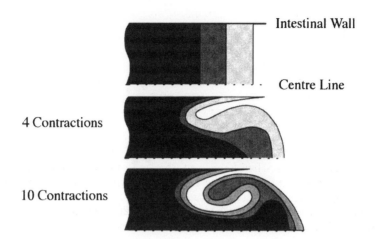

Figure 6.6 Laminar mixing produced by repetitive longitudinal contractions

ergic agonists such as bethanechol, whereas pure b-adrenergic agonists, such as isoprenaline, cause relaxation[13].

Scintigraphy often demonstrates accumulation or bunching of material at the ileocaecal junction, followed by spreading of material through the ascending colon[14]. Non-disintegrating matrices may remain at this location for some hours[15].

SMALL INTESTINAL TRANSIT TIMES
Methods for measuring small intestinal transit

There are several methods available for the measurement of small intestinal transit. The hydrogen breath test relies on metabolism of certain carbohydrates, e.g. lactulose, by microbial flora within the large bowel. The carbohydrate must be one which is not absorbed from the small intestine. The gas generated is detected in the expired air. Using this technique, it is possible to estimate the sum of gastric emptying and small intestinal transit times. This test assumes that the unabsorbed carbohydrate encounters fermentative bacteria only in the colon, however bacterial overgrowth into the small intestine will give erroneously short transit times.

Two-dimensional gamma scintigraphy can be used to measure stomach to caecum transit times, but cannot be used to measure the distance travelled by a unit through segments of the small intestine since it is highly coiled. Transit time through segments of the small intestine has been measured using a perspex capsule containing technetium-99m labelled 'Amberlite' resin[16]. External markers were placed on the front, back and sides of volunteers who were then imaged from the front, back and side. This enabled the three-dimensional movement of the capsule through the small intestine to be reconstructed and an estimate to be made of the velocity of the unit. After transit through the duodenum, which was too fast to be accurately measured, the capsule moved through the small intestine at between 4.2 and 5.6 cm per minute. There was no difference in transit times for two capsules with different specific gravities (1.0 and 1.6). The transit rate is in close agreement with the velocity of the migrating myoelectric potential down the small intestine (4.7 cm. min^{-1})[17] and that of 1 to 4 cm per minute for chyme[2].

Many older textbooks quote small intestinal transit times based on barium X-ray contrast measurements, but barium is not a good model of the intestinal contents. Measurements of transit from patients with some form of organic disease, such as those with ileos-tomies, should also be treated with caution.

Small intestinal transit times of food

A combination of scintigraphic, x-ray contrast and hydrogen breath techniques to follow the transit of a meal of sausages, baked beans and mashed potato showed that the residues left the small intestine between 2 and 12 hours after ingestion. This suggests that differential transit of meal components occurs[17 18]. There is however some controversy in the literature on this point, since another study failed to find a difference in the small intestinal transit time of the components of a mixed meal of cheese, biscuits, bran and water containing separately radiolabelled liquid and fibre[19]. In this experiment, differences in mouth-to-caecum time of the two labelled components were entirely explained by differences in rates of gastric emptying. A mean small intestinal transit time for a liquid test meal has been reported to be approximately 1.25 h[20]. Further intake of food appears to have little effect on the transit of material already in the small intestine[21].

Physiological and pathophysiological effects on small bowel transit

It has been reported that severe exercise delays the gastric emptying of food whereas moderate exercise accelerates it. In spite of these findings, exercise has little effect on the small intestinal transit of pellets given to fasted individuals[22]. Larger objects such as radio-opaque markers showed a marked reduction in whole gut transit time following moderate exercise (jogging and cycling)[23].

In cases of accelerated gastrointestinal transit, administration of a drug in a controlled release formulation instead of a conventional formulation may cause a higher fraction of the dose to escape absorption in the small intestine and enter the colon. This can reduce the availability of the drug either because of slow and erratic absorption or because of inactivation by colonic bacteria (Table 6.1). In contrast, diseases that retard small bowel transit could increase the bioavailability of drugs that are released slowly from controlled-release forms; however, conditions that encourage the overgrowth of bacteria in the small intestine could reduce the bioavailability of drugs susceptible to bacterial degradation (e.g. digoxin).

In patients with partial intestinal obstruction or a narrowed lumen, a single unit may lodge in the gut and expose the intestinal mucosa to high concentrations of drug which may lead to gastric irritation, bleeding, and even perforation[24-26]. For patients with this disease, multiparticulate formulations provide an advantage, because even if pellets lodged within the gut, they would do so over a wide area as they are well dispersed. In addition, each

Table 6.1 Disease causing accelerated and decreased small intestinal transit times (SITT)

Faster SITT	Slower SITT
Secretory diarrhoea	Constipation
Thyrotoxicosis	Myxoedema
Irritable bowel syndrome	Pseudo-obstruction
Chronic pancreatitis	Ileal resection
	Partial gastrectomy
	Jejuno-ileal bypass
	Autonomic neuropathy

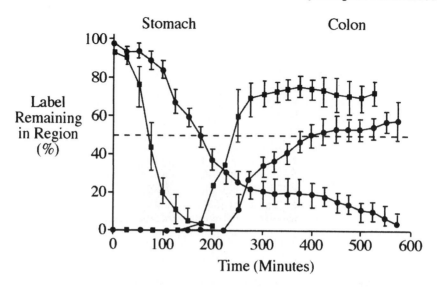

Figure 6.7 Effect of light (■) and heavy breakfast (●) on the gastric emptying and colon arrival of a co-administered multiparticulate formulation

pellet only contains a small fraction of the total dose administered so local concentrations of the drug would be small thus reducing mucosal damage.

Castor oil is believed to decrease the activity of the circular smooth muscle which is thought to produce an increase in intestinal transit. The mechanism by which castor oil produces its effect on the gut could involve inhibition of Na^+, K^+-ATPase, activation of adenylate cyclase, stimulation of prostaglandins and nitric oxide biosynthesis. Castor oil also changes the intestinal permeability and causes histological abnormalities.

Small intestinal transit time of dosage forms

During fasting, both monolithic and multiparticulate dosage forms will be swept rapidly through the small bowel by the migrating myoelectric complex. The action is propulsive and not mixing in nature, thus a capsule containing pellets given on an empty stomach may leave the stomach and pass down the small intestine as a bolus with minimal dispersal[27]. The increased dispersal of pelleted formulations within the small intestine when the formulations are taken with a meal occurs because the pellets become dispersed in the food mass within the stomach[28 29]. As their particle size is small, pellets will continue to be emptied from the stomach as part of the chyme, thus prolonging their delivery to the small intestine (Figure 6.7). Monolithic tablets, on the other hand, depending upon their size, will empty erratically from the stomach after food and as the single unit traverses the small bowel. Hence, the presentation of the drug to the small intestinal mucosa will depend solely upon its dissolution characteristics in each area. The degree of spread of a formulation within the small intestine is particularly important for drugs with poor solubility or for drugs which are slowly transported across the epithelium. Microparticulate dosage forms show longer and more reproducible median transit times compared with single unit tablets[30], giving rise to more predictable and uniform blood levels and reducing the risk of enlodgement and mucosal damage.

A review of data suggests that the small intestinal transit is around 4 hours for solutions, pellets and single unit formulations (Figure 6.8)[31]. Small intestinal transit of dosage

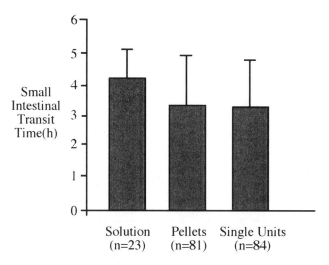

Figure 6.8 Small intestinal transit times of various dosage forms

forms is not affected by their physical state, size or the presence or absence of food, but high calorific loads may slow it slightly although the majority of the effect is on gastric emptying (Figure 6.9)[32]. Small intestinal transit time is remarkably resistant to pharmaceutical intervention and in man physical properties such as shape, density or putative bioadhesive properties are without significant effect on transit. In a study of the spread of controlled-release isosorbide-5-dinitrate within the gastrointestinal tract[33] (Figure 6.10), a deconvolution technique was used to calculate the drug absorption profile, and revealed that isosorbide-5-nitrate was well absorbed from the preparation whilst the pellets resided in the stomach and small intestine. However, absorption was reduced when the preparation entered the colon, hence the absorption window based on an average mouth-caecum transit time (6 - 8 hours) represents the maximum acceptable time for drug release from this oral controlled-release preparation. These studies suggest that if matrix tablets are designed to release their con-

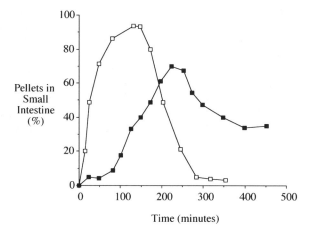

Figure 6.9 Delivery of multiparticulates from the stomach to the small intestine in fasted volunteers (□) after a heavy breakfast (■)

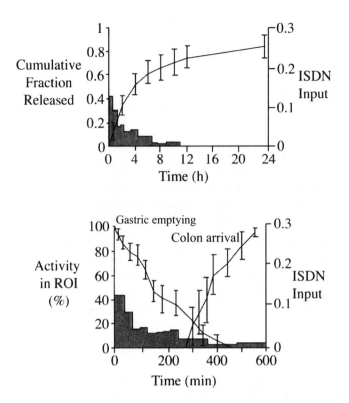

Figure 6.10 Gastrointestinal transit and absorption of isosorbide-5-dinitrate from controlled release pellets using combined gamma scintigraphy and blood sampling (ROI = region of interest)

tents over 12 h then colonic absorption of the drug is necessary and the drug must not be degraded by colonic bacteria.

Large amounts of unabsorbable carbohydrate or a large amount of fluid accelerates transit through the small bowel, and could therefore reduce the degree of absorption from a controlled-release formulation taken with the meal[34]. This principle has been used as the basis for a sustained release tablet containing riboflavin and myristyl tripalmitate[35]. Increasing the viscosity of the luminal contents by ingesting viscous polysaccharides such as guar gum or pectin will also prolong small bowel transit time, and may therefore increase the degree of absorption from slowly released or slowly absorbed drugs[36]. For example, the absorption of riboflavin is enhanced after being mixed with a viscous sodium alginate solution[37].

The prolonged mouth-to-caecum transit may explain why the recovery of hydrochlorthiazide in the urine is greater when a controlled-release formulation of the drug is given with food than when given to fasted subjects[38]. Controlled-release lithium preparations are thought to cause diarrhoea by an action on ion transport in the ileum but this does not occur when they are taken with food[39]. This may also be due to enhanced absorption of the drug in the upper part of the small intestine, which occurs with a more prolonged transit in this region produced by the food, thus reducing the amount of lithium reaching the ileum to induce diarrhoea.

Scintigraphy often demonstrates accumulation or bunching of material at the ileocaecal junction. Non-disintegrating matrices may remain at this location for some time[15] [40]. The stagnation at the ileocaecal junction may also cause problems for controlled-release dosage forms which are designed to release drug over a period of 9 to 12 hours, since the concentration of drug could build up within this localized area. This will have no effect on the absorption of most drugs, providing that the rate at which the drug is released from the dosage form is slower than the rate of uptake across the ileal epithelium, and the drug is not degraded by ileal bacteria.

Density and small intestinal transit

Early studies indicated that pellet density affected small intestinal transit in ileostomy patients[41], although subsequent studies were unable to confirm this finding in normal subjects[16 42]. A further scintigraphic study eventually confirmed that small intestinal transit in patients with ileostomies was not affected by density in the range 0.94 to 1.96 g cm^{-3} (Figure 6.11)[43]. Standard sized units (1.18-1.40 mm) of density 1.5, 2.0 and 2.4 g cm^{-3} administered to healthy volunteers all had similar small intestinal transit times[44].

Small particles with densities close to that of a meal will be emptied continuously with the meal[21 45]. This means that, for a well designed enteric coated multiparticulate formulation, there is little delay in the onset of plasma levels even when the drug is given with food. As has been discussed previously, buoyant materials and ultra-dense materials do show a slowed gastric emptying. This of course will affect the time course for which they are presented to the small intestine.

ABSORPTION OF DRUGS

The permeability of the epithelium to small ions and water-soluble organic molecules is greater in the duodenum and jejunum than it is in the ileum, which would indicate that there are larger and more numerous water-filled channels high in the small bowel. The variation in absorptive capacity can also, in part, be explained by the higher surface area per unit length in the upper intestine compared with the lower part. A few studies have been carried out to compare the absorption of drugs in the upper and lower small intestine. Human perfusion studies have demonstrated a proximal-to-distal small intestinal absorption

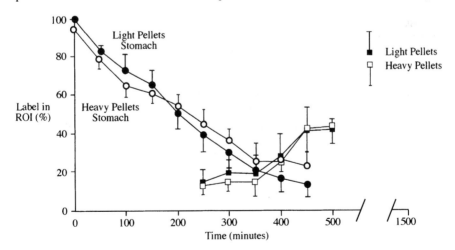

Figure 6.11 The transit of light and heavy pellets in ileostomy patients measured by gamma scintigraphy (ROI = region of interest)

gradient for hydrocortisone but not for triamcinolone[46]. Digoxin[47] and hydrochlorthiazide[38] have also been shown to be absorbed predominantly from the duodenum and upper jejunum. Although there is excellent absorption from the duodenum, transit through this area is extremely rapid, in the order of seconds[16] and hence the actual amount of drug absorbed from this region will be small.

Cell monolayers formed from the human colon cancer cell line Caco-2 have been widely used to study the absorption of drugs[48]. Caco-2 cells form confluent and polarized monolayers when maintained in culture and differentiate towards the mature small bowel enterocyte phenotype. Caco-2 cell monolayers mimic intestinal absorptive epithelium and represent a very useful tool for studying transepithelial drug transport. However, some enzymes and transport systems are expressed to a lesser extent in Caco-2 cells compared to normal enterocytes[49]. Caco-2 cells also express various cytochrome P450 isoforms and phase II enzymes such as UDP-glucuronosyltransferases, sulphotransferases and glutathione-S-transferases, and hence they have been used study presystemic drug metabolism[50].

Specific carriers for the transport of riboflavin and iron are found principally in the duodenum and jejunum, whereas carriers for bile acid and vitamin B_{12} are found mainly in the ileum. The acid microclimate is less obvious in the ileum, favouring the absorption of weak bases while discouraging the absorption of weak acids. Finally, the ileum contains more commensal bacteria than the duodenum and jejunum. In elderly subjects, the bacterial population in the ileum may be high enough to metabolize certain drugs thereby reducing their efficacy.

Absorption and delivery of macromolecules

It is generally accepted that macromolecules, particularly food proteins, do cross the mature small intestinal epithelium in small amounts and reach the systemic circulation. The potential as delivery route for orally administered macromolecular drugs including proteins is being widely explored[51]. There have been several studies on the mechanism and substrate structure-affinity relationship for this transport system. Rapid progress has been made recently in studies on the molecular basis of the intestinal peptide transport system. A protein apparently involved in peptide transport has been isolated from rabbit small intestine, and genes for human intestinal peptide transporters have been cloned, sequenced and functionally expressed[52]. The cellular uptake of small peptides such as di-, tri- and tetrapeptides and peptidomimetic drugs proceeds via specialized proton-coupled transporters[53]. The proton-dependent uptake at the apical cell membrane of the enterocytes results in subsequent exit of intact di- or tri-peptides across the basolateral membrane or, alternatively, intracellular hydrolysis and exit of component amino acids across the basolateral membrane[54]. The peptide carrier has a broad substrate specificity.

Lectins are resistant to digestion and binding to brush-border membranes, hence appreciable amounts of lectins and/or toxins of the general structure of A (toxin)-B(lectin), either free or included in liposomes, may be taken up by and transported through the epithelial cells of the small intestine. As a result tomato lectins have been explored as potential drug delivery agents[55].

Various strategies have been used to target vaccine antigens to the gut-associated lymphoid tissues, such as microspheres prepared from various polymers. Certainly in mice the size of the microspheres has to be less than 5 μm for them to be transported within macrophages through the efferent lymphatics [56]. Transcytosis through Peyer's patches is most suited for highly potent compounds since there are a limited number of Peyer's patches, hence the overall surface area is relatively small. Patch tissue is rich in lymphocytes, thus substances which interact with lymphocytes are best targeted to Peyer's patches when using the oral route[57].

It is known that a number of microorganisms are able to bind selectively to a receptor on the M-cell surface and thereby enter the host. Utilizing the microorganism's ligand could be beneficial for specific targeting to Peyer's patches, bypassing lysosomal degradation in absorptive cells. Moreover, transport of membrane-bound macromolecules by M cells is about 50 times more efficient than that of soluble, non-adherent macromolecules. The colonization of the small intestine by Escherichia coli strains is mediated by cell surface antigens called fimbriae which enable bacteria to adhere to the brush border of epithelial cells. Due to the very close contact between the epithelial cells and the bacteria an enhanced absorption of substances including peptides and proteins can occur. To use bacterial adhesion for the design of drug delivery and drug targeting systems the fimbrial antigenicity has to be reduced. One approach was to truncate the NH_2- terminal on K99-fimbrial proteins by recombinant DNA-technology[58].

Intestinal pH

A drug administered in a solid form must dissolve in gastrointestinal contents and pass out of the stomach into the small intestine. It then has to gain access to the epithelium by convection of the luminal contents and diffusion across the unstirred microclimate. Finally it must cross the epithelium either by partitioning into the lipid membrane, by passing through water-filled channels or by combining with specific membrane-bound carriers. The residence of the formulation in the small intestine has to be long enough for complete absorption to take place. The principal permeability barrier is represented by the luminal surface of the brush border. Most drugs are absorbed by passive diffusion in their unionised state. The pH of the small intestine determines the degree of ionisation and hence controls the efficiency of absorption; this is the basis of the pH-partition theory of drug absorption which was discussed in Chapter 1. Protein binding at the serosal side of the epithelium helps maintain a concentration gradient by binding the absorbed drug, which is then removed by blood flow from the absorption site.

Gastric pH has been relatively well defined since it is accessible using a Ryle's tube, but fewer studies have investigated intestinal conditions. Data obtained using pH telemetry capsules indicate that the lumen of the proximal jejunum usually lies within the pH range 5.0 to 6.5, rising slowly along the length of the small intestine to reach pH 6 to 7, although high values in the range 7 to 9 have occasionally been found[59].

Measurements using microelectrodes have shown that the pH in the mucosal fluid adjacent to the intestinal epithelium is between 4.5 and 6.0 depending on the luminal glucose concentration. This acid microclimate immediately adjacent to the intestinal epithelium contributes to the absorption of acidic drugs such as acetylsalicylic acid[60]. The majority of the drug is ionised at the pH of the intestinal contents but the molecule is less ionised immediately adjacent to the intestinal epithelium and hence absorption is rapid. Unfortunately, this hypothesis suggests that basic drugs would be poorly absorbed, which is not the case. Bases may be absorbed in an ionised form through the paracellular route, or they may interact with organic cations which have been found to be secreted from the blood into the lumen of the intestine.

Solvent drag and intestinal permeability

The intestine absorbs approximately 10 litres of water a day from the diet and digestive secretions, and only 100-200 ml of water is lost in the stools. The question of whether the water flux influences drug absorption has been raised by many authors. Rat perfusion experiments have shown that the disappearance of the drugs sulphanilamide, sulphisoxazole and metoclopramide from the lumen increases with increasing fluid absorption and decreases when the tonicity of the perfusate increases, which causes intestinal secretion[61].

In a slight variation of the technique which measured appearance of drug in the plasma, the absorption of both acidic (benzoic, salicylic) and basic drugs (amidopyrine, antipyrine) increased with increasing water absorption[62 63]. This phenomenon is known as solvent drag. It is proposed that it will affect paracellular drug absorption and may affect the absorption of small and hydrophilic drugs. In humans the intestinal steady state perfusion technique using a triple lumen tube passed into the small intestine, combined with simultaneous measurement of drug plasma concentration, has shown that transmucosal water fluxes affect the absorption of paracetamol and ranitidine[64 65].

P-glycoprotein

P-glycoprotein is an ATP-dependent transporter which is capable of transporting an extremely wide variety of drugs out of the cell. The potential role for P-glycoprotein for determining the oral bioavailability of some drugs has only recently been appreciated[66]. P-glycoprotein is expressed in a variety of normal human tissues including the liver, brain, adrenal gland, kidney and intestinal tract epithelia[67]. This suggests a common role as a protective mechanism. In the small intestine it is localised in the apical membranes of the cell, but is not detectable in crypt cells. It is composed of two blocks each containing six trans-membrane regions and a site for binding ATP on each half (Figure 6.12).

The mechanism by which such a wide range of compounds is transported is unknown, but it appears that the drug is effluxed by flipping the drug from the inner to the outer leaflet of the bilayer membrane[68]. This model is consistent with the ability of compounds to penetrate lipid and the common denominator is that the P-glycoprotein substrates are hydrophobic and amphipathic in nature. The number of drugs that can be effluxed from the cell by P-glycoprotein include the immunosuppressive agent cyclosporin A, vinca alkaloids, digoxin, ß-blockers[69], erythromycin, antibiotics and cimetidine. The molecular weight of the compounds transported varies enormously and encompasses a range between 250 to 1850 Daltons (Gramicidin D). P-glycoproteins were originally identified by their ability to transport cytotoxic drugs out of certain types of tumour cells thus conferring resistance. This mechanism appeared to work against a range of drugs and gave rise to the concept of "multi-drug resistance" (MDR).

The therapeutic potential of inactivating this receptor protein has led to the search for non-cytotoxic drugs with the ability to block transport and increase influx to the target cells.

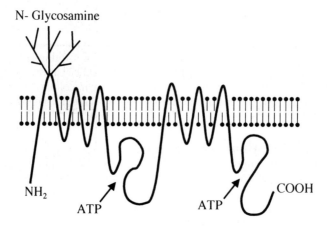

Figure 6.12 Structure of P-glycoprotein in the plasma membrane

It was soon realised that the wide diversity of compounds transported were mutual inhibitors, i.e. these compounds were also substrates for P-glycoprotein. Several of these reversal agents are now under trial in the treatment of acute myeloid leukaemia.

There is some speculation that P-glycoprotein may not prevent the complete absorption of a substrate but may simply control entry at a rate sufficient to ensure intestinal metabolism. The evidence for this is that the P-glycoprotein action appears to work in concert with cytochrome P450 3A4.

Cytochrome P450 3A4 (CYP3A4)

In the past, it was always assumed that the liver, rather than the intestine was the main guardian of the systemic circulation and that metabolism of xenobiotic compounds by the gut was functionally not so important. Although the importance of hepatic metabolism cannot be overstated, there is overwhelming evidence that the intestinal barrier provided by CYP3A4 is a major determinant of systemic bioavailability of orally administered drugs[70], for example, intestinal metabolism may account for as much as 50% of oral cyclosporine metabolism[71]. The cytochrome appears to be identical to that in hepatic cells and produces a similar pattern of Phase 1 metabolites[72].

It appears that CYP3A4 and P-glycoprotein are functionally integrated as there is a great overlap between the substrates for both systems. Secondly, the two complexes are co-localised in tips of the villus and not present in the crypts, and finally the CYP3A4 and P-glycoprotein genes appear to be close to each other on the same chromosome (Figure 6.13)[72].

The inter-relationship of P-glycoprotein and CYP3A4 operates in a complex manner. Firstly, P-glycoprotein limits the total drug transport across the membrane so that CYP3A4 in the enterocytes is not saturated. Secondly, the slowing of drug absorption by P-glycoprotein increases the duration of exposure of the drug to the CYP3A4 in the enterocyte, thus providing greater opportunity for metabolism. In addition, the metabolites generated by CYP3A4 are substrates for it. These metabolites are actively transported out of the cell by P-glycoprotein so that they do not compete with the metabolism of the parent drug.

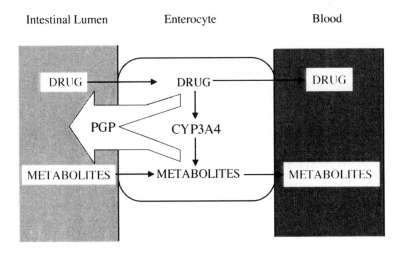

*Figure 6.13 Probable mechanism of interaction of P-glycoprotein
and cytochrome P4503A4 (CYP3A4)*

Intestinal reserve length

If the lumen of the small intestine is occluded by inflating a balloon a short distance below the pyloric sphincter, the plasma levels of glucose from a glucose drink are reduced when compared to levels obtained with free transit of the liquid[36]. Experiments of this type allowed an estimate to be made of the length of intestine required to absorb a particular material. Many nutrients are absorbed almost completely by the time the meal reaches a point 100 cm from the pylorus[73]. This formed the basis of the hypothesis that absorption of the drug from a particular formulation was completed in the upper part of the small intestine, and the remaining length was a "reserve", i.e. unused for drug absorption[74]. If the reserve length was long, this implied that the drug was rapidly absorbed.

In this model the reserve length is defined as the distance from the point at which 95% of the drug has been be absorbed (the absorption length), to the distal end of the small intestine. The drug concentration is assumed to decline continuously with distance from the pyloric sphincter as absorption takes place. If the absorption length is similar to the total intestinal length, then RL approaches zero and the drug will be completely absorbed. The choice of 95% absorption is arbitrary. This hypothesis may apply to some drugs, but it assumes that small bowel contents move down the small intestine at a relatively constant rate and that there are no differences in absorptive capacity along the gastrointestinal tract. This theory is also incorrect from a number of standpoints; there is considerable mixing in the small intestine and individual particles of food can move at independent and widely differing rates. Moreover, values for the median transit times of the same components of a meal in different subjects can show considerable variability. The liquid meals used in the earlier study contained nutrients which could be rapidly assimilated because they were in a simple and well-dispersed form. The intestinal reserve length theory would not necessarily apply to normal meals which are complex and semisolid. Analysis of the effluent from ileostomies, for example, shows that quite high proportions of ingested nutrient enter the terminal ileum. Studies in man and in experimental animals have shown that food may move more rapidly through the jejunum to collect in the lower ileum from where residues are propelled at a more gradual rate to the colon. Thus, it seems likely that most of the small intestinal length is used for the absorption of drugs, particularly when these are given with a meal, and the concept of small intestinal reserve length is not a generally applicable guide to bioavailability. This concept also cannot be applied to certain drugs which are incompletely absorbed; for example the b-blocker atenolol which is absorbed for 3-4 hours following administration. Absorption then stops abruptly, even though 50% of the dose remains unabsorbed, possibly on entry of the drug into the colon, where it is not absorbed. Similarly hydrochlorothiazide is poorly absorbed in the colon[75] and hence absorption stops abruptly as the bolus enters this region. Although intestinal reserve length is a useful guideline, it makes a number of physiological assumptions, primarily that there is no variation in the absorptive capacity of the small intestine along its length. This assumption may be true for some materials, but in other cases absorption may be carrier-mediated or occur at specific sites.

An alternative approach to the intestinal reserve length theory uses the calculation of the drug dissolution under sink conditions together with physiological variables such as the rate of gastric emptying[76]. The degree of absorption of a drug from the small intestine is directly related to the length of time that the drug remains in contact with the absorptive epithelium. Utilising measurements of drug dissolution under sink or non-sink conditions as appropriate, the time taken for the drug to be released from the formulation, i.e. disintegration and dissolution, can be calculated. This should be less than, or equal to the combined time available for absorption and transit through the potential absorption window in the small intestine. The latter terms will be highly influenced by the degree of colonic absorption since, in the absence of absorption from the proximal colon, only a maximum of

3-5 hours is available for absorption from the small intestine in the fasting state. Absorption from the proximal colon affords a further six hours of contact time. This model would predict a marked increase in bioavailability for formulations of poorly absorbed drugs such as frusemide taken with a heavy meal since the meal provides a slow input into the upper small intestine, the major site of absorption (Figure 6.14).

Interaction with food

The presence of food may influence the absorption of drugs and can either enhance, delay or reduce absorption[77]. The most serious problem with such studies is that variations in drug absorption may be due to several different effects. Primarily, the effect of food on gastric emptying is considerable, and variations in the rate at which food is presented to the small intestine will change the drug pharmacokinetics. Secondly, the drug can interact with the food in the intestinal lumen, adsorb to food or be or absorbed by it. Metal ions present in food such as milk can chelate drug, or the drug can bind to dietary proteins thus changing its bioavailability. The presence of viscous chyme can act as a physical barrier reducing drug access to the absorbing surface. Finally, food may influence the absorption process by direct interference with the epithelial biochemistry; for example the absorption of a drug that was taken up actively by a carbohydrate transport system would be slowed in the presence of a large carbohydrate meal which would compete for the transporter. In practice it is extremely difficult to disentangle these factors and so most studies simply report an overall effect.

The absorption of drugs such as penicillin V and G, theophylline and erythromycin is reduced by the presence of food, but food delays the absorption of other drugs (cimetidine, metronidazole and digoxin). The effect of food on drug absorption can be dependent on the type of dosage form used, the excipients and the form of the drug, for example erythromycin stearate in film coated tablets demonstrated reduced absorption with food, erythromycin estolate in suspension was unaffected by food, but absorption of erythromycin ethylsuccinate in suspension and erythromycin estolate in capsules was increased by the presence of food[77]. A co-administered meal decreases the oral absorption of bidisomide and does not influence the oral absorption of the chemically-related antiarrhythmic agent,

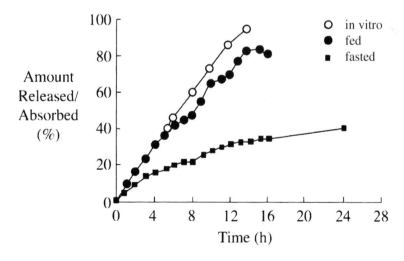

Figure 6.14 Absorption profile for a drug which is poorly absorbed from the colon when administered in a zero-order sustained release dosage form

disopyramide[78]. It was postulated that this was due to the bidisomide being well absorbed in the upper but not lower small intestine.

Certain components of food, notably fibre, have a particularly important effect on drug absorption. Fibre is known to inhibit the absorption of digoxin and entrap steroids. It is well accepted that foods such as milk products, which have a high content of polyvalent metals such as calcium, magnesium, iron, aluminium and zinc, inhibit the absorption of tetracycline and reduce availability. Doxycycline has a slightly lesser tendency to form chelates, thus milk reduces its bioavailability somewhat less than other tetracyclines.

Availability of many drugs is determined by their solubility at the local pH. In the stomach this is highly variable, depending on the presence of food, but the small intestine has a relatively constant pH around 7.0. Drug absorption may be modulated by the presence of food which alters the gastric pH, the viscosity and the transit time through various sections of the gut and a single clear effect may not be evident.

Grapefruit juice greatly increases the bioavailability of certain drugs such as lovastatin and simvastatin, but not pravastatin[79]. The increase in bioavailability probably results from downregulation of CYP3A4 in the small intestine[80]. Hence large amounts of grapefruit juice should be avoided, or the dose of affected drugs should be reduced accordingly. The effect appears to be specific to grapefruit juice, since it cannot be reproduced with other citrus juices such as orange juice. It has been suggested that the inhibitory effect of grapefruit juice may be partially counteracted as it may also activate P-glycoprotein efflux of some drugs[81]

Vitamin effects

The consumption of large amounts of certain vitamins (doses of 1g or more) has become popular with the general public. High doses of vitamin C do not materially affect the clearance of oral antipyrine which might suggest that vitamin C is without action on drug metabolism[82]; however, vitamin C is excreted by conjugation with sulphate. Drugs which are metabolised by sulphation such as ethinylestradiol would be likely to show competitive effects in their metabolism. Concomitant administration of ethinylestradiol with vitamin C resulted in a 50% increase in the steady state concentration of the drug, effectively converting a low dose oestrogen contraceptive pill to a high dose contraceptive pill[83].

Salt effects

It has been postulated that changes in dietary salt might alter metabolism[82]. Volunteers fed a high salt diet (400 mEq/day) compared to a low salt diet (10 mEq/day), during the administration of oral quinidine demonstrated that the bioavialability of quinidine was decreased on the high salt diet[84]. The mechanism of this interaction remains unclear although it could involve an effect on transit or P-glycoprotein status.

First-pass metabolism

Metabolism of drugs administered orally may occur either by gut wall enzymes or by the liver. Hepatic or gut wall enzymes have a limited capacity and the metabolizing enzymes may not necessarily be distributed evenly in the small intestinal epithelium. Estrone sulphokinases. for example, are more prevalent in the duodenal mucosa than the ileum[85]. Thus, oestrogens released lower down in the intestine may reach the blood at more rapid rates and in larger amounts, than the same compounds released in the duodenum and jejunum.

With the exception of the mouth and the terminal rectal area, the venous drainage of the gastrointestinal tract drains enters the liver via the portal vein. Thus, a fraction of the active agent undergoes biotransformation by the liver before reaching the systemic circulation and its site of action. Biotransformation generally inactivates drugs, but it can also transform drugs to active metabolites or compounds which have a different pharmacological action to the parent drug, or even to toxic metabolites. Extensive first-pass metabolism, that is inactivation of the parent drug in the liver, is often encountered with lipophilic bases, such as propranolol and amitryptiline, but rarely with lipophilic acids such as salicylic acid and penicillin. The exceptions are esters of lipophilic acids such as acetylsalicylic acid and pivampicillin which, are exclusively metabolized before they reach the systemic circulation[86].

Ingestion of food increases the bioavailability of drugs which are metabolized during first pass through the gut wall or liver[87]. Two mechanisms have been put forward to explain this effect. First, the enhanced splanchno-hepatic blood flow will increase the load of drug delivered to saturable enzyme systems so that a greater proportion escapes metabolism. Second, nutrients may compete for hepatic enzymes so that less drug is metabolized. Concurrent food intake particularly enhances the bioavailability of weak bases, including propranolol, metoprolol, labetalol, and hydralazine, which are metabolized by hydroxylation, glucuronidation and acetylation enzyme systems. It has little effect on the hepatic clearance of those weak bases which undergo presystemic dealkylation such as codeine, prazosin, and dextropropoxyphene[88]. Food is not expected to influence first-pass metabolism if drugs are given in sustained release preparations because the delivery of drug to the liver is limited by the release of the drug into the gut lumen and not by changes in blood flow.

RELATIONSHIP BETWEEN DRUG ABSORPTION AND POSITION OF DOSE FORM
Radio controlled capsule

In 1981, a capsule containing a balloon filled with drug was reported, which could be actuated in the gastrointestinal tract when required, by the application of a radio signal[89]. This technique has been used to study absorption at various sites in the gastrointestinal tract. To locate the capsule, it is swallowed with a small dose of barium sulphate to aid its localisation within the gut and is triggered when required. The absorption of frusemide was compared in 5 subjects using the device[90]. The drug was released in the ileo-caecal area in 3 subjects and in the ascending colon in the other two. Maximum plasma concentrations were lower after the release of the drug in the colon, and there was a forty-fold difference between absorption from the stomach and colon with bioavailabilities of 20% and 3% respectively. The capsule was also used to study the absorption of theophylline from the stomach, ileum and colon[91]. The mean relative bioavailability of theophylline was 86% after releasing the drug in the colon. Thus there was no evidence for a so called absorption window for theophylline which has previously been reported in the literature, suggesting that such a "window" might have been related to the pharmaceutical formulations used. The device provides a means of investigating drug absorption under normal physiological conditions but has limitations of single occasion use and the need for repeated x-rays[92].

Although in many studies there have been good correlations between the gamma scintigraphic data and the plasma concentration profile, there have been examples in the literature where the results have been completely inexplicable. For example, in a study of the transit and disintegration of acetylsalicylic acid from ^{51}Cr-labelled enteric-coated tablets, in four volunteers out of twelve, the absorption of acetylsalicylic acid was delayed more than 10 hours in spite of the fact that complete disintegration and gastric emptying of the tablet seemed to have occurred[93]. In three volunteers, this occurred in the in postprandial state and in one subject it occurred under fasting conditions. In the remaining eight of the twelve subjects, the time of onset of absorption correlated well with the time of disintegration.

Absorption of drugs and foreign substances through the lymphatic system

The lymphatic route has been suggested as a method of by-passing first-pass metabolism for extremely lipid soluble drugs. It has been argued that lipophilic drugs may become incorporated into lipid micelles and transformed into chylomicrons by the epithelium before being released into the lymphatic circulation. All the lymph from the lower part of the body flows up through the thoracic duct and empties into the venous system of the left internal jugular vein, thus avoiding the hepatic portal system. In order to be transported in the chylomicrons, the drug must be extremely lipophilic. The ratio of portal blood flow to intestinal lymph flow in the rat is approximately 500:1. Although lymph is the major transport route for fats, it only contains 1% lipids. The overall effect is to make systemic absorption 50,000 times more efficient than lymphatic absorption. In order for a drug to be transported at equal rates by both lymphatic and systemic circulations, the drug must be 50,000 times more soluble in the chylomicrons than the plasma, i.e have a partition coefficient of 50,000 (log P = 4.7)[94].

As expected, in practice the lymphatic route is of little importance, except for those materials which are extremely lipophilic, for example insecticides such as dichlorodiphenyltrichloroethane (DDT), in which the loading of drug in the chylomicrons is as high as 0.6 to 2% by weight[95 96]. These values are approximately 6 to 20% of the saturated solubility of DDT in triglycerides.

Studies of mesenteric lymph and blood plasma levels of p-amino salicylic acid delivered intra-duodenally to rats suggested that the drug was directly transported to the lymphatics[97]. In addition, tetracycline was found in the central lacteal of the villi after administration, but this route was insignificant compared to systemic absorption.

In the rat, the absorption of oestradiol-3-cyclopentyl ether administered in an aqueous solution was mainly via the bloodstream, but when the drug was given in sesame oil (primarily linoleic and oleic acid triglycerides) a greater proportion of the drug was absorbed by the lymphatic route[98]. Addition of glyceryl mono-oleate to the sesame oil augmented this effect. The lymphatic absorption of griseofulvin, a systemic antifungal agent, and probucol, a lipid-lowering agent, is also enhanced by food with high fat content, presumably by dissolution of the drug in the fat prior to absorption[99 100]. The natural extension of this is to dissolve the drug in a lipid administered as an emulsion, an approach which has proven useful with griseofulvin[101].

DRUG INDUCED DAMAGE

All commonly used non-steroidal anti-inflammatory drugs (NSAIDs), apart from aspirin and nalbumetone, are associated with increased intestinal permeability in man. Whilst reversible in the short term, it may take months to improve following prolonged NSAID use[102]. NSAIDs cause quite distinct and severe biochemical damage during drug absorption, with the uncoupling of mitochondrial oxidative phosphorylation proving to be most important. Different NSAIDs and different preparations of the same NSAID may have different effects on small bowel permeability[103]

Small bowel ulceration connected to the use of slow-release potassium chloride tablets has been reported[104]. Most were associated with of 1-2 cm of stenosis, and a significant fraction with perforation of the bowe,l and the mortality rate was 27%. These problems many be reduced if wax-matrix or microencapsulated preparations of potassium chloride are used which slowly release potassium and chloride ions over time[105].

REFERENCES

1. Bryan AJ, Kaur R, Robinson G, Thomas NW, Wilson CG. Histological and physiological studies on the intestine of the rat exposed to solutions of Myrj 52 and PEG 2000. *Int. J. Pharmaceut.* 1980;7:145-156.
2. Granger DN, Barrowman JA, Kvietys PR. The small intestine. *Clin. Gastroint. Physiol.* Philadelphia: Saunders, 1985:141-207.
3. Yoffey JM, Cortice FC. Lymphatics, Lymph and the lymphomyeloid complex. *Academic Press, New York and London* 1970.
4. Tasker RR. The collection of intestinal lymph from normally active rats. *J. Physiol (Lond)* 1951;115:292-295.
5. Borgström B, Laurell C-B. Studies on lymph and lymph-protein during absorption of fat and saline in rats. *Acta Physiol. Scand.* 1953;29:264-280.
6. Simmonds WJ. The relationship between intestinal motility and the flow and rate of fat output in thoracic duct lymph in unaneasthetised rats. *Quart. J. Exp. Physiol.* 1954;42:205-221.
7. Harms V, Wright EM. Some characteristics of Na/K ATPase from rat intestinal basal lateral membrane. *J. Memb. Biol.* 1980;53:119-128.
8. Uzel C, Conrad ME. Absorption of heme iron. *Semin. Hematol.* 1998;35:27-34.
9. Umbreit JN, Conrad ME, Moore EG, Latour LF. Iron absorption and cellular transport: The mobilferrin/paraferritin paradigm. *Semin. Hematol.* 1998;35:13-26.
10. Kellow JE, Borody TJ, Phillips SF, Tucker RL. Human interdigestive motility: variations in pattern from esophagus to colon. *Gastroenterol.* 1986;91:386-395.
11. Phillips SF. Transit across the ileocolonic junction. In: *Drug Delivery and the Gastrointestinal Tract.* Wilson CG, Hardy JG, Davis SS (eds) Chichester: Ellis Horwood, 1989:63-74.
12. Phillips SF. Diarrhea: role of the ileocecal sphincter,. In: *New Trends in Pathophysiology and Therapy of the Large Bowel.* Barbara L, Migioli M, Phillips SF (eds) Amsterdam: Elsevier Science Publishers BV, 1983.
13. Pahlin P-E. Extrinsic nervous control of the ileo-cecal sphincter in the cat. *Acta Physiol. Scand. Suppl.* 1975;426:1-32.
14. Munjeri O, Collett JH, Fell JT, Sharma HL, Smith A-M. *In vivo* behavior of hydrogel beads based on amidated pectins. *Drug Deliv. J. Deliv.Targeting Therap. Agents* 1998;5:239-241.
15. Marvola M, Aito H, Pohto P, Kannikoski A, Nykanen S, Kokkonen P. Gastrointestinal transit and concomitant absorption of verapamil from a single-unit sustained-release tablet. *Drug Dev. Ind. Pharm.* 1987;13:1593-1609.
16. Kaus LC, Fell JT, Sharma H, Taylor DC. The intestinal transit of of a single non-disintegrating unit. *Int. J. Pharmaceut.* 1984;20:315-323.
17. Kerlin P, Phillips SF. Diffential transit of liquids and solid residue through the human ileum. *Am. J. Physiol.* 1983;245:G38-G43.
18. Read NW, Al-Janabi MN, Holgate AM, Barber DC, Edwards CA. Simultaneous measurement of gastric emptying, small bowel residence and colonic filling of a solid meal by the use of the gamma camera. *Gut* 1986;27:300-308.
19. Malagelada JR, Robertson JS, Brown ML, Remmington M, Duenes JA, Thomforde GM, et al. Intestinal transit of solid and liquid components of a meal in health. *Gastroenterol.* 1984;87:1255-1263.
20. Caride CJ. Scintigraphic determination of small intestinal transit time: comparison with the hydrogen breath technique. *Gastroenterol.* 1984;86:714-720.
21. Mundy MJ, Wilson CG, Hardy JG. The effect of eating on transit through the small intestine. *Nucl. Med. Commun.* 1989;10:45-50.
22. Ollerenshaw KJ, Norman S, Wilson CG, Hardy JG. Exercise and small intestinal transit. *Nucl. Med. Commun.* 1987;8:105-110.
23. Oettle GJ. Effect of moderate exercise on bowel habit. *Gut* 1991;32:941-944.

24. McMahon FG, Ryan JR, Akdamar K, Ertan A. Upper gastrointestinal lesions after potassium chloride supplements: a controlled clinical trial. *Lancet* 1982;2:1059.
25. Shaffer JL, Higham C, Turnberg LA. Hazards of slow-release preparations in patients with bowel strictures. *Lancet* 1980;2:487.
26. Whittington RM, Thompson IM. Possible hazard of plastic matrix from slow release tablets [letter]. *Lancet* 1983;1:184.
27. Hunter E, Fell JY, Sharma H. The gastric emptying ot pellets contained in hard gelatin capsules. *Drug Dev. Ind. Pharm.* 1982;8:751-757.
28. Feinblatt TM, Ferguson Jr EA. Timed disintegration capsules: an *in vivo* roentgenographic study. *N. Engl. J. Med.* 1956;254:940-945.
29. Green MA. One year's experience with sustained release antihistamine medication: experimental and clinical study. *Ann. Allergy* 1954;12:273-276.
30. Conrad JM, Robinson JR. Sustained drug release from tablets and particles through coating. In: *Pharm. Dosage Forms Tablets*. Lieberman, H A, Lachman, L (eds) Marcel Dekker New York: , 1982:149-163.
31. Davis SS, Hardy JG, Fara JW. Transit of pharmaceutical dosage forms through the small intestine. *Gut* 1986;27:886-892.
32. Davis SS, Khosla R, Wilson CG, Washington N. The gastrointestinal transit of a controlled release pellet formulation of tiaprofenic acid. *Int. J. Pharmaceut.* 1987;34:253-258.
33. Fischer W, Boertz A, Davis SS, Khosla R, Cawello W, Sandrock K, Cordes G. Investigation of the gastrointestinal transit and *in vivo* drug release of isosorbide-5-dinitrate pellets. *Pharmaceut. Res.* 1987;4:480-485.
34. Read NW, Miles CA, Fisher D, Holgate AM, Kime ND, Mitchell MA. Transit of a meal through the stomach, small intestine and colon in normal subjects and its role in the pathogenesis of diarrhoea. *Gastroenterol.* 1980;79:1276-1282.
35. Groning R, Huen G. Oral dosage forms with controlled gastrointestinal transit. *Drug Dev. Ind. Pharm.* 1984;10:527-539.
36. Blackburn NA, Holgate AM, Read NW. Does guar gum improve post-prandial hyperglycaemia in humans by reducing small intestinal contact area? *Br. J. Nutr.* 1984;52:197-204.
37. Levy G, Rao BK. Enhanced intestinal absorption of riboflavin from sodium alginate solution in man. *J. Pharmaceut. Sci.* 1972;61:279-280.
38. Beerman B, Grochinsky-Grind M. Gastrointestinal absorption of hydrochlorothiazide enhanced by concomitant intake of food. *Europ. J. Clin. Pharm.* 1978;13:125-128.
39. Jeppsson J, .Sjogren J. The influence of food on side effects and absorption of lithium. *Acta Psychiatr. Scand.* 1975;51:285-288.
40. Wilson CG. Washington N. Assessment of disintegration and dissolution of dosage forms *in vivo* using gamma scintigraphy. *Drug Dev. Ind. Pharm.* 1988;14:211-218.
41. Bechgaard H, Ladefoged K. Distribution of pellets in the gastrointestinal tract. The influence on transit time exerted by the density or diameter of pellets. *J. Pharm. Pharmacol.* 1978;30:690-692.
42. Bogentoft C, Appelgren C, Jonsson U, Sjorgren J, Alpsten M. Intestinal transit time of ^{51}Cr-labelled pellets of different densities. In: *Radionuclide Imaging in Drug Research*. Wilson CG, Hardy JG, Frier M, Davis SS (eds). London: Croom Helm, 1982:p294.
43. Bechgaard H, Christensen FN, Davis SS, Hardy JG, Taylor M, Whalley DR, Wilson CG. Gastrointestinal transit of pellet systems in ileostomy subjects and the effect of density. *J. Pharm. Pharmacol.* 1985; 37:718-21.
44. Clarke GM, Newton JM, Short MB. Comparative gastrointestinal transit of pellet systems of varying density. *Int. J. Pharmaceut.* 1995;114:1-11.
45. Meyer JH, Elashoff J, Porter- Fink V, Dressman J, Amidon GL. Human postprandial gastric emptying of 1-3 mm spheres. *Gastroenterol.* 1988;94:1315-25.
46. Schedl HP, Cllfton JA. Cortisol absorption in man. *Gastroenterol.* 1963;44:134-145.

47. Beerman B, Hellstrom K, Rosen A. The absorption of orally administered 12 alpha H-digoxin in man. *Clin. Sci.* 1972;43: 507-510.

48. Delie F, Rubas W. A human colonic cell line sharing similarities with enterocytes as a model to examine oral absorption: advantages and limitations of the Caco-2 model. *Crit. Rev.Therap. Drug Carrier Syst.* 1997;14:221-286.

49. Hidalgo IJ, Li J. Carrier-mediated transport and efflux mechanisms of Caco-2 cells. *Adv. Drug Deliv. Rev.* 1996;22:53-66.

50. Meunier V, Bourrie M, Berger Y, Fabre G. The human intestinal epithelial cell line Caco-2; pharmacological and pharmacokinetic applications. *Cell Biol. Toxicol.* 1995;11:187-194.

51. Pusztai A. Transport of proteins through the membranes of the adult gastro- intestinal tract - A potential for drug delivery? *Adv. Drug Deliv. Rev.* 1989;3:215-228.

52. Yang CY, Dantzig AH, Pidgeon C. Intestinal peptide transport systems and oral drug availability. *Pharmaceut. Res.*1999;16:1331-1343.

53. Nussberger S, Steel A, Hediger M. Structure and pharmacology of proton-linked peptide transporters. *J. Cont.Rel.* 1997;46:31-38.

54. Smith PL, Eddy EP, Lee C-P, Wilson G. Exploitation of the intestinal oligopeptide transporter to enhance drug absorption. *Drug Deliv J. Deliv.Target. Therap. Agents* 1996;3:117-123.

55. Naisbett B, Woodley J. The potential use of tomato lectin for oral drug delivery: 2. Mechanism of uptake *in vitro. Int. J. Pharmaceut.*1994;110:127-136.

56. Eldridge JH, Hammond CJ, Meulbroek JA, Staas JK, Gilley RM, Tice TR. Controlled vaccine release in the gut-associated lymphoid tissues. I. Orally administered biodegradable microspheres target the Peyer's patches. *J. Cont. Rel.* 1990;11:205-214.

57. Hastewell J, Williamson I, Mackay M, Rubas W, Grass GM. Gastrointestinal lymphatic absorption of peptides and proteins. *Adv. Drug Deliv. Rev.* 1991;7:15-69.

58. Bernkopf-Schnurch A, Gabor F, Szostak MP, Lubitz W. Gentechnologische herstellung adhasiver arzeistofftrager (Production of adhesive drug carriers using recombinant DNA-technology). *Scientia Pharmaceutica* 1995;63:159-166.

59. Hardy JG, Evans DF, Zaki I, Clark AG, Tønnesen HH, Gamst ON. Evaluation of an enteric-coated naproxen tablet using gamma scintigraphy and pH monitoring. *Int. J. Pharmaceut.* 1987;37:245-250.

60. Lucas M. The surface pH of the intestinal mucosa and its significance in the permeability of organic anions. In: Csáky T.Z. ed, *Pharmacology of Intestinal Permeation II*, Springer-Verlag, Berlin. 1984:119-163.

61. Kitizawa S, Ito H, Sezak H. Transmucosal fluid movementand its effect on drug absorption. *Chem. Pharm. Bull.* 1975;23:1856-1865.

62. Ochensfahrt H, Winne D. The contribution of solvent drag to the intestinal absorption of the acidic drugs benzoic acid and salicyclic acid from the jejunum of the rat. *Naunyn. Schmiedebergs Arch. Pharmacol.* 1974;281:175-196.

63. Ochensfahrt H, Winne D. The contribution of solvent drag to the intestinal absorption of the basic drugs amidopyrine and antipyrine from the jejunum of the rat. *Naunyn. Schmiedebergs Arch. Pharmacol.* 1974;281:197-217.

64. Gramatte T, Richter K. Paracetamol absorption from different sites in the human small intestine. *Br. J. Clin. Pharmacol.* 1994;37:608-611.

65. Gramatte T, El Desoky E, Klotz U. Site-dependent small intestinal absorption of ranitidine. *Eur. J. Clini. Pharmacol.* 1994;46:253-259.

66. Watkins P. The barrier function of CYP3A4 and P-glycoprotein in the small bowel. *Adv. Drug Deliv. Rev.* 1997;27:161-170.

67. Thiebaut F, Tsuruo T, Hamada H, Gottesman M, Pastan I, Willingham MC. Cellular localisation of the multi-drug resistant gene product in normal human tissues. *Proc. Natl. Acad. Sci. USA* 1987;84:7735-7738.

68. Schinkel AH. P-glycoprotein, a gate-keeper in the blood-brain barrier. *Adv. Drug Deliv. Rev.* 1999;36:179-194.

69. Gramatte T, Oertel R. Intestinal secretion of intravenous talinolol is inhibited by luminal R-verapamil. *Clin. Pharmacol. Therap.* 1999;66:239-245.

70. Wacher VJ, Silverman JA, Zhang Y, Benet LZ. Role of P-glycoprotein and cytochrome P450 3A in limiting oral absorption of peptides and peptidomimetics. *J. Pharmaceut. Sci.* 1998;87:1322-1330.

71. Hebert M. Contributions of hepatic and intestinal metabolism and P-glycoprotein to cyclosporine and tacrolimus oral drug delivery. *Adv. Drug Deliv. Rev.* 1997;27:201-214.

72. Watkins P. The barrier function of CYP3A4 and P-glycoprotein in the small bowel. *Adv. Drug Deliv. Rev.* 1987;27:161-170.

73. Borgstrom B, Dahlovist A, Lunh G, Sjovall J. Studies of the intestinal digestion and absorption in the human. *J. Clin. Invest.* 1957;36:36.

74. Ho NFH, Merkle HP, Higuchi WI. Quantitative, mechanistic and physiologically realistic approach to the biopharmaceutical design of oral drug delivery systems. *Drug Dev. Ind. Pharm.* 1983;9:1111-1184.

75. Taylor DC, Lynch J, Leahy DE. Models for intestinal permaeability to drugs. In: *Drug Delivery to the Gastrointestinal Tract.* Hardy JG, Davis SS, Wilson CG, eds. Chichester: Ellis Horwood, 1989:133-145.

76. Dressman J. Kinetics of drug absorption from the gut. *Drug Delivery to the Gastrointestinal Tract.* Hardy JG, Davis SS, Wilson CG, eds. Chichester: Ellis Horwood, 1989:195-219.

77. Toothaker RD, Welling PG. The effect of food on drug bioavailability. *Ann Rev. Pharmacol. Toxicol.* 1980;20:173-199.

78. Pao L-H, Zhou SY, Cook C, Kararli T, Kirchhoff C, Truelove J, et al. Reduced systemic availability of an antiarrhythmic drug, bidisomide, with meal co-administration: Relationship with region-dependent intestinal absorption. *Pharmaceut. Res.* 1998;15:221-227.

79. Lilja JJ, Kivisto KT, Neuvonen PJ. Grapefruit juice increases serum concentrations of atorvastatin and has no effect on pravastatin. *Clin. Pharmacol. Therap.* 1999;66:118-127.

80. Lown KS, Bailey DG, Fontana RJ, Janardan SK, Adair CH, Fortlage LA, Brown MB, Guo W, Watkins PB. Grapefruit juice increases felodipine oral availability in humans by decreasing intestinal CYP3A protein expression. *J. Clin. Invest.* 1997;99:2545-2553.

81. Soldner A, Christians U, Susanto M, Wacher VJ, Silverman JA, Benet LZ. Grapefruit juice activates P-glycoprotein-mediated drug transport. *Pharmaceut. Res.* 1999;16:478-485.

82. Wilkinson GR. The effects of diet, aging and disease states on presystemic elimination and oral drug bioavailability in humans. *Adv. Drug Deliv. Rev.* 1997;27:129-159.

83. Briggs MH. Megadose vitamin C and metabolic effects of the pill. *Br. Med. J.* 1981;283:1547.

84. Darbar D, Dell'Orto S, Morike K, Wilkinson GR, Roden D. Dietary salt increases the first pass elimination of oral quinidine. *Clin. Pharmacol. Therap.* 1997;61:292-300.

85. Bostrom H, Bromster D, Nordenstram H, Wengle B. On the occurrence of phenol and steroid sulphokinases in the human gastrointestinal tract. *Scand. J. Gastroenlerol.* 1968;3:369-374.

86. Melander A, McLean A. Influence of food intake on the presystemic clearance of drugs. *Clin. Pharmacokinet.* 1983;8:286-295.

87. Melander A. Influence of food on the bioavailability of drugs. *Clin. Pharmacokinet.* 1978;3:337-341.

88. Read NW, Sugden K. Gastrointestinal dynamics and pharmacology for the optimum design of controlled-release oral dosage forms. *CRC Crit. Rev. Ther. Drug Carr.* 1987;4:221-267.

89. Zimmer A, Roth W, Hugemann B, Spieth W, Koss, FW. A novel method to study drug absorption. Evaluation of the sites of absorption with a capsule for wireless controlled drug liberation in the GI tract. Aiche JM, Hirtz J, (eds). *First Europ. Congress Biopharmaceut. Pharmacokinet.*; 1981.p211.

90. Graul EH, Loew D, Schuster O. Voraussetzung fur die Entwicklung einer sinnvollen Retard- und Diuretika-Komination. *Therapiewoche* 1985;35:4277-4291.
91. Staib AH, Loew D, Harder S, Graul EH, Pfab R. Measurement of theophylline   absorption from different regions of the gastro-intestinal tract using a remote controlled drug delivery device. *Eur. J .Clin. Pharmacol.* 1986;30:691-697.
92. Bieck PR. Drug absorption from the human colon. In: *Drug Delivery to the Gastrointestinal Tract*. Wilson CG, Hardy JG, Davis SS. (eds) Chichester: Ellis Horwood, 1989:147-160.
93. Bogentoft C, Alpsten M, Ekenved G. Absorption of acetylsalicylic acid from enteric-coated tablets in relation to gastric emptying and *in vivo* disintegration. *J. Pharm. Pharmacol.* 1984;36:350-351.
94. Noguchi T, Charman WNA, Stella VJ. The effect of lipophilicity and lipid vehicles on the lymphatic transport of various testosterone esters. *Int. J. Pharmaceut.* 1985;24:173-184.
95. Vost A, Maclean N. Hydrocarbon transport in chylomicrons and high density lipoproteins in the rat. *Lipids* 1984;19:423-435.
96. Charman WNA, Stella VJ. Effects of lipid class and lipid vehicle volume on the intestinal lymphatic transport of DDT. *Int. J. Pharmaceut.* 1986;33:165-172.
97. DeMarco TJ, Levine RR. Role of lymphatics in the intestinal absorption and distribution of drugs. *J. Pharmacol. Exp. Therap.* 1969;169:142-151.
98. Gianninna T, Steinetz BG, Meli A. Pathway of absorption of orally administered ethynyl estradiol-3-cyclopentyl ether in the rat as influenced by vehicle of administration. *Proc. Soc. Exp. Biol. Med.* 1966;121:1175-1179.
99. Palin KJ, Wilson CG, Davis SS, Phillips AJ. The effects of oils on the lymphatic absorption of DDT. *J. Pharm. Pharmacol.* 1982;34:707-710.
100. Palin KJ, Wilson CG. The effect of different oils on the absorption of probucol in the rat. *J. Pharm. Pharmacol.* 1984;36:641-643.
101. Bates TR, Sequeira JA. Bioavailability of micronised griseofulvin from corn oil-in-water emulsion, aqueous suspension and commercial tablet dosage forms in humans. *J. Pharmaceut. Sci.* 1975;64:793-797.
102. Bjarnason I, Peters TJ. Influence of anti-rheumatic drugs on gut permeability and on the gut associated lymphoid tissue. *Baillieres Clin. Rheumatol.* 1996;10:165-176.
103. Choi VMF, Coates JE, Chooi J, Thomson ABR, Russell AS. Small bowel permeability - a variable effect of NSAIDS. *Clin. Invest.Med.- Med. Clin. Exp.* 1995;18:357-361.
104. Leijonmarck CE, Raf L. Ulceration of the small intestine due to slow-release potassium chloride tablets. *Acta Chir. Scand.*1985;151:273-278.
105. Skoutakis VA, Acchiardo SR, Wojciechowski NJ. The comparative bioavailability of liquid, wax-matrix and microencapsulated preparations of potassium chloride. *J. Clin. Pharmacol.* 1985;25:619-621.

Chapter Seven

Drug Delivery to the Large Intestine and Rectum

INTRODUCTION

The large intestine is responsible for the conservation of water and electrolytes, formation of a solid stool, and storage of faeces until a convenient time for defaecation. Its function is quite distinct from that of the small intestine whose primary role is the digestion of food and absorption of simple nutrients.

Administration by the rectal route is preferable for drugs which produce emesis or are irritant when given orally. For the purposes of drug delivery, the colon has to be considered as two regions; the distal colon, which can be reached from the anus, and the proximal colon, which is only accessible via the oral route. The splenic flexure limits the area of exposure of drugs administered by the anal route to the descending and sigmoid colon, rectum and anus. Instillation of large volumes to overcome this restriction triggers the defaecation reflex. Nevertheless the rectal route is popular in Europe, though not in the U.S.A! Formulations targeted to the proximal colon have to be delivered via the oral route and must be protected against the hostile environment of the stomach and small intestine. Transit through the colon is slower than other areas of the gastrointestinal tract and so there is an opportunity for sustained drug delivery from the ascending and first part of the transverse colon.

ANATOMY AND PHYSIOLOGY OF THE COLON

The colon extends from the ileo-caecal junction to the anus and is approximately 125 cm long *in vivo*. The large intestine is wider and shorter than the small intestine. The lumen progressively diminishes from a maximum diameter at the caecum (about 8.5cm) to the sigmoid segment (about 2.5 cm). It can be divided into the caecum, ascending, transverse, descending, and sigmoid colon, rectum and anus (Figure 7.1).

The caecum is the widest part of the colon and is a downward pointing blind pouch approximately 8.5 cm long with the appendix attached to its apex, and its base at the ileo-caecal junction. It is attached to the floor of the right iliac fossa by the peritoneum, within the folds of which lies the appendix. It receives undigested food material from the small intestine and is considered the first region of the large intestine. It is separated from the ileum (the final portion of the small intestine) by the ileocecal valve (also called Bauhin's valve). The ileocaecal valve limits the rate of food passage into the caecum and may help prevent material from returning to the small intestine. In humans, the caecum's main functions are to absorb fluids and salts that remain after the completion of intestinal digestion and absorption, and to mix its contents with mucus for lubrication. The internal wall is composed of a thick mucous membrane beneath which is a deep layer of muscle tissue that produces churning and kneading motions.

The ascending colon is approximately 20 cm long and extends from the caecum to the hepatic flexure, which lies lateral to the right kidney and in contact with the inferior surface of the liver. The transverse colon is normally over 45 cm in length and hangs loosely between the hepatic and the splenic flexures, often following the greater curvature of the stomach. The splenic flexure is usually located higher than the hepatic flexure. The

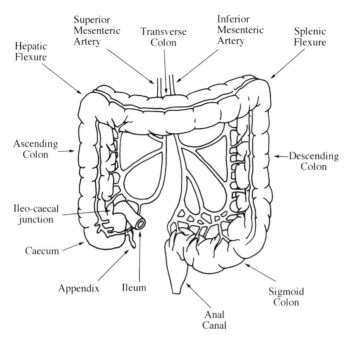

Figure 7.1 Anatomy and perfusion of the colon

descending colon extends downwards from the splenic flexure to the pelvic brim and is approximately 30 cm long. The colon then turns towards the midline to form the coiled sigmoid colon, which is about 40 cm in length. This in turn joins the rectum in front of the third part of the sacrum and travels for approximately 12 cm before joining the anal canal. This is 3 cm long and its diameter is narrower than that of the rectum to which it connects. It is identified by the presence of the anal sphincters which replace the muscular coats of the rectum. The sling of the puborectales muscle supports the ano-rectal junction.

In humans the rectum is formed by the last 15 to 20 cm of the large intestine. The internal cavity of the rectum is divided into three or four chambers; each chamber is partly segmented from the others by permanent transverse folds (valves of Houston) that apparently help to support the rectal contents. A sheath of longitudinal muscle surrounds the outside wall of the rectum, making it possible for it to shorten in length.

Interspecies differences in structure

The variation in relative dimension of the large intestine is largely correlated with diet. In herbivores, such as horses and rabbits, which depend largely on microbial fermentation for nutrition, the large intestine is very large and complex. Omnivores like pigs and humans have a substantial but smaller large intestine. Carnivores such as dogs and cats have a small and simple large intestine. The structure and function of the caecum varies in many animals. Vertebrates such as rabbits and horses, which live on a diet composed only of plant life, have a larger caecum that is an important organ of absorption, since it contains bacteria that help digest cellulose. Animals that eat only meat have a reduced or absent caecum. In cats and dogs, muscle contractions of the caecum are much more vigorous and are reversible. Materials already passed to the next region of the large intestine can be brought back to the caecum for mixing with new food substances.

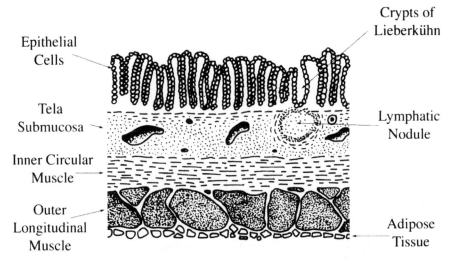

Figure 7.2 Structure of the colon wall

Colonic structure

The wall of the colon is divided into four layers: the serosa, external muscular region (muscularis externa), submucosa and mucosa (Figure 7.2). The squamous epithelium of the serosa is covered with adipose tissue which forms distended fat pouches of peritoneum, known as appendices epiploicae. These are larger and more numerous in the distal half of the colon and are one of its distinguishing features. The serosa is absent from the rectum and anal canal.

The muscularis externa consists of an inner circular muscle layer and an incomplete outer longitudinal layer composed of three separate 0.8 cm wide, longitudinal strips known as teniae coli. These bands converge in the caecum at the root of the appendix. They travel the length of the colon and eventually widen and join to form a continuous outer longitudinal muscle layer which covers the rectum. Between the teniae coli is a thin layer of longitudinal muscle which allows the inner circular muscle layer to bulge outwards. This outward bulge is interrupted at intervals by contractions of the circular muscle, giving the colon its characteristic sacculated appearance. These sacculae are also known as haustra and are more pronounced in the proximal half of the colon. Their size and shape varies with the contractile activity of the circular muscle.

Colonic mucosa

The colonic mucosa is divided into three layers: the muscularis mucosae, the lamina propria and the epithelium. The muscularis mucosae is a layer of smooth muscle approximately 10 cells thick which separates the submucosa from the lamina propria. The lamina propria supplies structural support for the epithelium and is well supplied with blood vessels and lymphatics. It also contains numerous T lymphocytes, macrophages, plasma cells and some lymph nodules. These cells play an important role in the immune function of the colon, and help to protect it from bacterial invasion and attack.

There are many histological similarities in the structure of the mucosa in the large and small intestine. The most obvious difference is that the mucosa of the large intestine is devoid of villi. The colonic epithelium consists of a single layer of columnar cells lining the lumen, and is punctuated by numerous crypts, termed crypts of Lieberkühn. These are responsible for the production and differentiation of the absorptive, goblet and endocrine cells that make up the colonic epithelial layer. The goblet cells are responsible for the production of mucus which is important in minimising friction between the mucosal surface and the semi-solid luminal contents.

The mucosa is thrown into irregular folds known as plicae semilunares which, along with the microvilli of the absorptive epithelial cells, serve to increase the surface area of the colon by 10 to 15 times that of a simple cylinder of similar dimensions. The terminal portion of the digestive tract in most animals is distinguished from the rectum because of the transition of its internal surface from a mucous membrane layer (endodermal) to one of skin-like tissue (ectodermal). The anal opening is keratinized skin that has several folds while contracted. When open, the folds allow the skin to stretch without tearing. In the skin around the anal opening but not immediately adjacent to it are glands that give off perspiration. Both the upper and lower portions of the anal canal have circular and longitudinal muscle layers that allow expansion and contraction of the canal. The luminal surface of the rectum is covered by a membrane formed from columnar epithelial, endocrine and goblet cells.

Very few Paneth cells are found in the colon, although some exist in the caecum and ascending colon. It is believed that Paneth cells are involved in a variety of functions including secretion of digestive enzymes, production of trophic factors and elimination of heavy metals. They have abundant zinc-rich secretory granules which contain lysozyme, glycoprotein and other proteins.

The gut associated lymphoid tissue (GALT) is unevenly distributed throughout the GI tract. The lymphoepithelial regions of the colon are known as lymphoglandular complexes (LGC). They resemble sites in the small intestine which are associated with antigen sampling, but very little is known about this tissue.

Mucus

Mucus is produced by goblet cells and acts as a lubricant protecting the colon from abrasion from solid matter, particularly in the distal colon. Mucins are degraded by colonic bacterial flora. Much of the colonic mucin is sulphated, the degree of sulphation being greater in the distal colon and decreasing proximally towards the terminal ileum[1]. Histochemical studies have shown a relative depletion of colonic sulphomucins in both ulcerative colitics and patients with Crohn's disease[2]. Desulphation of the mucus will alter the net charge on the mucin and therefore change its physical properties, rendering it more susceptible to bacterial sialase attack[3].

Gut wall metabolism

The colon and small intestine resemble each other in the spectrum of metabolizing enzymes, but since the mucosal surface area is much higher in the upper gut, the total metabolic activity of the colonic wall is much lower. Thus enzyme systems should be easier to saturate than in the jejunum and ileum, and the problem of enzymatic degradation of drugs should be reduced.

Blood supply

The blood supply to the colon and upper rectum derives from the superior and inferior mesenteric arteries, and venous return is via the superior and inferior mesenteric veins (Figure 7.1). These join the splenic vein as part of the portal venous system to the liver. Thus any drugs absorbed from the colon and upper rectum are subjected to first pass elimination by the liver. Measurement of blood flow through the colon is difficult and reported values range from 8 to 75 ml. min^{-1} [4]. Blood flow through the colon is considerably less than that to the small intestine, and the proximal colon receives a greater share of the blood flow than the more distal part[5].

The anal canal connects with the rectum at the point where it passes through a muscular pelvic diaphragm. The upper region of the anal canal has 5 to 10 vertical folds in the mucous membrane lining, called the anal, or rectal, columns; each column contains a small artery and vein. These are the terminal portions of the blood vessels that furnish the rectal and anal areas; they are susceptible to enlargement, commonly known as haemorrhoids. The mucous membrane of the upper portion of the rectum is similar to that in the rest of the large intestine; it contains mucus-producing and absorptive cells. Drugs absorbed from the lower rectum and anal canal are transported via these haemorrhoidal plexuses and internal iliac veins to the vena cava, and thus have the advantage of avoiding first pass elimination. However, not all rectally absorbed drug passes through this route, as the veins in this region are heavily anastomosed, causing a fraction of the blood flow to return via the hepatic portal vein to the liver. In cases of portal hypertension, this effect is reduced and a larger proportion of a rectally administered drug can avoid first pass metabolism.

Nervous and humoral control

Parasympathetic supply to the colon is provided by the vagi to the proximal colon and pelvic nerves to the distal colon, whereas sympathetic supply is via the splanchnic and lumbar colonic nerves which supply the proximal and distal colon respectively. Axons from both branches of the autonomic nervous system impinge on the neurons of the myenteric plexus. Vagal stimulation initiates segmental contractions in the proximal colon, whereas pelvic nerve stimulation causes tonic propulsive contractions in the distal colon. Stimulation of either the splanchnic or lumbar sympathetic nerves causes the colonic muscles to relax.

Plexuses of Auerbach, involved with colonic motility, and Meissner, associated with mucus secretion, have an integrated system enabling stimuli to be detected and the appropriate response produced. The muscle of the large intestine can be stimulated by stretching, and a number of chemical substances such as acetylcholine and histamine can cause contraction or enhance motility. Adrenaline and noradrenaline can depress smooth muscle activity.

The central nervous system (CNS) modifies many functions of the gastrointestinal tract. In cats, stimulation of the cerebrum, midbrain and hypothalamus increases colonic motility. The colon appears to receive impulses from the CNS and upper gastrointestinal tract via the spinal cord. This is supported by the association of thoracic spinal cord injury with intractable constipation[6]. If the proximal region of the colon is distended, contraction distally is inhibited by impulses passing along intermesenteric neurons between pre- and para- vertebral ganglia and then via splanchnic or lumbar colonic nerves. With extrinsic regulation the parasympathetic neurons appear to be excitatory and the sympathetics inhibitory in the musculature of the colon.

A number of hormones influence colonic motility. Gastrin can intensify contractions and may decrease the evacuation time of the colon. Cholecystokinin has been proposed as a mediator of the lipid generated increase in rectosigmoid motor activity. However infusion of cholecystokinin at physiological concentrations does not reproduce the complex milieu of events that occur postprandially. Neurotensin is present in the myenteric plexus and mucosa of the colon and may also play a part in the increase in colonic motility seen on ingestion of fat as the serum levels rise. Substance P appears to stimulate the circular smooth muscle, unlike progesterone, which acts an inhibitor of muscle contraction, thus perhaps accounting for some of the changes seen in colonic motility during the menstrual cycle and pregnancy. Secretin and glucagon also inhibit colonic motility. Despite the influ-

Table 7.1 Comparison of the environment in different parts of the gastrointestinal tract

Region	Length (m)	Surface Area (m²)	pH	Residence Time	Micro-organisms
Oesophagus	0.3	0.02	6.8	>30 seconds	unknown
Stomach	0.2	0.2	1.8-2.5	1-5 hours	$\leq 10^2$
Duodenum	0.3	0.02	5-6.5	>5 minutes	$\leq 10^2$
Jejunum	3	100	6.9	1-2 hours	$\leq 10^2$
Ileum	4	100	7.6	2-3 hours	$\leq 10^7$
Colon	1.5	3	5.5-7.8	15-48 hours	$\leq 10^{11}$

ence of hormonal and neural mechanisms on colonic motility, the major control for the transit of luminal contents is exerted by the smooth muscle itself.

Colonic environment

The colonic environment markedly differs from other parts of the gastrointestinal tract as illustrated in Table 7.1. The absorptive capacity of the colon is much less than that of the small intestine, due mainly to the reduced surface area. The mucosal surface of the colon is similar to that of the small intestine at birth, but rapidly changes by losing villi leaving a flat mucosa with deep crypts. As the gut ages there is a decrease in the number of non-goblet crypt cells and this is related to an increase in faecal water[7].

Water and electrolytes

The colon has a very high absorptive capacity; for every 2 litres of water entering the colon, the residual water in the stools will be less than 200 ml. The flow of chyme from the ileum to the colon in healthy human beings is 1 - 2 litres.h⁻¹. The colon is capable of absorbing up to 4 L of water per day and can withstand an infusion rate of 6 ml.min⁻¹ before there is any increase in faecal water[8 9]. The large capacity of the colon to absorb fluid may, however, be overwhelmed by a large fluid input and unabsorbed solutes, such as bile acids, fatty acids, or carbohydrates can also impair this adaptive capacity, possibly resulting in diarrhoea. Absorption of water and sodium is negligible from the rectum. Solids are consolidated to 200-300g of wet material which is equivalent to 30–40 g of dry matter, which is mainly bacterial in origin but contains undigested organic matter and fibre.

The colon is responsible for the absorption of sodium ions, chloride ions and water from the lumen in exchange for bicarbonate and potassium ions. The absorption of sodium is an active process and involves its diffusion across the apical membrane of epithelial cells via water filled channels. Sodium absorption in the colon is enhanced by the hormone aldosterone. A sodium-potassium exchange pump system in the baso-lateral membrane then moves sodium against steep concentration (14 mM to 140 mM) and electrical (-30 mV to +20 mV) gradients into the intercellular space. This movement of sodium creates an osmotic gradient which causes a net movement of water from the colonic lumen via the epithelial cells, through the tight junctions between epithelial cells into the intercellular spaces.

In healthy individuals, approximately 10 mEq of potassium enters the colon each day whilst 5 to 15 mEq are lost in the faeces during the same time period. Potassium secretion is determined by the luminal concentration of potassium, with concentrations of below 15 mEq leading to net secretion. This is accomplished by passive movement of potassium ions along an electrochemical gradient from plasma to lumen, and is facilitated by the tight junctions between epithelial cells which are highly permeable to potassium ions. The sodium-potassium pump in the basolateral membrane of epithelial cells creates a high intracellular potassium concentration (80 mM), of which only a small proportion is lost to the colonic lumen, since the apical epithelial membrane is essentially impermeable to potassium.

pH

Studies using a pH sensitive radiotelemetry capsule in normal, ambulatory volunteers have shown that the mean pH in the colonic lumen is 6.4 ± 0.6 in the ascending colon, 6.6 ± 0.8 in the transverse colon and 7.0 ± 0.7 in the descending colon[10].

Many factors such as disease, diet, pharmaceutical formulations or therapeutic agents may alter the pH or the difference in pH between the ascending and descending colon. For example, administration of the laxative disaccharide lactulose causes the production of large amounts of lactic acid by the caecal bacteria, acidifying the proximal colon to $5.5 - 5.0$. Less pronounced decreases are produced by guar gum and isphagula. Evidence exists suggesting that there are substantial changes in gastrointestinal pH in patients with malabsorption due to cystic fibrosis and in ulcerative colitis the pH may drop below 5[11]. Current dosage forms designed for release in the proximal bowel employ enteric coatings, and are therefore dependent on luminal pH. Alteration of the pH profile of the gastrointestinal tract in various disease states may be an important factor influencing the bioavailability of drugs delivered in this form.

Bacteria

The gastrointestinal tract is sterile at birth, but colonization typically begins within a few hours of birth, starting in the small intestine and progressing caudally over a period of several days. In most circumstances, a "mature" microbial flora is established by 3 to 4 weeks of age. The colonic microflora contain up to 400 different species of both aerobic and anaerobic bacteria and make up approximately 30% of faecal dry weight. The most prevalent anaerobes are *Bacteroides* sp. and *Bifidobacterium* whilst the most numerous aerobes are *Escherichia coli*, enterococci and *Lactobacillus*. The major site of bacterial activity is the caecum where the anaerobic bacteria ferment substrates in a liquid mixture. The principal sources of nutrition for the bacteria are complex carbohydrates including starches, non-starch polysaccharides including dietary fibre (celluloses, gums and pectins) and smaller saccharides such as lactose, sorbitol and xylitol. It is thought that 2 - 20% of dietary starch escapes absorption in the small bowel. Synthesis of vitamin K by colonic bacteria provides a valuable supplement to dietary sources and makes clinical vitamin K deficiency rare.

Cellulose is a common constituent in the diet of many animals, including man, but no mammalian cell is known to produce a cellulase. Several species of bacteria in the large bowel synthesize cellulases and digest cellulose, and the major end products of digestion of this and other carbohydrates are volatile fatty acids, lactic acid, methane, hydrogen and carbon dioxide. Fermentation is thus the major source of intestinal gas. Volatile fatty acids (acetic, proprionic and butyric acids) generated from fermentation can be absorbed by passive diffusion in the colon and metabolised in the epithelial cells and liver. Short chain fatty acids remaining in the colon are neutralised by bicarbonate ions which are secreted into the lumen.

In man, the metabolic activity of the caecal bacteria can be demonstrated by ingestion of lactulose or baked beans which are fermented by the caecal bacteria, causing a rise in breath hydrogen. This is used as a method of estimating the time of mouth to caecal transit.

Colonic bacteria possess exocellular lipases which are able to hydrolyse fatty acid esters at the 1 and 3 positions of the triglyceride molecule. They also produce enzymes capable of metabolising long chain fatty acids. Approximately 25% of faecal fatty acids are hydroxylated by colonic bacteria, for example oleic acid is hydroxylated to form hydroxystearic acid. The presence of hydroxylated fatty acids in the colon has an inhibitory effect on colonic electrolyte and water transport, and at high concentrations they cause net secretion of water and electrolytes, which results in diarrhoea and therefore a significantly increased colonic transit rate. Infusion of oleic acid (4.3 g per 100 ml) into the mid-ascending colon accelerated colonic transit rate and defaecation when compared to a control infusion[12].

The microbial population exerts a profound effect on the structure and function of the digestive tract, as the morphology of the intestine of germ-free animals differs considerably from normal animals. Villi of the small intestine are remarkably regular, the rate of epithelial cell renewal is reduced and, as one would expect, the number and size of Peyer's patches is reduced. The caecum of germ-free rats is roughly 10 times the size of that in a conventional rat.

Colonic motility

Patterns of motility

The colon is an intermittently active organ and three patterns of motility are observed:

(i) segmental contractions which chop and mix the contents, increasing contact with the mucosa where absorption can occur.

(ii) antiperistaltic contractions which propagate toward the ileum. These serve to retard the movement of contents through the colon, allowing additional opportunity for absorption of water and electrolytes to occur. Peristaltic contractions, in addition to influx from the small intestine, facilitate movement of contents through the colon.

(iii) mass movements constitute a type of motility not seen elsewhere in the digestive tube. They are also known also as giant migrating contractions; this pattern of motility resembles a very intense and prolonged peristaltic contraction which strips an area of large intestine clear of contents.

Segmental activity consists of local contractions which are usually effected by circular muscle and lead to the mixing of luminal contents, whereas propulsive activity is largely due to contraction of longitudinal muscle. In the colon, the predominant activity is segmental, with the propulsive type of movement occurring infrequently (3-4 times daily in normals)(Table 7.2).

Table 7.2 Patterns of colonic motility[13]

Type of movement	Frequency of occurrence		Distance Travelled	Rate (cm. min)
	At rest %	Postprandial %		
Haustral shuttling	38	13	0	0
Haustral propulsion	36	57	5 - 10 cm	2.5
Haustral retropulsion	30	52	5 - 20 cm	2.5
Multihaustral propulsion	9	17	Variable	2.5 - 5
Peristalsis	6	8	18 - 20 cm	1 - 2
Mass	Rare	12	> 30 cm	5 – 35

Once food waste reaches the sigmoid colon, it remains there until it is ready to be excreted from the body. As the faecal material enters the rectum, the walls distend to accommodate it. When sufficient pressure occurs within the distended rectal cavity, the urge to eliminate wastes begins. When receptors of the nervous system within the rectal wall are stimulated by its stretching, they send impulses to the anal canal, chest and abdominal-wall muscles, and the medulla of the brain, which makes the individual conscious of the need to defaecate.

Electrical activity

Changes in the electrical potential of the smooth muscle coat are often used to assess gastrointestinal motility. Two types of electrical activity have been recorded in the colon i) slow wave activity and ii) spike potentials. The former consist of regular phasic depolarisations of the cell membrane which originate in the circular muscle layer of the transverse colon[14]. When compared with that of the stomach and small intestine, colonic slow wave activity is of low frequency and irregular. The slow wave pacemaker in the proximal or transverse colon maintains co-ordinated regular activity throughout the colon, and appears, at least in the cat, to migrate towards the caecum[15 16]. The retrograde propagation of slow waves in the proximal segment allows longer mucosal exposure for the intraluminal contents resulting in more complete absorption[17]. In man, the dominant slow wave frequency is 11 cycles per minute in the transverse and descending colon, slightly less in the caecum, ascending and sigmoid colon, whilst that in the rectum is the highest observed in the gastrointestinal tract at 17 cycles per min.

Spike potentials may be superimposed on the slow waves or may exist as bursts unrelated to slow wave activity, and are thought to initiate functional colonic contractions. Spike bursts of long duration (>10s) increase after eating and may increase luminal transit. Short duration spike bursts (<3.5s) are seen in patients with constipation and are not associated with movement of the intestinal contents. Such contractions only occur when the membrane potential rises above a prevailing threshold level which is set by both neural and humoral mechanisms.

Gastrocolic reflex

After eating, there is a rapid increase in spike and contractile activity in the colon[18-20]. The calorific content appears to have a more important effect on the degree of motility than the size or pH of the meal. Fat is a more important stimulant of motility than either carbohydrate or protein. Ingestion of fat alone produces both an early (10 to 40 min) and late (70 to 90 min) increase in colonic motility[19]. The late response can be abolished by the simultaneous ingestion of protein, and both responses are inhibited by the ingestion of amino acids. This colonic response to feeding is known as the gastrocolic reflex, and must be an integrated response to both fat and protein induced mediators. The gastrocolic response is initiated by a sensory receptor in the gastroduodenal mucosa[20].

Three components have been identified in the response of the colon to the ingestion of a meal: an initial cholinergic propulsive reflex, followed by a cholinergic segmenting reflex and finally a noradrenergic segmenting reflex[21]. Intravenous infusion of anticholinergic drugs prior to a meal abolishes the early colonic effects, thus supporting a cholinergic neural mechanism for mediation of the early response to eating. It is possible that there may also be a humoral component to this early response, in that the release of gastrointestinal hormones may be responsible for stimulating the cholinergic neural pathways. The late response, however, is unaffected by pre-treatment with anticholinergic drugs, thus implicating an essentially humoral pathway which may involve release of gastrin, cholecystokinin (CCK) or another gastrointestinal hormone. A postprandial increase in gastrin levels has been observed and CCK is released from the duodenum in the presence of fat. CCK stimulates gall bladder contraction and increases motility in both the small intestine and colon. Gastrin, in the G17 short chain form, and CCK stimulate colonic motility at serum concentrations within the physiological range[22]. Intravenous and intraduodenal amino acids stimulate the release of pancreatic glucagon, which has been shown to be a potent inhibitor of colonic myoelectric and motor activity. Enkephalins, endogenous pentapeptides, have been implicated since the response to a meal can be blocked by naloxone, an opiate antagonist[20]. Met-enkephalin analogues inhibit colonic motility through a peripheral mechanism thought to involve the myenteric cholinergic plexus whereas leu-enkephalins stimulate motility through a centrally-acting mechanism[20 23].

Despite this almost immediate colonic motor response to eating in normal subjects, the right colon does not empty soon after a meal, although this phenomenon can be seen in patients with the irritable bowel syndrome[24]. Studies to elucidate this apparent anomaly have shown that non-propagating motor activity increases in all colonic segments immediately after eating a 1000 kcal meal. When propagating contractions do occur postprandially these are associated with a rapid movement of intraluminal contents[25]. The greatest increase in motor activity is seen in the descending colon[26] and this is often associated with retrograde movement of colonic contents from the descending to the transverse colon[25].

Defaecation

The characteristic brown colour of faeces is due to stercobilin and urobinin, both of which are produced by bacterial degradation of bilirubin. Faecal odour results from gases produced by bacterial metabolism, including skatole (3-methylindole), mercaptans, and hydrogen sulphide. In most individuals, dietary and social habits condition the time of defaecation. The majority of adults defaecate once a day, although frequencies from 2 per day to once every 2 days are considered normal.

Several times each day, mass movements push faeces into the rectum, which is usually empty. Distension of the rectum stimulates the defecation reflex. This is largely a spinal reflex mediated via the pelvic nerves, and results in reflex relaxation of the internal anal sphincter followed by voluntary relaxation of the external anal sphincter and defaecation. Colonic emptying occurs during defaecation, which is not only a process of rectal evacuation[27]. In humans and house-trained animals, defaecation can be prevented by voluntary constriction of the external sphincter. When this happens, the rectum soon relaxes and the internal sphincter again contracts, a state which persists until another bolus of faeces is forced into the rectum.

Physiological factors affecting colonic motility

Eating and morning awakening appear to be the major stimuli in eliciting colonic motility. There is also evidence that the menstrual cycle and pregnancy cause disturbances in gastrointestinal function. Transit is delayed in the luteal phase of the cycle, i.e. when serum progesterone levels are highest, and thus progesterone may depress colonic motility[28].

There are studies showing that no difference exists in colonic transit rates between men and women[29 30], whilst other studies have reported a prolonged colon transit in women[28] [31 32]. A study aimed specifically to resolve this dispute has failed to find any difference in colonic transit of radiopaque markers in 10 women in the follicular phase, in 10 women in the luteal phase of the menstrual cycle, in 5 women on oral contraceptives and in 11 males[33]. A wide variation in stool weight exists between subjects on a standard diet and response to wheat fibre[34]. This variation is significantly related to sex but not to age, height or weight. Stool weight in men (162 ± 11 g. day^{-1} mean $\pm$ se) was approximately double that in women

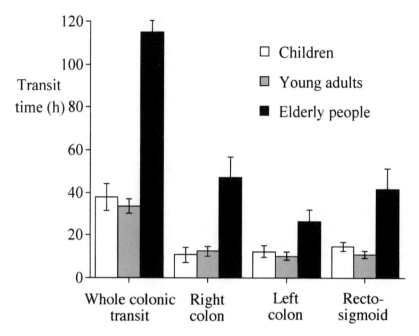

Figure 7.3 The effect of age on transit thriugh the colon

$(83 \pm 11$ g. day^{-1} mean $\pm$ se) and could be explained entirely by differences in transit. The increase in stool weight with fibre was significantly related to dose with approximately 1 g of non-starch polysaccharides (the main component of dietary fibre) increasing stool weight by 5 g per day. Smaller increases in stool weight were seen in females, persons with initially low stool weights and small people. Faecal pH was lower in men than in women and was related to methane production. Methane producers had higher faecal pH than non-producers (7.06 compared to 6.65), lower stool weight (93 ± 12 g. day^{-1} compared to 156 ± 13 g. day^{-1}) and slower transit times (84.6 ± 11.7 h compared to 48.6 ± 6.6 h). These studies show that, when on similar diets, women have much lower stool weights and slower transit times than men. Children appear to have similar colonic transit times to adults, although colonic transit is significantly delayed in the elderly (Figure 7.3).

The effect of stress on gastrointestinal transit remains controversial. Colonic motility can be increased by emotional stress[35]. It is generally recognized that abdominal pain increases and bowel function becomes irregular in patients with the irritable bowel syndrome in periods of emotional stress, and that the symptoms often improve as the anxiety diminishes.

Although exercise is often recommended as therapy for constipation, the relationship between gastrointestinal transit and exercise is unclear[36]. Certainly immobility leads to constipation, but increased exercise above the norm appears to have no effect. However, one study reported that moderate exercise decreases whole gut transit time from a mean of 51 hours to 37 hours when riding and 34 hours when jogging[37].

The effect of diet

Whole bowel transit time is generally between 24 and 36 hours in healthy individuals, but values ranging from 0.4 to 5 days have been reported in the literature[38][39]. Transit through the large bowel is highly influenced by the pattern of daily activity. The highest calorie intake in the western world occurs in the evening and colonic motility decreases at night.

Dietary fibre in the form of bran and wholemeal bread, fruit and vegetables, increases faecal weight by acting as a substrate for colonic bacterial metabolism. This increased faecal bulk is associated with a reduced colonic transit time, although the mechanism is uncertain. In the healthy colon, an additional 20 g per day of bran increases faecal weight by 127% and decreases the mean transit time from 73±24 h to 43±7 h[40]. Not all fibres produce an equal effect on the colon, since the same quantity of fibre as cabbage, carrot or apple produced a smaller effect. The disparate effect of fibre provided as either rice bran or wheat bran was also demonstrated by a two-fold increase in faecal mass and stool frequency with rice bran over wheat bran, despite a similar accelerating effect on transit time with both types of fibre[41]. These differences almost certainly depend upon differing metabolism of the fibre by colonic bacteria.

Dietary fibre is either soluble and viscous, i.e. resistant starch, gums, mucilages and pectins, which amounts to approximately 30% of ingested fibre, or insoluble fibre such as cellulose. The relationship between bacterial degradation of fibre and the effect on faecal mass and whole gut transit time is complex. Three viscous polysaccharides, guar gum, ispaghula and xanthan gum varied in their responses to bacterial degradation *in vitro*[42]. Guar gum was rapidly fermented *in vitro* by faecal bacteria with concomitant loss of viscosity and reduction in pH; ispaghula maintained its viscosity during incubation, but the pH fell significantly, and xanthan gum incubations showed considerable individual variation. Faecal mass was increased only by ispaghula. Whole-gut transit time was reduced by gum feeding to a significantly greater extent in those subjects whose faecal bacteria reduced the viscosity of that gum, than in those subjects where the viscosity was maintained. The rate of proximal colonic transit is directly influenced by the presence and the metabolism of polysaccharides[43]. Using a lactulose-induced catharsis model of accelerated proximal colonic transit in healthy volunteers, ispaghula husk was found to significantly delay proximal colonic transit, whilst guar gum, being more rapidly degraded by bacterial metabolism, caused an accelerated proximal colonic transit (Figure 7.4).

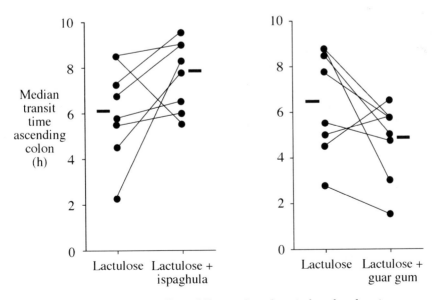

Figure 7.4 The effect of fibre on lactulose-induced catharsis

The diet of an individual is closely linked with the proliferation of the colonic mucosa. Food deprivation and "elemental diets' can result in intestinal atrophy and decreased cell production[44 45]. Refeeding of starved rats with a fibre-free elemental diet supplemented with fermentable fibre stimulates colonic and small intestinal epithelial cell proliferation, whilst the addition of inert bulk to the elemental diet has no such effect[46]. This proliferative effect of fermentable fibre on the gut epithelium was not observed in germ free rats, suggesting that epithelial proliferation is effected by the products of bacterial fermentation rather than the presence of fermentable fibre.

Colonic intraluminal pressure decreases after eating either wheatbran or cellulose[47], however, the physical characteristics of the dietary fibre may be important since coarse bran ingestion decreases colonic motility whereas ingestion of fine bran increases intracolonic pressure[48].

Normal constituents of the colonic lumen include some unmetabolised carbohydrate, protein and bile salts, but very little fat. A considerable amount of starch enters the colon to contribute further substrate for bacterial fermentation. Fermentation produces short-chain fatty acids (SCFA's), notably acetate, propionate and butyrate. SCFA's, whilst being normal constituents of the colon, are not found in the terminal ileum except under conditions of colo-ileal reflux. The effect of SCFA's on the ileum is to stimulate propulsive motility, causing the ileum to be emptied[49] and subsequent return of the SCFA's to the right colon where they aid water absorption. This reflux may be important in preventing bacterial overgrowth in the terminal ileum. Accumulation of SCFAs causes the pH to fall[50].

Long-chain fatty acids (LCFA's) should not normally reach of the colonic lumen and generally are only found in patients with fat malabsorption. LCFA's are cathartic, a fact which may further contribute to the lack of fat metabolism, and have been shown to stimulate unusual motor patterns; an emulsion of oleic acid infused into the ascending colon accelerated colonic transit by induction of high amplitude, prolonged, propagating pressure waves originating near the ileocaecal junction[12]. This was associated with a narrowing of the ascending colon with a reduced reservoir function and may be the mechanism by which diarrhoea is produced in patients with fat malabsorption.

Coffee produced an increase in the motility of distal colon within four minutes of ingestion of both regular and decaffeinated coffee in 8 responders, but not in 6 non-responders[51]. The increase in rectosigmoid motility lasted at least 30 minutes.

Influence of drugs

Although constipation is associated with a slow transit through the left colon in most patients, right colon transit is essentially normal. By contrast, accelerated proximal colonic transit is a common feature of many diseases and treatment is often designed to reduce the transit rate to allow sufficient absorption of nutrients and electrolytes. An increased intestinal transit time is associated with a decreased stool weight and bacterial mass[52].

Codeine phosphate or loperamide are commonly employed to produce a reduction in stool volume and correction of accelerated colonic transit in patients with diarrhoea[53]. These drugs exert their antidiarrhoeal effect through a change in the gastrointestinal motor function, leading to an increased capacitance of the proximal gut, and a delay in the passage of fluid through the gastrointestinal tract [54 55].

Morphine delays transit in the caecum and ascending colon, increases colonic capacitance and reduces bowel movements in man[56 57]. The potency of opiates may be due to their action to modulate the normal neural controls via the enkephalinergic neurones in the colon. The possible role of endogenous opioids has been explored using naloxone, an opiate receptor antagonist. This has been shown to cause an accelerated transit through the colon in cats and in man, but without increasing the number of bowel movements[56 58].

Loxiglumide is a specific and highly potent CCK-receptor antagonist which inhibits postprandial gall bladder contraction and causes an accelerated gastric emptying[59-61]. The effect of CCK-receptor antagonists on the colon is uncertain since loxiglumide shortens colonic transit time in healthy controls[61], but prolongs colonic transit time in patients with accelerated colonic transit.

Drug absorption from the colon

The transport pathways of the colon allow rapid and specific active bi-directional transport of ions across the epithelial layer. Unlike the small intestine, there are no documented active transporters for organic nutrients in the mature organ and, therefore, no chances for drug molecules to be absorbed in a piggy-back fashion[62]. The apparent lack of organic nutrient transporters may limit the potential for drug design with respect to carrier mediated transport across the colon, hence drug absorption is a consequence of the general properties and features of the colon. These include transmucosal and membrane potential differences and the bulk water absorption which may allow drug absorption via osmotic solvent drag.

Animal models suggest that sugars such as sucrose and glucose, and amino acids, are poorly absorbed from the adult colon[63 64], but the relevance to humans has to be demonstrated, since diet has a major effect on colonic physiology and these studies were carried out in the rat and horse. An *in vitro* study of the permeability of the rat colonic mucosa suggests that the colon excludes molecules on the basis of size and charge[65]. It has been calculated that the pore size is 2.3Å in the human colon compared to 8Å in the jejunum and 4Å in the ileum[66].

The dissociation of a drug at the absorption site will depend on the pH of the microclimate at the mucosal wall and not the pH of the bulk phase. It is estimated that the unstirred microclimate near the mucosal wall has a thickness or extent of about 840 μm[67]. The concentration of K^+ is lower in the microclimate than the luminal contents, and it is independent of bulk K^+ concentration.

The fluidity of the caecal and ascending colon is gradually reduced as the water is reabsorbed. The reduction in the water content means that there is less mixing in the bulk phase and therefore less access to the mucosal surface, along with less water available for drug dissolution. Gas bubbles present in the colon also will reduce contact of drug with the mucosa.

Some viscous soluble dietary fibres may increase the thickness of the unstirred water layer by reducing intraluminal mixing[68]. Dietary fibres such as pectin and chitosan have cation-exchange properties which may bind drug molecules. These physical factors will all act to slow drug absorption in the colon, with increasing effect as water is removed and the transport properties of the faecal mass are reduced.

DRUG DELIVERY

A wide range of colonic transit times must be taken into consideration during the design of drug delivery systems. Rapid transit will allow little time for the drug to be released before the dosage form is excreted, whilst prolonged colonic residence may result in the accumulation of drug from multiple doses.

After the hepatic flexure, the consolidation of faecal matter gradually increases the viscosity of the luminal contents. This results in increasing difficulty of drug diffusion to the absorbing membrane. Only the ascending colon is sufficiently fluid to present a favourable environment for drug absorption. Absorption of even the most water-soluble drugs is reduced after the mid-transverse colon, due to the lack of water. For example, ciprofloxacin demonstrates a clear reduction in drug uptake with a more distal delivery[69]. On rare occa-

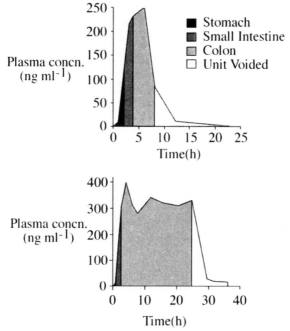

*Figure 7.5 Plasma concentration-time profiles for oxprenolol delivered from an Oros®
device in an individual with a short (top diagram) and long (bottom diagram) colon
transit time*

sions, drug absorption can be seen from the distal regions due to the drug affecting the
fluidity of the contents of the transverse and descending colon.

Current knowledge suggests that it is possible to optimise delivery systems for topical release of drugs to the colon, since transit through the small intestine is relatively predictable and independent of diet. The major problems for colonic absorption are reduced
surface area, wider lumen, sluggish movement, low volume of available dissolution fluid
and the reduced permeability of the colonic epithelium to polar compounds. Thus it would
be expected that the absorption of most drugs from the colon would be slower than from the
small intestine. This is balanced by the slower transit through the colon. The potential of
the colon as an area for drug absorption is illustrated in Figure 7.5, which shows the plasma
concentration-time profiles of oxprenolol delivered in an Oros® device for two individuals
with differing colonic transit times. The effect of the extended colon residence on the
plasma drug concentration is clearly illustrated. An additional advantage for colonic delivery may lie in the much lower activity of proteinases in the colon, which is 20 – 60 fold less
than in the small intestine, suggesting that absorption of labile peptides might be possible.
Achieving therapeutically relevant doses of proteins and peptides when administered via
the colon still remains a major challenge.

Transit

The data available concerning movement of material through the colon was previously confined to measurements of whole gut transit time, However, gamma scintigraphy
now enables transit to be followed in each section of the colon (Table 7.3).

Table 7.3 Colonic transit of single unit dose forms

Time of dosing	Morning	Morning	Morning	Evening
	Fasted	Light Breakfast	Heavy Breakfast	
Ascending colon	3.6 ± 1.2	2.48 ± 1.45	4.8 ± 3.9	8.9 ± 4.34
Transverse colon	5.8 ± 2.9	-	-	11.25 ± 3.24

There is a large variability in the data, but in general, units administered prior to retiring for the night have a slower colonic transit than those dosed in the morning, which is in keeping with the suppressed electrical and contractile activity[70-73], and decreased tone in the colon overnight[74]. There are conflicting values in the literature for the average transit time from caecum to splenic flexure; in one study it was reported to be 14 hours[31]; however another study reported that 50% of large units reach the splenic flexure within 7 hours of entering the colon, and the size and density of such units had little effect on the transit times[75]. Steady state experiments, conducted by repeated daily administrations of technetium-99m labelled resin, demonstrate that the transverse colon remains relatively empty during the day.

Studies examining the transit of different sized particles through the colon have suggested that large objects move more rapidly than smaller ones. In a study on a limited number of healthy volunteers (n=6), a pressure sensitive radiotelemetry device (25 x 9 mm) was seen to move ahead of dispersed pellets (0.5-1.8 mm) in the ascending and transverse colon (Figure 7.6)[76]. Similarly a tendency for transit rates to increase with increasing unit volume (0.3 to 0.8 to 1.8 cm[3]) has also been demonstrated[75]. Differential transit rates have also been noted between 0.5-1.8 mm pellets and 6 mm plastic markers[77]. In contrast, others have found no difference in the passage of 0.2mm and 5mm particles[78] or between 0.2mm,

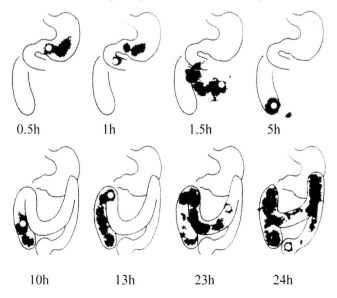

| 0.5h | 1h | 1.5h | 5h |

| 10h | 13h | 23h | 24h |

Figure 7.6 Transit of a large non-disintegrating unit and pellets through the gastrointestinal tract - a scintigraphic study

5mm, and 8.4mm particles[79] through the ascending colon. Interestingly, in this latter study, there was a trend towards a shorter residence time within the ascending colon for 0.2mm compared to 5mm particles, which became significant following laxative administration. Selective retention of small particles is known as colonic sieving and may be important in drug delivery, although the upper cut-off size limit for retention of particles has yet to be established. The sieving behaviour in disorders such as ulcerative colitis, where the degree of haustration is reduced, may influence the upper size limit for retention.

If units become too large, they can have prolonged transit due to periods of stasis at the ileo-caecal junction, hepatic and splenic flexures. Care should be taken when using large rigid units to study drug absorption from the colon, since an unphysiologically long colonic transit time would suggest an erroneously long time for drug absorption. The absorption times would then be significantly reduced when the drug was administered in a more normally sized dosage form.

The sieving effect causes dispersible dosage forms such as pellets to become widely distributed in the colon, whilst large single units or fragments of tablets travel rapidly through the colon ahead of the smaller pellets (Figure 7.7). This phenomenon is related to the observation that batches of markers of increasing sizes given with successive meals become interdispersed within the large intestine[80] which could be explained by the larger particles moving fastest. In the descending colon, the particles come together before defaecation. This data suggests that optimisation of drug delivery to the proximal colon may be achieved with a multiparticulate preparation which remains intact for approximately the first 5 hours after administration to the fasted patient. This would allow time for gastric emptying and transit through the small intestine. The drug preparation should then disperse allowing release of the material over the following 10 to 12 hours in the ascending and transverse colon. Extending the release profile over a longer period would not be an added advantage due to the variability of excretion patterns and the slower diffusion through consolidating faecal material.

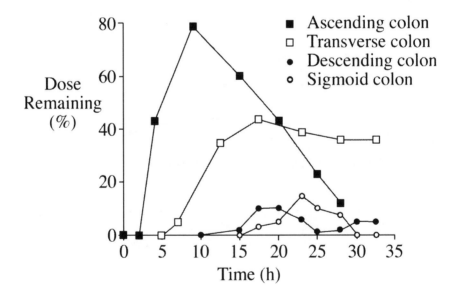

Figure 7.7 Distribution of pellets within the colon following pulse release at the ileocaecal junction

Dietary factors

Diet, in particular dietary fibre, could play a significant role in the absorption of drugs from the colon. Individuals ingesting a vegetarian diet or taking stool bulking agents may possibly show a difference in colonic drug absorption when compared with individuals ingesting a relatively low fibre diet. However, increased dietary fibre leads to decreased gastrointestinal transit times, which may offset any absorptive benefit gained by increasing the mucosal surface area in the colon[81]. Since fibre alters the transit through the colon it would be expected to have the greatest influence on the absorption of drugs from sustained release preparations. In young vegetarians the mouth to anus transit of a single unit can be less than 6 hours, indeed, for one "normal" subject, the total transit time was 2 hours (Washington et al, unpublished observation).

Temporal factors

Once-a-day dosing for a sustained release medication is usually taken to mean administration in the morning, and for a typical individual, housekeeper sequences clear the stomach of material by 1100 hours. The formulation would then arrive in the ascending colon by 1300-1400 hours. Intake of a light lunch will increase colonic motility via activation of the gastrocolic reflex. This has the effect of shortening the time of contact with the ascending colon. If the same once-a-day medication is administered between 1600 and 1700 hours, the unit will leave the stomach before the main meal at night and will be in the ascending colon by the time the patient has retired to bed. At night, the motility of the ascending colon will become quiescent. Motility increases in the first 30 minutes after waking, with the initiation of high amplitude contractions. In the majority of the population, this is causes an urge to void, and the colonic activity moves the contents of the proximal region to the distal colon. Consequently, afternoon dosing results in prolonged contact with the proximal colon compared to morning dosing.

Targeting the proximal colon

The proximal colon is relatively inaccessible. Even large volume enemas will only just reach the transverse colon[82]. Any substance administered orally has to pass through the hostile environment of the stomach and through the small intestine where it is likely to be digested and absorbed. Protecting the drug from these factors and releasing it at the base of the ascending colon to optimise colonic exposure has been the subject of much research.

Several approaches have been expored to achieve site specific delivery to the colon. These most commonly include:

  i) utilizing the pH change which occurs on transit from the small to the large intestine[83]
  ii) providing release of a drug after a pre-determined time [84-86]
  iii) colon-targeting lectins[87]
  iv) utilizing degradation mechanisms of bacteria specific to the colon[88 89]

pH

Eudragit and other enteric coatings are widely used to produce acid resistant formulations, and with appropriate control of dissolution time may be reasonably effective in achieving release of drug in the ascending colon. For colonic delivery, Eudragits L and S, which are anionic copolymers of methacrylic acid and methyl methacrylate, have been widely used. These polymers are insoluble at low pH but form salts and dissolve above pH 6 and 7, respectively. Eudragit LI00-55, a copolymer of methacrylic acid and ethyl acrylate, is water soluble which avoids the need for organic solvents in the coating process[90].

The first study which employed Eudragit S for colon-targeting used sulphapyridine as a marker for drug release[84]. Hard gelatin capsules containing the drug, and barium sulphate to aid radiological visualisation, were coated with the polymer and administered to 6 subjects who each swallowed 6 capsules. Twelve hours after administration, 4 capsules had broken in the distal ileum, 23 in the colon and 9 remained intact. The same approach was used with 5-aminosalicylic acid (5-ASA) but the thickness of the polymer coating was reduced from 120 to 80 μm[91]. This formed the basis of the commercial formulation of 5-ASA tablet. There has been at least one report of patients taking 5-ASA and reporting the transit of intact tablets in their stools. This is probably a result of the high pH at which the Eudragit S-based coatings dissolve.

The study of Eudragit S coated tablets (10 mm diameter) in 7 volunteer subjects using gamma scintigraphy yielded some interesting results[92]. In some subjects, stasis at the ileocaecal junction was noted. Other subjects had rapid transit through the colon, leading the authors to speculate whether the variability in transit meant that a pH-based coating was an unreliable means of delivery to the colon.

Recently the potential for pH-sensitive dextran hydrogels to be used as colon-specific delivery systems has been investigated *in vitro*[93 94].

Time

The constancy of transit of dosage forms through the small intestine has been well established. It has been speculated that if a unit could be timed to release drug around four hours after leaving the stomach, the unit should be at the base of the ascending colon at the time of drug release. Approaches to achieve targeted colonic delivery based on hydrogel technology, exemplified by the Pulsincap™ delivery system (Figure 7.8), appear to largely succeed. The Pulsincap comprises an impermeable capsule body containing the drug formulation, sealed at the neck edge with a hydrogel polymer plug[95]. On ingestion, the capsule becomes exposed to gastric fluids and the water soluble gelatin cap dissolves, allowing the hydrogel plug to hydrate. At a pre-determined and controlled time point after ingestion, the swollen plug is ejected from the capsule body thereby enabling the drug formulation to be released. The time of plug ejection is controlled by the length of the hydrogel plug and its position relative to the neck of the capsule body.

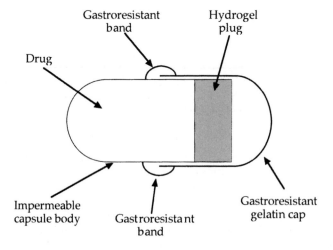

Figure 7.8 Enteric-coated Pulsincap™ dosage form

Other devices employing time-dependent erosion have been utilized; for example a system termed the 'Time Clock' is composed of a solid core coated with a mixture of hydrophobic material (waxes), surfactant, and water-soluble polymer (HPMC). The coating is designed to slowly erode away and after a predetermined interval the drug is released. Another approach is to use a dosage form coated with an outer enteric polymer and an inner layer of HPMC. The outer layer dissolves exposing the inner layer of HPMC, which gels and slowly erodes away. When erosion has reached a critical level, the drug is released from the inner core of the dosage form.

Finally, a variant of the osmotic pump has been patented which provides colon-specific drug delivery. The enteric-coated pump is activated on leaving the stomach. A drug-free layer adjacent to the delivery port exhausts over the first 3-4 hr following activation. The units then begin to release drug within the colon.

Bioadhesives

Lectins from fruits and vegetables have emerged as possible candidates for site-specific bioadhesion. They are readily available and, with the exception of kidney bean lectin, are considered non-toxic. The majority of studies have been conducted with lectins from *Lycopersicon esculentum*, the tomato, since these are resistant to intraluminal digestion and do not change the integrity of the cell upon binding[96]. Lectins show potential for uptake by endocytosis; however the amount that reaches the blood stream is minimal as they may accumulate in the interior of the cell. The specificity of lectin-based systems to target the colon has yet to be demonstrated.

Bacterially triggered systems

Sulphasalazine (salicylazosulphapyridine) was one of the earliest prodrugs used in the treatment of inflammatory bowel disease. It contains 5-aminosalicyclic acid (mesalazine) linked covalently to sulphapyridine. 5-aminosalicyclic acid (5-ASA) is not effective orally because it is poorly absorbed, and is inactivated before reaching the lower intestine; therefore prior to its administration as a prodrug, its was only effective when given as a suppository or a rectal suspension enema. The prodrug sulphasalazine is similarly poorly absorbed after oral administration, but it is reduced to its active components by bacterial azoreductase in the colon. Additional prodrugs which rely on bacterial activation have also been introduced, including olsalazine (sodium azodisalicylate, a dimer of 5-aminosalicylate linked by an azo bond), ipsalazine (5-ASA:p-aminohippurate) and balsalazine (5-ASA:4-amino benzoylglycine) (Figure 7.9).

Bacterial metabolism includes enzymatic systems unique to a small region of the bowel, the most widely investigated being the bacterial azoreductase system, and several polymers have been devised which should be degraded by these enzymes. Hydrogels based on acrylic acid, N,N-dimethylacrylamide and N-terbutyl-acrylamide cross-linked with azo-aromatic groups show pH-dependent swelling. At low pH the polymer does not swell. As it passes out of the stomach into the higher pH of the small intestine swelling occurs and, on reaching the colon, the hydrogel becomes sufficiently swollen to allow access to bacterial azoreductase. However, *in vitro* studies suggest that the polymer swelling is too slow to be successful *in vivo*. Alternative approaches have been described using azo-polymers containing different ratios of methylmethacrylate and hydroxyethyl methacrylate (HEMA)[97 98]. Hydrophilic polymers, those with a high HEMA content, showed the greatest susceptibility to colonic degradation. It was concluded that a balance needed to be achieved between hydrophilicity, to ensure effective reduction, and hydrophobicity, to provide adequate resistance to gastric and intestinal fluid. Early data suggested that oral delivery of peptides

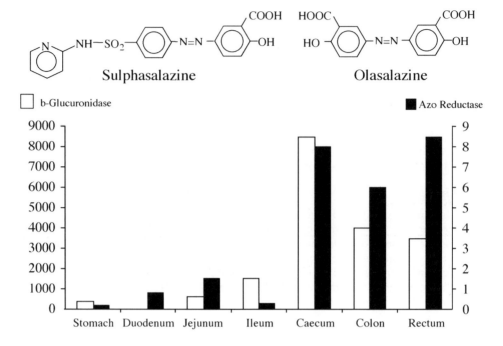

Figure 7.9 Azo prodrugs and enzyme activity in the gastrointestinal tract

such as vasopressin and even insulin was possible using these polymers to protect the peptide[99]although later investigations with these materials were less successful.

Concentrated senna extract contains anthracene derivatives in the form of glycosides which can be hydrolysed to anthraquinones, anthranols and oxanthrones. When sennosides are delivered directly to the colon no laxative activity occurs, but incubation of the compound with faeces or *E. coli* liberates free anthraquinones which promote peristalsis. More recently, drug glycosides have been synthesized and tested for their ability to deliver drugs, such as glucocorticosteroids and spasmolytic agents, to the large intestine. Glucuronide prodrugs of the budesonide and menthol have been tested in animal models with promising results[100].

Complex carbohydrates are metabolized by caecal bacteria, hence matrices and coatings based on pectin, guar gum and starch have received extensive study for colon specific delivery systems[101 102]. Guar gum, locust bean gum, tragacanth, and xylan have been mixed with methacrylate copolymers (Eudragit O) and used to coat tablets. The beta-1,4- or alpha-1,6-glycosidic links in locust bean galactomannan and dextran are biodegraded quickly in the human colon, but these carbohydrates are quite water-soluble and they must be transformed into insoluble derivatives[103]. Cyclodextrins are fermented to small saccharides by colonic microflora, whereas they are only slightly hydrolyzable and thus are not easily absorbed in the stomach and small intestine[104].

Pectin and calcium pectate have been evaluated by several groups as colon-specific coatings and matrices[105-107]. Tablets prepared from calcium pectate mixed with indomethacin were compressed into tablets and the release of drug was evaluated *in vitro*[108]. Under controlled conditions, release of indomethacin into pH 7 buffer was minimal (< 10% after 24 h). Adding caecal contents from rats that had been induced to produce pectinolytic enzymes to the dissolution medium resulted in a significant increase in indomethacin re-

Table 7.4 Bacterial metabolism of some drugs

Enzyme	Micro-organism	Example of metabolic reaction
Nitroreductase	*Bacteriodes sp.*	Reduction of aromatic and heterocyclic nitrocompounds
Azoreductase	*Clostridia, lactobaccilli*	Reductive scission of azo-bonds
Sulphoxide reductase	*E. coli*	Removal of oxygen from sulphoxides
Glucosidase	*Strep. Faecalis, eubacteria*	Hydrolysis of β-glycosides
Glucuronidase	*E. coli A. aerogenes*	Hydrolysis of β-gluronides of phenols and alcohols
Sulphatase	*Streptococci, cloistridia*	Cleavage of O-sulphates
Amdases & Esterases	*Enerobacter sp.*	Hydrolysis of amides or esters of carboxylic acids

lease (approximately 60% after 24 h). Similarly, a dissolution experiment in the presence of a bacterium able to hydrolyze pectin resulted in a significant increase in indomethacin release, although the total amount released after 6 h was only about 20%.

Bacterial degradation of drug

Once a drug has been released into the colonic lumen it is possible for it to be metabolised by colonic bacteria, which may result in the release of toxic products or the metabolism of the active drug to an inactive metabolite. For example, the bioavailability of digoxin from a delayed release formulation is reduced when compared with its bioavailability from conventional formulations, due to its degradation by colonic bacteria to the inactive dihydro-digoxin[109].

Drugs such as stilboestrol, morphine and indomethacin are excreted in the bile as inactive sulphate or glucuronic acid conjugates. These conjugates are metabolized by bacterial enzymes (Table 7.4) to release the active form of the drug, which can then be reabsorbed and prolong pharmacological action.

Effect of disease and co-medication on colonic drug absorption

Gastrointestinal diseases are known to have a significant effect on the absorption of some orally administered drugs. Enteric coated formulations designed for release in the colon have been shown to release their contents in the stomach of achlorhydric patients. Such patients may have bacterial overgrowth in the small intestine which could lead to the premature release of drugs such as sulphasalazine or sennosides, thus rendering the therapy ineffective, as the drug would be absorbed before reaching the colon.

Increased permeability of the mucosal lining, allowing entry of microbial or dietary antigens, has been proposed as a possible cause in the pathophysiology of chronic inflammatory bowel disease. Interestingly, in Crohn's disease of the colon, there is abnormal permeability in apparently uninvolved proximal small intestine as well as in the colon[110]. Patients with Crohn's disease are subject to gastrointestinal strictures where a controlled release matrix may lodge and cause epithelial damage due to the release of concentrated drug at one site over a prolonged period of time[111].

Normal subjects have rapid diffuse spread of water soluble radioisotopes through the colon, with the majority of activity being lost to faeces after 24 h[112]. In patients with intractable constipation, some will show normal transit, but in those with colonic inertia the major site of isotope hold-up is the transverse colon and splenic flexure. Other constipated patients show delay of label at a later stage and accumulation of activity in the descending and rectosigmoid colon. Diarrhoea causes changes in the electrolyte and water content of the colonic lumen which therefore alters luminal pH, resulting in changes in the rate of absorption of drugs from the lumen. As a result the effectiveness of colonic delivery may be unpredictable in patients with constipation or diarrhoea. The increased rate of transit would also be responsible for the premature voiding of sustained release formulations, and would also be expected to alter the sieving function of the colon. Diarrhoeal diseases are known to cause decreased gut transit time, and hence incomplete metabolism, of pro-drugs such as sulphasalazine. To date, however, little detailed information exists in the literature concerning the effect of motility disorders on colonic delivery.

RECTAL ADMINISTRATION OF DRUGS

The rectal route of drug administration offers several advantages, including
a) a relatively large dosage form can be accommodated in the rectum
b) the rectal route is safe and convenient for elderly and young patients
c) drug dilution is minimized as the residual fluid volume is low
d) the rectum is generally empty
e) absorption adjuvants have a more pronounced effect than in the upper gastrointestinal tract
f) degradative enzymes in the rectal lumen are at relatively low concentrations
g) therapy can easily be discontinued
h) first-pass elimination of drug by the liver is partly avoided

The rectal route is often used when administration of dosage forms by mouth is inappropriate, for example, in the presence of nausea and vomiting, in unconscious patients, if upper gastrointestinal disease is present which could affect the absorption of the drug, or if the drug is unpleasant tasting or acid-labile.

Drug absorption and avoidance of first-pass metabolism

Several factors have to be overcome for a drug to be absorbed after rectal administration. If the drug is administered as a suppository, melting or liquefaction of the base has to occur and the degree of this will partly determine the spreading of the dose through the rectum. The drug must then dissolve in the limited rectal fluid available, which has been estimated to be between 1 and 3 ml. The amount of drug available for absorption can be further reduced by degradation by luminal contents, adsorption to luminal contents and defaecation. The drug must then diffuse across the unstirred water and mucous layers adjacent to the epithelium.

Drugs may be absorbed across the epithelial cell or via tight junctions, and it is believed that only passive transport occurs. Venous return from the colon and upper rectum is via the portal vein to the liver. If a drug is delivered to the upper part of the rectum, it is transported into the portal system (Figure 7.10), and is therefore subject to first pass metabolism in the liver. The only way of avoiding first-pass metabolism is to deliver the drug to the lower part of the rectum. This simple principle is complicated by the presence of anastomoses which do not allow a precise definition of the areas which drain to the portal and systemic circulation. A 100% increase in the availability of lignocaine was demonstrated when administered rectally rather than orally, and it was calculated that the mean fraction of the rectally administered dose escaping first-pass metabolism was 57%[113]. Other drugs with high first pass metabolism, such as salicylamide and propranolol, did not demonstrate as large an increase in bioavailability when administered rectally. However, this may be due to incomplete absorption since these drugs exhibited a much larger bioavailability when administered rectally rather than orally to rats[114].

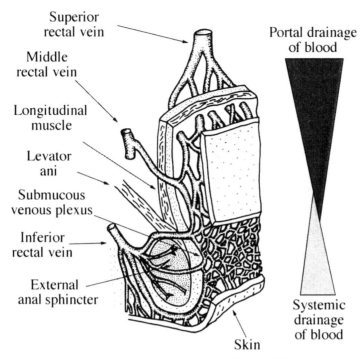

Figure 7.10 Structure and perfusion of the rectum

Dosage forms for rectal delivery

Drugs can be administered in several formulations via the rectal route. Suppositories are normally either solid suspensions or solid emulsions, whereas rectally administered gelatin capsules can contain liquid formulations. Micro-enemas have a volume of between 1 and 20 ml, and macro enemas 50 ml or more, both of which may be administered as either solutions or suspensions. The suspension suppository is the most widely used formulation, and it has been demonstrated that the release characteristics are dependent upon physiological factors, physicochemical properties of the drug, the suppository base and local environment within the rectum. In general, aqueous solutions of drugs are absorbed more quickly from the rectal route than the oral route, but absorption is usually slower with non-aqueous formulations, due to the limited amount of water available for drug dissolution.

There has been some work exploring the use of controlled release to the rectum, to achieve prolonged and sustained drug delivery. The studies were performed using an osmotically driven device with zero-order release characteristics. It appears to be a promising delivery system for drugs such as nifedipine which effectively reduced blood pressure without the unwanted side effect of increased heart rate[115]. Hydrogel systems with near zero-order delivery have also been used to deliver morphine intrarectally[116].

Adjuvants and enhancers

Transport from the rectal epithelium primarily involves two transport processes: paracellular and transcellular routes. As in other parts of the gut, the opening of tight junctions by absorption enhancers has been extensively investigated. Putative enhancers include enamine derivatives, salicylates, calmodulin inhibitors, surfactants, chelating agents, fatty acids and lectins. It is generally agreed that the rectum is potentially an important

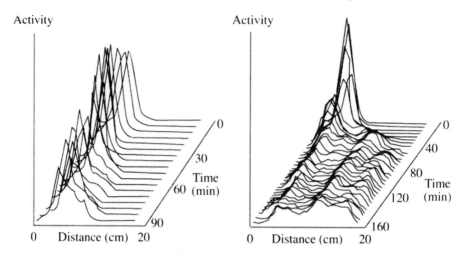

Figure 7.11 Spreading of a Witepsol suppository expressed as activity-distance plots as a function of time without (left) and with neostigmine (right)

route for peptide absorption, although enhancers would be required to increase flux through this region. For example, bioavailability of a small peptide such as vasopressin is increased to nearly 30% in the presence of sodium taurodihydrofusidate. It should always be borne in mind that the enhancement via the paracellular route is non-selective, with the risk of absorption of bacterial endotoxins caused by lysis of bacterial cell walls.

Spreading of rectal dosage forms

In order to treat the colon via the rectal route, rather than simply aiming for rectal absorption, the preparation must spread efficiently. This limits topical treatment of the colon to areas distal to the splenic flexure. A number of attempts have been made to increase penetration through the use of novel formulations, using scintigraphy to evaluate the distribution of the formulation.

Tukker et al studied the spreading of suppositories and the effect of added surfactant (Witepsol H-15) in recumbent dogs[117]. The addition of surfactants markedly increased the penetration into the colon. Similarly pre-administration of neostigmine, which increases colonic motility, markedly increased the spreading of the suppository (Figure 7.11).

The spreading behaviour of suppository bases and incorporated suspensions has also been studied in humans[118]. The bases, Witepsol H15 and Labrafil WL2514 were labelled by the incorporation of small amounts of iodine-123 labelled oily markers (arachis oil and Labrafil WL2700 respectively). The suspension consisted of micronized cationic exchange resin incorporated throughout the base at a disperse phase loading of 10% w/v. Most of the spreading of both base and suspension occurred in the first hour after administration, and the area of spreading was small, with a maximum of 8 to 10 cm. The time from defaecation to administration of the suppository appeared to affect the degree of spreading, with the greatest spreading occurring when defaecation occurred immediately prior to dosing[119].

Disease activity in ulcerative colitis had no effect on the spreading behaviour of different volumes of mesalazine enemas, but the adminstered volume had a significant effect[120]. A 30 ml enema remained mainly in the sigmoid colon (99%), a 60 ml enema was distributed through the rectum (9%), the sigmoid (61%) and the descending colon (15%) and a 100 ml enema was distributed between the sigmoid (66%) and descending colon

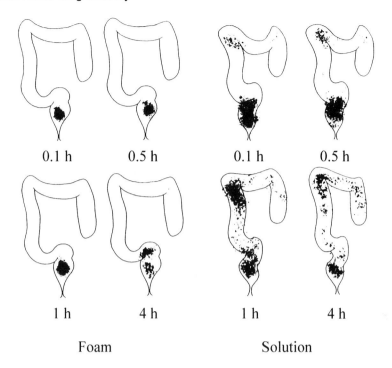

0.1 h   0.5 h   0.1 h   0.5 h

1 h   4 h   1 h   4 h

Foam   Solution

Figure 7.12 Spreading of liquid and foam enema after rectal administration

(25%). Consequently it appears that increasing the administered volume causes the dose to spread more effectively into the colon.

In an attempt to increase the penetration of small volumes of liquid, foam enemas have been studied[121]. However retrograde spreading of foams was lower than solution enemas, being limited to the sigmoid colon (Figure 7.12).

Therapeutic agents administered rectally

Anticonvulsants

Traditionally the need for rapid attainment of a therapeutic blood concentration of a drug has meant that intravenous drug delivery has been the only method available for the treatment of status epilepticus or serial seizures. However, the technical problems associated with intravenous administration have prompted the evaluation of rectal dosage forms as a practical alternative.

Diazepam is rapidly absorbed from rectally delivered solution in propylene glycol-water-ethanol in healthy volunteers[122]. Suppository formulations of diazepam appear to be effective and safe in the prevention of recurrent febrile convulsions in children, suggesting that formulations with non-instantaneous release may be adequate for prophylactic therapy[123]. In adult epileptic patients, 10mg of diazepam in 2ml of an intravenous solution was administered rectally, and this resulted in serum concentrations comparable with those obtained after oral administration of a 10mg tablet; absolute rectal bioavailability amounted to 81%[124]. 'Valium' suppositories however have a bioavailability of just less than 70%, but have a very slow rate of absorption, with a T_{max} ranging from 90 to 480 mins[125].

Clonazepam, rectally administered as a suspension in 2.2 to 3.8ml of a propylene glycol-water mixture, also containing acetic acid, ethanol and benzylalcohol (Rivotril) demonstrated rapid absorption. However, the intersubject variability was substantial. Sodium valproate is completely, although not rapidly, absorbed from an aqueous microenema (T_{max} = 2.2h) in healthy volunteers, whereas the absorption from a Witepsol H15 suppository was lower (T_{max} = 3.3h, bioavailability 89%). The rectal bioavailability of sodium valproate appears to be better than that of enteric coated tablets which are erratically absorbed.

Rectal absorption of phenobarbital and its sodium salt from aqueous microenemas and suppositories is relatively slow[126]. The sodium salt, dissolved in a vehicle containing 10% alcohol and 75% propylene glycol, resulted in a rectal bioavailability of 90% relative to intramuscular administration. However, rectal absorption was delayed compared to intramuscular delivery (T_{max} = 4.4 h compared to 2.1 h). Consequently, this formulation could be considered as an alternative to intramuscular injection, but is not appropriate for the treatment of status epilepticus.

An aqueous suspension of carbamazepine, which also contained propylene glycol, sorbitol and sucrose, resulted in slow absorption of carbamazepine at a dose of 400 to 600mg, with a mean T_{max} of 6.3 h and C_{max} of 5.1 mg.L^{-1}. This can probably be explained by the poor water solubility of the compound. The bioavailability was 80% and 67% relative to oral tablets and oral suspensions respectively. Hence the rectal suspension was useful in maintaining administration in case of interrupted oral therapy. Unfortunately it was highly irritant, indicating the need to optimise the formulation[127]. An aqueous suspension of 200 mg of carbamazepine containing 30% sorbitol showed a rectal bioavailability of 80% relative to the same suspension delivered orally[128]. However, this formulation was difficult to retain, possibly because of a laxative effect of sorbitol.

Preoperative medication and induction of anaesthesia

Preoperative medication is usually administered parenterally; however a more acceptable delivery route, particularly for children, is being sought. Rectal administration of midazolam produced a satisfactory sedative action 30 minutes after administration in children[129]. Rectal instillation of a solution of midazolam hydrochloride (5 g.L^{-1}: 0.3 mg.kg^{-1}) in healthy volunteers produced a bioavailability of about 50%, however metabolic studies suggested that complete rectal absorption of the parent drug had occurred with substantial first-pass metabolism[130]. Absorption was rapid, the mean T_{max} being 31 min and C_{max} reaching 120 µg.L^{-1}.

Diazepam may also be used for preoperative medication. In adult patients, one study reported that premedication with a rectal diazepam solution was considered less effective than oral dosing. However the oral dose used was 50% higher than the rectal dose (15 vs. 10 mg)[131]. Rectally administered diazepam has been used in children for sedation for dental operations[132].

The use of rectal methohexital to induce anaesthesia in children has received considerable interest in recent literature. In children aged between 2 and 7 years, anaesthesia was induced with rectal administration of 15 mg.kg^{-1} of methohexital solution. Peak plasma concentrations ranged between 1 and 6 mg.L^{-1} and were reached in 7 to 15 min. indicating very rapid absorption[133]. Although the bioavailability ranged between 8 and 32%, satisfactory induction of anaesthesia was reached in 90% of children. It has been suggested that the variability in methohexital plasma levels is due the depth to which the drug is inserted, thereby altering the amount of drug which avoids first-pass metabolism. No clear correlation exists between rectal pH and absorption, suggesting that the variability in the extent of first-pass metabolism has a greater effect than the effect of luminal pH on drug uptake[134].

Atropine is administered prior to inhalation anaesthetics to reduce salivation and the production of bronchopulmonary secretions. Absorption from a rectal saline solution was slower and less complete than with intramuscular administration[135]. Atropine sulphate in a HPMC base had a bioavailability of approximately 30%, but absorption was fast, reaching a T_{max} after 15 minutes[136].

Analgesics and antiarthritics

Oral administration of narcotic analgesics in the treatment of postoperative and cancer pain is often limited by nausea and vomiting, or poor patient condition. Studies indicate that rectally administered morphine has a variable bioavailability compared to an intramuscular injection, 30-70% when administered in a starch-containing gel and 40-88% from a hard fatty suppository. Increasing the pH of a rectal morphine microenema from 4.5 to 7.4 significantly increased the extent of absorption[137]. Hydrogels have also been used to successfully deliver morphine, producing a lower and more sustained plasma concentration than intramuscular morphine given on demand[116].

Methadone administered rectally has a similar rate of uptake to an oral solution, but with a lower bioavailability. The use of the solvent glycofurol increased the rate and extent of absorption of methadone from a microenema (Figure 7.13)[138].

Rectal absorption of acetylsalicylic acid is strongly dependent upon the type of formulation in which it is administered, with an aqueous microenema (20 ml at pH 4) giving the best results. In contrast, the pH of the paracetamol microenema was unimportant. Paracetamol is well absorbed when administered intrarectally, although absorption is slower than from an oral solution.

Indomethacin is rapidly absorbed when delivered rectally, however the bioavailability is less than from oral capsules and there is great intersubject variation. Naproxen, ibuprofen and ketoprofen are all well absorbed when rectally delivered.

Diflunisal (Figure 7.14) had a bioavailability of 55% as a rectal suspension, but this could be inproved to 70-80% by either using a cosolvent (glycofural) or by buffering the pH

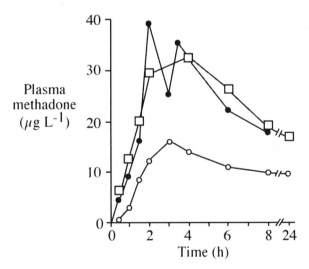

Figure 7.13 Plasma concentration of methadone after oral solution (●), Witepsol H-15 suppository (○) and PEG 1540 suppository (□)

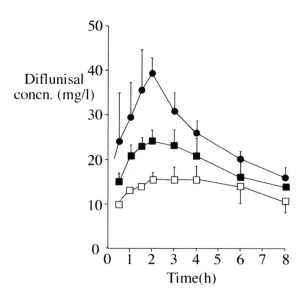

Figure 7.14 Plasma concentration versus time curves of 250 mg diflunisal after oral administration as a suspension in water (●) and after rectal administration in methylcellulose solution at pH 4.5 (□) and 7 (■)

to 7.0. Control of pH appears to be important to optimize the solubility of a number of drugs; for example codeine, when delivered in solution at pH 9, produced better absorption than at pH 4.3[139]. When delivered in 'Witepsol' H15, codeine phosphate can exhibit a plasma concentration profile almost identical to the oral formulation[140].

Natural or hydrogenated soya lecithin added to diclofenac suppositories prolonged absorption from about 1 h to 6 h in healthy volunteers, without affecting the extent of absorption[141]. Interestingly, this study reported that absorption was not affected by defaecation.

Antiemetics

Orally administered antiemetics suffer from quite obvious drawbacks and hence rectal administration of alizapride, promethazine and metoclopramide have been investigated. Rectal administration of alizapride as a suppository in an unspecified base resulted in a mean bioavailability of 61% relative to an intravenous bolus dose[142]. Both alizapride and promethazine have considerably slower absorption profiles from rectal administration compared to either oral or intramuscular administration. In addition, promethazine produces significant rectal irritation.

In human subjects, an aqueous microenema containing metoclopramide resulted in rapid absorption and complete absolute bioavailability. Another advantage of delivering metoclopramide rectally is that when given orally, it undergoes extensive first-pass metabolism.

Antibacterial agents

Metronidazole is used extensively in the prophylaxis and treatment of anaerobic infections. For practical and economical reasons, attempts have been made to develop rectal metronidazole formulations. It is absorbed rapidly but incompletely from aqueous suspension formulations.

Ampicillin is poorly absorbed from the rectum and despite many formulation attempts, currently the problem has not been overcome. In addition the drug can produce mucosal irritation and diarrhoea.

Xanthines

Theophylline absorption from a rectal solution is similar to absorption from oral solutions, and generally occurs rapidly and completely. However, absorption from suppositories may be variable and incomplete. Interestingly, theophylline was well absorbed when delivered in a rectal osmotic delivery device, despite the fact that the level of water available in the rectum is very low[143].

The absorption of enprofylline, a bronchodilating xanthine drug which is poorly metabolised, shows somewhat slow absorption from rectal administration of an aqueous solution compared with oral intake. Oral absorption was complete, whereas urinary data indicated an absolute rectal bioavailability of about 89%[144].

Drugs in inflammatory bowel disease

Mesalazine is the locally active moiety of sulphasalazine used in the treatment of inflammatory bowel disease. It is liberated from the orally administered parent drug in the colon by bacterial splitting of an azo bond. It is frequently delivered by enema, particularly in patients with ulcerative colitis of the distal colon. As the adverse effects of oral sulphasalazine are ascribed to the sulphapyridine moiety, colon specific formulations have been developed which have low systemic bioavailability without the sulphapyridine group.

Rectal instillation of corticosteroids is a well-established approach for the treatment of inflammatory bowel disease. Corticosteroids which show high efficacy and low systemic drug concentrations are preferred, in order to minimise adrenal suppression and other adverse effects inherent in steroid therapy. Rectal prednisolone, budesonide, tixocortol pivalate and beclomethasone diproprionate appear to interfere less with adrenocortical function than hydrocortisone acetate, prednisolone-2l-phosphate and betamethasone. In clinical practice, steroid enemas prove to be difficult to retain because of their large volume, and hence foams are used.

Cardiovascular active drugs

Rate-controlled rectal drug delivery of nifedipine by an osmotic delivery device in healthy volunteers resulted in a steady-state plasma concentration, with the low input rate resulting in a lowering of blood pressure without concurrent reflex tachycardia.

Rectal irritation and damage

Long term rectal application of drugs has been reported to produce irritation, rectal bleeding pain and even ulceration. Ergotamine tartrate suppositories used at a dose range of 1.5 to 9 mg over a period of between 1 and 8 years can produce rectal damage, probably due to mucosal ischaemia produced by the alkaloid[145].

Rectal ulceration and stenoses have also been reported in patients using suppositories containing dextropropoxyphene[146], paracetamol, aspirin, caffeine, carbromal, bromisoval and codeine phosphate[147]. Rectal damage only appears to occur after long term daily suppository use and aspirin, ergotamine and paracetamol appear to cause the most common problems.

Local irritation can be elicited by rectal application of various drug in humans, for example oxprenolol solution, diazepam preparations, promethazine suppositories and carbamazepine suspension, hence tolerability represents an important consideration in the development of rectal formulations. Interestingly, epithelial cell loss and local inflammatory reactions have been observed after administration of plain suppository bases, e.g. Suppocire AP, Witepsol H12, H15 and H19, and polyethylene glycols in rats[148 149]. However, since these materials are well accepted in clinical practice, the occurrence of mucosal damage does not necessarily preclude their use in humans, if the damage is reversible.

CONCLUSIONS

Reliable delivery of drugs to the proximal colon is one of the key areas of research in drug delivery at the present time. It is hampered by the relative inaccessibility and the difficulty in producing *in vitro* models which mimic the environment of the colon. Results from the studies of sustained release dosage forms using pharmacokinetic and scintigraphic techniques indicate that, for once a day dosing to be successful, the drug must be absorbed from the ascending colon to maintain therapeutic levels.

Oral dosing is the preferred route of administration for drug delivery to the proximal colon. Consequently the design of peroral controlled-release dosage forms has to take into account a plethora of factors which may influence the transit of the delivery system and the consequent degree of drug absorption.

REFERENCES

1.   Filipe MI. Mucins in the gastrointestinal epithelium: a review. *Invest. Cell Pathol.* 1979;2:195-216.
2.   Ehsanullah M, Filipe MI, Gazzard B. Mucin secretion in inflammatory bowel disease; correlation with disease activity and dysplasia. *Gut* 1982;23:485-489.
3.   Rhodes JM, Gallimore R, Elias E, Kennedy JF. Faecal sulphatase in health and in inflammatory bowel disease. *Gut* 1985;26:466-469.
4.   Kvietys PR, Granger DN. Regulation of colonic blood flow. *Fed. Proc.* 1982;41:2100-2110.
5.   Grandison AS, Yatres J, Shields R. Capillary blood flow in the canine colon and other organs at normal and raised portal pressure. *Gut* 1981;22:223-227.
6.   Glick ME, Meshkinpour H, Haldeman S, Bhatia NN, Bradley WE. Colonic dysfunction in multiple sclerosis. *Gastroenterol.* 1982;83:1002-1007.
7.   Braaten B, Madara JL, Donowitz M. Age related loss of non-goblet cells parallels decreased secretion in rat descending colon. *Am. J. Physiol.* 1988;255:G72-G84.
8.   Debongie JC, Phillips SF. Capacity of the human colon to absorb fluid. *Gastroenterol.* 1978;74:698-703.
9.   Palma R, Vidon N, Bernier JJ. Maximal capacity for fluid absorption in human bowel. *Dig. Dis. Sci.* 1981;26:929-934.
10. Evans DF, Pye G, Bramley R, Clark AG, Dyson TJ, Hardcastle JD. Measurement of gastrointestinal pH profiles in normal, ambulant human subjects. *Gut* 1988;29:1035-1041.
11. Gilbert J, Kelleher J, Littlewood JM, Evans DG. Ileal pH in cystic fibrosis. *Scand. J. Gastroenterol.* 1988;23(Suppl. 43):132-134.
12. Spiller RC, Brown ML, Phillips SF. Decreased fluid tolerance, accelerated transit and abnormal motility of the human colon induced by oleic acid. *Gastroenterol.* 1986;91:100-107.
13. Granger DN, Barrowman JA, Kvietys PR. Clinical Gastrointestinal Physiology. W.B. Saunders Company, Philadelphia 1985.
14. Christensen J, Caprilli R, Lund GF. Electrical slow waves in the circular muscle of cat colon. *Am. J. Physiol.* 1969;217:771-776.
15. Christensen J, Anuras S, Hauser RL. Migrating spike bursts and electrical slow waves in the cat colon: effect of sectioning. *Gastroenterol.* 1974;66:240-247.
16. Christensen J, Hauser RL. Longitudiinal axial coupling of slow waves in the proximal cat colon. *Am. J. Physiol.* 1971;221:246-250.
17. Devroede G, Soffie M. Colonic absorption in ideopathic constipation. *Gastroenterol.* 1973;64:552-561.

18. Holdstock DJ, Misiewicz JJ. Factors controlling colonic motility: Colonic pressures and transit after meals in patients with total colonic gastrectomy, pernicious anaemia and duodenal ulcer. *Gut* 1970;11:100-110.

19. Wright RA, Snape WJ, Battle W, Cohen S, London RL. Effect of dietary components on the gastrocolic response. *Am. J. Physiol.* 1980;238:G228-G232.

20. Sun EA, Snape WJ, Cohen S, Renny A. The role of opiate receptors and cholinergic neurones in the gastrocolic response. *Gastroenterol.* 1982;82:689-693.

21. Tansy MF, Kendell CsFM. Experimental and clinical aspects of gastrocolic reflexes. *Am. J. Dig. Dis.* 1973;18:521-531.

22. Snape Jr WJ, Matarazzo SA, Cohen S. Effect of eating and gastrointestinal hormones on human colonic myoelectrical and colon activity. *Gastroenterol.* 1978;75:373-378.

23. Vizi SE, Ono K, Adam-Vizi V, Duncalf D, Foldes FF. Presynatic inhibitory effect of met enkephalin on [14C] acetylcholine release from the myenteric plexus and its interaction with muscarinic negative feedback inhibition. *J. Pharmacol. Exp. Ther.* 1984;230:493-499.

24. Jian R, Najean Y, Bernier JJ. Measurement of intestinal progression of a meal and its residues in normal subjects and patients with functional diarrhoea by a dual isotope technique. *Gut* 1984;25:728-731.

25. Moreno-Osset E, Bazzocchi G, Lo S, Trombley B, Ristow E, Reddy SN, et al. Association between postprandial changes in colonic intraluminal pressure and transit. *Gastroenterol.* 1989;96:1265-1273.

26. Bassotti G, Betti C, Imbimbio BP, Pelli MA, Morelli A. Colonic motor response to eating: A manometric investigation in proximal and distal portions of the viscus in man. *Am. J. Gastroenterol.* 1989;84:118-122.

27. Lubowski DZ, Meagher AP, Smart RC, Butler SP. Scintigraphic assessment of colonic function during defecation. *Int. J. Colorect. Dis.* 1995;10:91-93.

28. Davies GJ, Growder M, Reid B, Dickerson JWT. Bowel function measurements of individuals with different eating patterns. *Gut* 1986;27:164-169.

29. Arhan P, Devroede G, Jehannin B, et a. Segmental colonic transit time. *Dis. Colon Rectum* 1981;24:625-629.

30. Wyman JB, Heaton KW, Manning AP. Variability of colonic function in healthy subjects. *Gut* 1978;19:146-150.

31. Metcalf AM, Phillips SF, Zinsmeister AR, MacCarty RL, Beart RW, Wolff BG. Simplified assessment of segmental colonic transit. *Gastroenterol.* 1987;92:40-47.

32. Abrahamsson H, Antov S, Bosaeus I. Gastrointestinal and colonic segmental transit time evaluated by a single abdominal x-ray in healthy subjects and constipated patients. *Scand. J. Gastroenterol.* 1988;23:72-80.

33. Hinds JP, Stoney B, Wald A. Does gender or the menstrual cycle affect colonic transit? *Am. J. Gastroenterol.* 1989;84:123-126.

34. Stephen AM, Wiggins HS, Englyst HN. The effect of age, sex and level of intake of dietary fibre from wheat on large-bowel function in thirty healthy subjects. *Br. J. Nutr.* 1986;56:349-361.

35. Narducci F, Snape WJ, Battle WM, London RL, Cohen S. Increased colonic motility during exposure to a stressful situation. *Dig. Dis. Sci.* 1985;30:40-44.

36. Keeling WF, Martin BJ. Gastrointestinal transit during mild exercise. *J. Appl. Physiol.* 1987;63:978-981.

37. Oettlé GJ. Effect of moderate exercise on bowel habit. *Gut* 1991;32:941-944.

38. Hinton JM, Lennard-Jones JE, Young AC. A new method for studying gut transit times using radio-opaque markers. *Gut* 1969;10:847-857.

39. Kirwan WO, Smith AN. Gastrointestinal transit estimated by an isotope capsule. *Scand. J. Gastroenterol.* 1974;9:763-766.

40. Cummings JH, Branch W, Jenkins DJA, Southgate DAT, Houston H, James WPT. Colonic response to dietary fibre from carrot, cabbage, apple, bran and guar gum. *Lancet* 1978;1:5-9.

41. Tomlin J, Read NW. Comparison of the effects on colonic function caused by feeding rice bran and wheat bran. *Eur. J. Clin. Nutr.* 1988;42:857-861.

42. Tomlin J, Read NW. The relation between bacterial degradation of viscous polysaccharides and stool output in human beings. *Br. J. Nutr.* 1988;60:467-475.

43. Barrow L, Steed KP, Watts PJ, Melia CD, Davies MC, Wilson CG, et al. Scintigraphic demonstration of lactulose-induced accelerated proximal colon transit. *Gastroenterol.* 1991;103:1167-1175.

44. Janne P, Carpenter Y, Willems G. Colonic mucosal atrophy induced by a liquid elemental diet in rats. *Am. J. Dig. Dis.* 1977;22:808-812.

45. Goodlad RA, Wright NA. The effects of the addition of cellulose or kaolin to an elemental diet on intestinal cell proliferation in the mouse. *Br. J. Nutr.* 1983;50:91-98.

46. Goodlad RA, Lenton W, Ghatei MA, Bloom SR, Wright NA. Effects of an elemental diet, inert bulk and different types of dietary fibre on the response of the intestinal epithelium to refeeding in the rat and the relationship to plasma gastrin, enteroglucagon and PYY levels. *Gut* 1987;28:171-180.

47. Findlay JM, Smith AN, Mitchell WD, Anderson AJD, Eastwood MA. Effects of unprocessed bran on colonic function in normal subjects and in diverticular disease. *Lancet* 1974;i(7849):146-149.

48. Kirwan WO, Smith AN, McConnell AA, Mitchell WD, Eastwood MA. Action of different bran preparations on colonic function. *Br. Med. J.* 1974;4:187-189.

49. Fich A, Phillips SF, Hakim NS, Brown ML, Zinsmeister AR. Stimulation of ileal emptying by short-chain fatty acids. *Dig. Dis. Sci.* 1989;34:1516-1520.

50. Pye G, Crompton J, Evans DF, Clarke AG, Hardcastle JD. Effect of dietary fibre supplementation on colonic pH in healthy individuals (abstract). *Gut* 1987:A1328.

51. Brown SR, Cann PA, Read NW. Effect of coffee on distal colon function. *Gut* 1990;31:450-453.

52. Stephen AM, Wiggins HS, Cummings JH. Effect of changing transit time on colonic microbial metabolism in man. *Gut* 1987;28:601-609.

53. O'Brien JD, Thompson DG, McIntyre A, Burnham WR, Walker E. Effect of codeine and loperamide on upper intestinal transit and absorption in normal subjects and patients with postvagotomy diarrhoea. *Gut* 1988;29:312-318.

54. Schiller LR, Davis GR, Santa Ana CA, Morawski SG, Fordtran JS. Studies of the mechanism of the antidiarrheal effect of codeine. *J. Clin. Invest.* 1982;70:999-1008.

55. Schiller LR, Santa Ana CA, Morawski SG, Fordtran JS. Mechanism of the antidiarrheal effect of loperamide. *Gastroenterol.* 1984;86:1475-1480.

56. Kaufman PN, Krevsky B, Malmud LS, Maurer AH, Somers MB, Siegel JA, et al. Role of opiate receptors in the regulation of colonic transit. *Gastroenterol.* 1988;94:1351-1356.

57. Kamath PS, Phillips SF, O'Connor MK, Brown ML, Zinsmeister AR. Colonic capacitance and transit in man: modulation by luminal contents and drugs. *Gut* 1990;31:443-449.

58. Krevsky B, Libster B, Maurer AH, Chase BJ, Fisher RS. Effects of morphine and naloxone on feline colonic transit. *Life Sciences* 1989;44:873-879.

59. Konturek JW, Konturek SJ, Kurek A, Bogdal J, Olesky J, Rovati L. CCK receptor antagonism by loxiglumide and gall bladder contractions in response to cholecystokinin, sham feeding and ordinary feeding in man. *Gut* 1989;30:1136-1142.

60. Corazziari E, Ricci R, Biliotti D, Bontempo I, De'Medici A, Pallotta N, et al. Oral administration of loxiglumide (CCK antagonist) inhibits postprandial gallbladder contraction without affecting gastric emptying. *Dig. Dis. Sci.* 1990;35:50-54.

61. Meyer BM, Werth BA, Beglinger C, Hildebrand P, Jansen J, Zach D, et al. Role of cholecystokinin in regulation of gastrointestinal motor functions. *Lancet* 1989;2(8653):12-15.

62. Mackay M, J. P, J. H. Peptide drug delivery: Colonic and rectal absorption. *Adv. Drug Deliv. Rev.* 1997;28:253-273.

63. Schanker LS. Absorption of drugs from the rat colon. *J. Pharmacol.* 1959;126:283-290.

64. Slade L, Bishop R, Morris JG, Robinson DW. Digestion and absorption of 15N labelled microbial protein in the large intestine of the horse. *Br. J. Vet.* 1971;11:127-130.

65. Kathpalia SC, Favus MJ, Coe JL. Evidence for the size and charge permselectivity of rat ascending colon. Effect of ricinoleate and bile salts on oxalic acid and neutral sugar transport. *J. Clin. Invest.* 1984;74:805-811.

66. Fordtran JS, Restor FC, Ewton MF, Soter N, Kinney J. Permeability characteristics in the human small intestine. *J. Clin. Invest.* 1965;44:1935-1944.

67. McNeil NI, Ling KLE, Wager J. Mucosal surface pH of the large intestine of the rat and of normal and inflamed large intestine in man. *Gut* 1987;28:707-713.

68. Johnson IT, Gee JM. Effect of gel forming food gums on the intestinal unstirred layer and sugar transport *in vitro. Gut* 1981;22:398-403.

69. Staib AH, Beermann D, Harder S, Fuhr U, Liermann D. Absorption differences of ciprofloxacin along the human gastrointestinal tract determined using a remote-control drug delivery device (HF-capsule). *Am. J. Med.* 1989;87:66S-69S.

70. Bassotti G, Gaburri M. Manometric investigation of high-amplitude propagated contractile activity of the human colon. *Am. J. Physiol.* 1988;255:G660-G664.

71. Bassotti G, Betti C, Fusaro C, Morelli A. Colonic high-amplitude propagated contractions (mass movements): repeated 24-h manometric studies in healthy volunteers. *J. Gastrointest. Mot.* 1992;4:187-191.

72. Narducci F, Bassotti G, Gaburri M, Morelli A. Twenty four hour manometric recording of colonic motor activity in healthy man. *Gut* 1987;28:17-25.

73. Frexinos J, Bueno L, Fioramonti J. Diurnal changes in myoelectrical spiking activity of the human colon. *Gastroenterol.* 1985;88:1104-1110.

74. Steadman CJ, Phillips SF, Camilleri M, Haddad AC, Hanson RB. Variation of muscle tone in the human colon. *Gastroenterol.* 1991;101:373-381.

75. Parker G, Wilson CG, Hardy JG. The effect of capsule size and density on the transit through the proximal colon. *J. Pharm. Pharmacol.* 1988;40:376-377.

76. Hardy JG, Wilson CG, Wood E. Drug delivery to the proximal colon. *J. Pharm. Pharmacol.* 1985;37:874-877.

77. Proano M, Camilleri M, Phillips SF, Brown ML, Thomforde GM. Transit of solids through the human colon: regional quantification in the unprepared bowel. *Am. J. Physiol.* 1990;258:G856-G862.

78. Barrow L, Steed KP, Spiller RC, Maskell NA, Brown JK, Watts PJ. Quantitative, noninvasive assessment of antidiarrheal actions of codeine using an experimental model of diarrhea in man. *Dig. Dis. Sci.* 1993;38:996-1003.

79. Watts PJ, Barrow L, Steed KP, Wilson CG, Spiller RC, Melia CD. The transit rate of different-sized model dosage forms through the human colon and the effects of a lactulose-induced catharsis. *Int. J. Pharmaceut.* 1992;87:215-2.

80. Halls J. Bowel shift during normal defaecation. *Proc. Roy. Soc. Med.* 1965;58:859-860.

81. Cummings JH. Constipation, dietary fibre and the control of large bowel function. *Postgrad. Med. J.* 1984;60:811-819.

82. Hardy JG, Lee SW, Clark AG, Raynolds JR. Enema volume and spreading. *Int. J. Pharmaceut.* 1986;31:151-155.

83. Healey JNC. Enteric coatings and delayed release. *In: Drug Delivery to the Gastrointestinal Tract,* Hardy, J.G., Davis, S.S., Wilson, C.G. (eds) Ellis Horwood, Chichester 1989;Chapter 7:83-96.

84. Dew MJ, Hughes PJ, Lee MG, Evans BK, Rhodes J. An oral preparation to release drugs in the human colon. *Br. J. Clin. Pharmacol.* 1982;14:405-408.

85. Wilson CG, Bakhashaee M, Stevens HNE, Perkins AC, Frier M, Blackshaw PE, et al. An evaluation of a gastro-resistant pulsed release delivery system (Pulsincap) in man. *Drug Delivery* 1997;4:201-206.

86. Sangalli ME, Maroni A, Busetti C, Zema L, Giordano F, Gazzaniga A. *In vitro* and *in vivo* evaluation of oral systems for time and site specific delivery of drugs (Chronotopic technology). *Bollettino Chimico Farmaceutico* 1999;138:68-73.

87. Duchene D, Ponchel G. Colonic administration, development of drug delivery systems, contribution of bioadhesion. *STP Pharma Sciences* 1993;3:277-285.
88. Rubinstein A. Microbially controlled drug delivery to the colon. *Biopharm. Drug Disposition* 1990;11:465-487.
89. Van Den Mooter G, Samyn C, Kinget R. Azo polymers for colon-specific drug delivery. *Int. J. Pharmaceut.* 1992;87:37-46.
90. Khan M, Prebeg Z, Kurjakovic N. A pH-dependent colon targeted oral drug delivery system using methacrylic acid copolymers. I. Manipulation Of drug release using Eudragit L100-55 and Eudragit S100 combinations. *J. Cont. Rel.* 1999;58:215-222.
91. Dew MJ, Ryder REJ, Evans N, Evans N, Rhodes J. Colonic release of 5-aminosalicylic acid from an oral preparation in active ulcerative colitis. *Br. J. Clin. Pharmacol.* 1983;16:185-187.
92. Ashford M, Fell JT, Attwood D, Sharma HL, Woodhead PJ. Colonic drug delivery via the use of pH dependent polymers (abstract). *J. Pharm. Pharmacol. (Suppl.)* 1991;43:60.
93. Chiu HC, Hsiue GH, Lee YP, Huang LW. Synthesis and characterization of pH-sensitive dextran hydrogels as a potential colon-specific drug delivery system. *J. Biomater. Sci., Polymer Edition* 1999;10:591-608.
94. Brondsted H, Andersen C, Hovgaard L. Crosslinked dextran—a new capsule material for colon targeting of drugs. *J. Cont. Rel.* 1998;53:7-13.
95. Rashid A. Dispensing Device. *British Patent Application* 1990;2230441A:15 February, 1990.
96. Kilpatrick DC, Pusztai A, Grant G, Graham C, Ewen SWB. Tomato lectins resists digestion in the mammalian alimentary canal and binds to intestinal villi without deleterious effects. *FEBS letters* 1985;185:299-305.
97. Schacht E, Gevaert A, Kenawy ER, Molly K, Verstraete W, Adriaensens P, et al. Polymers for colon specific drug delivery. *JJ. Cont. Rel.* 1996;39:327-338.
98. Van Den Mooter G, Offringa M, Kalala W, Samyn C, Kinget R. Synthesis and evaluation of new linear azo-polymers for colonic targeting. *S.T.P. Pharma Sciences* 1995;5:36-40.
99. Saffran M, Kumar GS, Savariar C, Burnham GS, Williams F, Neckers DC. A new approach to the oral administration of insulin and other peptide drugs. *Science* 1986;233(4768):1081-1084.
100. Friend DR. Glycoside prodrugs: Novel pharmacotherapy for colonic diseases. *S.T.P. Pharma Sciences* 1995;5:70-76.
101. Krishnaiah YS, Satyanarayana S, Rama Prasad YV, Narasimha Rao S. Gamma scintigraphic studies on guar gum matrix tablets for colonic drug delivery in healthy human volunteers. *J. Cont. Rel.* 1998;55:245-252.
102. Krishnaiah YS, Satyanarayana S, Prasad YV. Studies of guar gum compression-coated 5-aminosalicylic acid tablets for colon-specific drug delivery. *Drug Develop. Indust. Pharm.* 1999;25:651-657.
103. Bauer KH, Kesselhut JF. Novel pharmaceutical excipients for colon targeting. *S.T.P. Pharma Sci.* 1995;5:54-59.
104. Uekama K, Minami K, Hirayama F. 6A-O-[(4-biphenylyl)acetyl]-alpha-, -beta-, and -gamma-cyclodextrins and 6A-deoxy-6A-[[(4-biphenylyl)acetyl]amino]-alpha-, -beta-, and -gamma-cyclodextrins: potential prodrugs for colon-specific delivery. *J. Med. Chem.* 1997;40:2755-2761.
105. Ashford M, Fell J, Attwood D, Sharma H, Woodhead P. An evaluation of pectin as a carrier for drug targeting to the colon. *J. Cont. Rel.* 1993;26:213-220.
106. Radai R, Rubinstein A. *In vitro* and *in vivo* analysis of colon specificity of calcium pectinate formulations. 1993:330-331.
107. Wakerly Z, Fell JT, Attwood D, Parkins D. Pectin/ethylcellulose film coating formulations for colonic drug delivery. *Pharmaceut. Res.* 1996;13:1210-1212.
108. Rubinstein A, Radai R. *In vitro* and *in vivo* analysis of colon specificity of calcium pectinate formulations. *Europ. J. Pharmaceut. Biopharmaceut.* 1995;41:291-295.
109. Magnusson JO, Bergdahl B, Bogentofot C, Jonsson UE. Metabolism of digoxin and absorptive site. *Br. J. Clin. Pharmacol.* 1982;14:284-285.
110. Olaison B, Sjödahl R, Leandersson P, Tagesson C. Abnormal intestinal permeability pattern in colonic Crohn's disease. *Scand. J. Gastroenterol.* 1989;24:571-576.

111. Shaffer Saitt JL, Higham C, Turnberg LA. Hazards of slow release preparations in patients with bowel strictures. *Lancet* 1980;30:2(8192):487.

112. Roberts JP, Newell MS, Deeks JJ, Waldron DW, Garvie NW, Williams NS. Oral [In-111] DTPA scintigraphic assessment of colonic transit in constipated subjects. *Dig. Dis. Sci* 1993;38:1032-1039.

113. De Boer AG. First-pass elimination of some high clearance drugs following rectal administration to humans and rats. PhD. Thesis, University of Leiden, The Netherlands. 1979.

114. De Boer AG, Breimer DD, Pronk FJ, Gubbens-Stibbe JM. Rectal bioavailability of lidocaine in rats: absence of significant first-pass elimination. *J. Pharmaceut. Sci.* 1980;69: 804-807.

115. Kleinbloesem CH, van Harten J, de Leede LGJ. Nifedipine kinetics and dynamics during rectal infusion to steadt state with an osmotic system. *Clin. Pharmacol. Therapeut.* 1984;36:396-401.

116. Hanning CD, Vickers AP, Smith G, Graham NB, McNeil ME. The morphine hydrogel suppository. *Br. J. Anaesthesiol.* 1988;61:221-227.

117. Tukker J. Biopharmaceutics of fatty suspension suppositories: The influence of physiological and physical parameters of spreading and bioavailability in dog and man: PhD thesis, University of Leiden, The Netherlands. 1983.

118. Hardy JG, Feely LC, Wood E, Davis SS. The application of gamma-scintigraphy for the evaluation of the relative spreading of suppository bases on rectal hard gelatin capsules. *Int. J. Pharmaceut.* 1987;38:103-108.

119. Sugito K, Ogata H, Noguchi M, Kogure T, Takano M, Maruyama Y, et al. The spreading of radiolabelled fatty suppository bases in the human rectum. *Int. J. Pharmaceut.* 1988;47:157-162.

120. Vanbodegraven AA, Boer RO, Lourens J, Tuynman HARE, Sindram JW. Distribution of mesalazine enemas in active and quiescent ulcerative-colitis. *Aliment. Pharmacol. Therapeut.* 1996;10:327-332.

121. Wood E, Wilson CG, Hardy JG. The spreading of foam and solution enemas. *Int. J. Pharmaceut.* 1985;25:191-197.

122. Moolenaar F, Bakker S, Visser J, Huizinga T. Comparative biopharmaceutics of diazepam after single rectal, oral, intramuscular and intravenous administration in man. *Int. J. Pharmaceut.* 1980;5:127-137.

123. Shrirai H, Miura H, Sunaoshi W. A clinical study on the effectiveness of intermittent therapy with rectal diazepam suppositories for the prevention of recurrent febrile convulsions and the development of epilepsy during the study period. *Brain and Development* 1988;10:201-202.

124. Dhillon S, Oxley J, Richens A. Bioavailability of diazepam after intravenous, oral and rectal administration in adult epileptic patients. *Br. J. Clin. Pharmacol.* 1982;13:427-432.

125. Milligan N, Dhillon S, Richens A, Oxley J. Absorption of diazepam from the rectum and its effect on interrictal spikes in the EEG. *Epilepsia* 1982;23:323-331.

126. De Boer AG, Moolenaar F, de Leede LGJ, Breimer DD. Rectal drug administration: clinical pharmacokinetic considerations. *Clin. Pharmacokinet.* 1982;7:285-311.

127. Graves NM, Kriel RL, Jones-Saete C, Cloyd JC. Relative bioavailability of rectally administered carbamazepine suspension in humans. *Epilepsia* 1985;26:429-433.

128. Neuvonen PJ, Tokoia O. Bioavailability of rectally administered carbamazepine mixture. *Br. J. Clin. Pharmacol.* 1987;24:839-841.

129. Saint-Maurice C, Meistelman C, Rey E, Esteve C, de Lauture D. The pharmacokinetics of rectal midazolam for premedication in children. *Anaesthesiol.* 1986;65:536-538.

130. Clausen TG, Wolff J, Hansen PB, Larsen F, Rasmussen SN. Pharmacokinetics of midazolam and α-hydroxy-midazolam following rectal and intravenous administration. *Br. J. Clin. Pharmacol.* 1988;25:457-463.

131. Ravnborg M, Hasselstrøm L, Østengard D. Premedication with oral and rectal diazepam. *Acta Anaesthesiol. Scand.* 1986;30:132-138.

132. Lundgren S, Ekman A, Blomback U. Rectal administration of diazepam in solution. *Swed. Dent. J.* 1979;2:161-166.

133. Kraus G, Frank S, Knoll R, Prestele H. pharmakokinetische Untersuchungen nach intravenoser, intermuskularar und rektaler. Applikation von Methohexital bei Kindern. *Anaesthesist* 1984;33:266-271.

134. Jantzen JPAH, Erdmann K, Witton PK, Klein AM. Der Einfluss der rekalen pH-Wertes auf die Resorption von Methohexital. *Anaesthesist* 1986;35:469-499.

135. Olsson GL, Bejersten A, Feychting H, Palmer L, Petterson B-M. Plasma concentrations of atropine after rectal administration. *Anaesthesia* 1983;38:1179-1182.

136. Michel P, Benoit I, Grellet J, Saux MC, Hazane C. Evaluation pharmacocinétique en pédiatrie d'un gel rectale hydrophile de sulfate d'atropine. *J. Pharmacie Clin.* 1988;7:4-19.

137. Moolenaar F, Yska JP, Visser J, Meijer DKF. Drastic improvement in the rectal absorption profile of morphine in man. *Europ. J. Clin. Pharmacol.* 1985;29:119-121.

138. Moolenaar F, Kauffmann BG, Visser J, Meijer DKF. Rectal absorption of methadone from dissolution-prmotong vehicles. *Int. J. Pharmaceut.* 1986;33:249-252.

139. Moolenaar F, Grasmeijer G, Visser J, Meijer DKF. Rectal versus oral absorption of codeine phosphate in man. *Biopharmaceut. Drug Disposit.* 1986;4:195-199.

140. Moolenaar F, Cox HLM. Rectaal absorptieprofiel van codeine vanuit zetpillen bereid met codeinefosfaat en acetylsalicylzuur. *Pharm. Weekblad* 1983;118:818-821.

141. Nishihata T, Sudho M, Kamada A, Keigami M, Fujimoto T. Investigation of sustained-release suppository of sodium diclofenac in humans. *Int. J. Pharmaceut.* 1986;33:181-186.

142. Houin G, Barre J, Tillement JP. Absolute intramuscular, oral and rectal bioavailability of alizapride. *J. Pharmaceut. Sci.* 1984;73:1450-1453.

143. De Leede LGJ, De Boer AG, Van Velzen SL, Breimer DD. Zero order rectal delivery of theophylline in man with an osmotic system. *J. Pharmacokinet. Biopharmaceut.* 1982;10:525-527.

144. Lunell E, Andersson K-E, Borga O, Fagerstrom P-O. Absorption of enprofylline from the gastrointestinal tract in healthy subjects. *Europ. J. Clin. Pharmacol.* 1984;27:329-333.

145. Eckardt VF, Kanzler G, Remmele W. Anorectal ergotism: another cause of solitary rectal ulcers. *Gastroenterol.* 1986;91:1123-1127.

146. Rotenberg A, Chauveinc L, Rault P, Rozenberg H, Nemeth J, Potet F. Lesions rectales secondaires a l'abus de suppositoires de dextropropoxyphene et paracetamol. *Presse Medicale* 1988;17:1545-1551.

147. Lanthier P, Detry R, Debognie JC, Mahieu P, Vanheuverzwyn R. Lésions solitaires du rectum dues a des suppositoires associant acide acetylsalicylique et paracetamol. *Gastroenterol. Cliniq. Biologiq.* 1987;11:250-253.

148. Reid AS, Thomas NW, Palin KJ, Gould PL. Formulation of fenbufen suppositories. I: quantitative histological assessment of the rectal mucosa of rates following treatment with suppository bases. *Int. J. Pharmaceut.* 1987;40:181-185.

149. Van Hoogdalem EJ, Vermeij-Keers C, De Boer AG, Breimer DD. Topical effects of absorption enhancing agents on the rectal mucosa of rats *in vivo*. *J. Pharmaceut. Sci.* 1990;79:866-870.

Chapter Eight

Transdermal Drug Delivery

INTRODUCTION

The skin, or integument, of the human body both provides protection and receives sensory stimuli from the environment. The skin is the most extensive and readily accessible organ of the body. In an average adult, it covers a surface area of over 2m² and receives about one-third of the blood circulation; this blood drains into the venous circulation and so avoids first-pass metabolism. It is normally self-regenerating.

Although it is well known that drugs can be applied to the skin for local treatment of dermatological conditions, the advantages of accessibility and the avoidance of first-pass metabolism make it attractive for the systemic delivery of drugs. The objective of a transdermal delivery system is to provide a sustained concentration of drug for absorption, without breaching the barrier function of the skin, and avoiding local irritation. However, the slow transport of many drugs across the skin limits this technique to potent drugs which require plasma concentrations of only a few µg per ml.

Generally, the higher the lipid solubility of a drug and the lower its melting point, the faster it will penetrate the skin. Several drugs can be successfully administered by this route, notably scopolamine, glycerine trinitrate, clonidine and oestradiol. Nicotine patches are becoming common in smoking cessation programmes. Nonsteroidal anti-inflammatory drugs (NSAIDs) are also being administered increasingly by transdermal delivery for the treatment of local muscle inflammation. Recently some attention has been focused on the delivery of acetylcholinesterase inhibitors for the treatment of Alzheimer's disease[1]. Other potential candidates are ß-blockers, antihistamines and testosterone.

STRUCTURE OF THE SKIN

The skin is elastic and quite rugged despite the fact that it is only approximately 3 mm thick. It consists of three anatomical layers, the epidermis, the dermis and a subcutaneous fat layer (Figure 8.1).

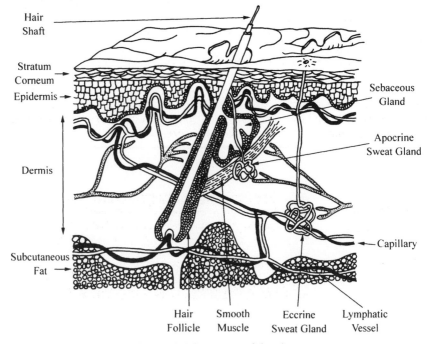

Figure 8.1 Structure of the skin

Epidermis

The epidermis is a thin, dry and tough outer protective outer layer. It forms a barrier to water, electrolyte and nutrient loss from the body, and at the same time is also responsible for limiting the penetration of water and foreign substances from the environment into the body. Damage or removal of the epidermis allows diffusion of small water-soluble non-electrolytes to occur approximately 1000 times faster than in the intact skin[2].

The epidermis is made up of two layers; a basal layer known as the stratum germinativum, which is living, and an outer dead layer called the stratum corneum. The primary cell type in the stratum germinativum is the corneocyte or keratinocyte, which grows from the basal layer outwards to the skin surface. The journey to the surface takes between 12 to 14 days, during which time the cells synthesise the various proteinaceous materials called keratin, they become thin, hard and dehydrated and begin to die. The lifespan of such a cell on the surface is two to three weeks. These cells, together with intercellular lipids synthesized by the keratinocyte, form the outer stratum corneum or horny layer, which is dead. The stratum corneum is the primary protective layer and consists of eight to sixteen layers of flattened, stratified and fully keratinised dead cells. Each cell is about 34 to 44 μm long, 25 to 36 μm wide and 0.15 to 0.20 μm thick, and they are continuously replaced from the basal layer. The water content of the normal stratum corneum is 15 to 20% of its dry weight, but when it becomes hydrated it can contain up to 75% water.

Because the stratum corneum is the main barrier to drug absorption its structure has been closely studied. The most widely used description is the 'bricks and mortar' model (Figure 8.2) in which the keratinocytes form the hydrophilic bricks and the intercellular lipid is the mortar, so that there is a continuous hydrophobic path through the stratum corneum. There is no direct hydrophilic path since the lipid effectively 'insulates' the keratinocytes from each other, and techniques such as electroporation (q.v.) are required to form a continuous hydrophilic path. The lipids consist mainly of ceramides, fatty acids, and cholesterol. Alkanes are commonly present although they are almost certainly derived from environmental sources. It is particularly difficult to study the intercellular lipids since they are easily contaminated with lipids from the sebaceous glands (squalane and triglycerides) or from epidermal fat[3].

The basal layer also contains melanocytes which produce the pigment melanin, which imparts colour to the skin and also protects it from the effects of ultraviolet radiation. Other cells found in the epidermis include Langerhans cells, which play a role in the body's immune defences, and Merkel cells, which are involved in sensory reception. Structures such as hair follicles, nails, and sweat and sebaceous (oil-producing) glands are appendages that develop from the epidermis and extend into the dermis.

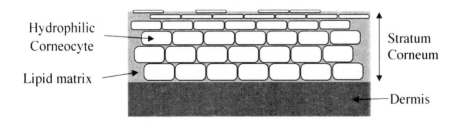

Figure 8.2 Bricks and mortar model of drug absorption through the skin

Dermis

The dermis is a fibrous layer which supports and strengthens the epidermis. It ranges from 2 to 3 mm thick and in man constitutes between 15% to 20% of the total body weight. The dermis consists of a matrix of loose connective tissue composed of fibrous protein collagen, embedded in an amorphous ground substance. The ground substance consists primarily of water, ions, and complex carbohydrates such as glycosaminoglycans that are attached to proteins (proteoglycans). The ground substance helps to hold the cells of the tissue together and allows oxygen and nutrients to diffuse through the tissue to cells.

There are two distinct layers in the dermis; the papillary layer, which is adjacent to the epidermis, which contains mainly reticulin fibres, with smaller amounts of collagen and elastin, and the reticular layer, which provides structural support since it has extensive collagen and elastin networks, and few reticulin fibres. Elastin is more flexible than collagen and it serves to anchor the epidermis to the dermis, which helps the skin return to its original form after it has been stretched.

The dermis contains blood vessels, nerves, hair follicles, sebum and sweat glands. A deep plexus of arteries and veins is found in the subcutaneous tissue, and this sends out branches to the hair follicles and various glands. A second network of capillaries is located on the sub-papillary region of the dermis. From this plexus, small branches are sent towards the surface layers of the skin. The capillaries do not enter the epidermis, but they come within 150 to 200 μm from the outer surface of the skin. In man, dermal blood flow is approximately 2.5 ml.min^{-1}.100 g^{-1}, but it can reach 100 ml.min^{-1}.100 g^{-1} in the fingers.

Three different types of cells are scattered throughout the dermis. These are fibrocytes which synthesize collagen, elastin, and ground substance, histiocytes which are a type of macrophage, and mastocytes, or mast cells which are located near blood vessels; they release histamine in response to irritation, fever, oedema, and pain.

Subcutaneous fat layer

The subcutaneous fat layer acts as an insulator, a shock absorber, reserve depot of calories and supplier of nutrients to the other two layers. This subcutaneous tissue or hypodermis is composed of loose, fibrous connective tissue which contains fat and elastic fibres. The base of the hair follicles are present in this layer, as are the secretory portion of the sweat glands, cutaneous nerves and blood and lymph networks. It is generally considered that the drug has entered the systemic circulation if it reaches this layer; however the fat deposits may serve as a deep compartment for the drug and this can delay entry into the blood.

Hair and nails

Unlike other large land mammals, humans lack extensive body hair apart from epigamic areas which are concerned with social and sexual communication, either visually or by scent from glands associated with the hair follicles. The hair shaft consists of differentiated horny cells and it is the only part which breaks the surface of the skin. Hair follicles have a diameter of approximately 70 μm and occur at fixed intervals, and hence their separation increases during growth. The density of hair varies over the body surface and it is normally absent from certain areas such as the lips and palms. The extent of hair growth plays an important role in fastening a transdermal delivery system to the skin.

Nails are a modification of the epidermal structure. They are plates of hard keratin which lie along a nail bed, which is composed of modified skin and is very vascular.

Sebaceous glands

Sebaceous glands vary in size from between 200 to 2000 μm in diameter and are found in the upper third of the hair follicle. Sebaceous glands secrete sebum into the hair follicle, which eventually ends up on the surface of the skin. Sebum consists, on average, of 58% triglycerides, 26% waxy esters, 12% squalene, 3% cholesteryl esters and 1% cholesterol. The lipids maintain a pH of about 5 on the skin surface, and can cause problems for the adhesives in transdermal delivery systems.

Eccrine sweat glands

Eccrine sweat glands are simple tubular glands which possess a coiled section located in the lower dermis. There are approximately 3,000,000 on the body. The normal diameter of the surface opening is 70 μm, but the average width of the ducts is between 5 and 14 μm. They make up 1/10,000 of the total body surface area. Eccrine sweat glands secrete fluid which consists of 99% water with other minor components such as proteins, lipoproteins, lipids and several saccharides. The pH of the secretion is about 5. Apocrine sweat glands are ten times larger than eccrine sweat glands and they open into the hair follicle; however, the apocrine glands secrete a lower volume of sweat than the eccrine glands.

Surface characteristics

The characteristic features of skin change from the time of birth to old age. In infants and children it is velvety, dry, soft, and largely free of wrinkles and blemishes. The sebaceous glands in children up to the age of two years function minimally and hence they sweat poorly and irregularly. Adolescence causes sweating and sebaceous secretions to increase dramatically and the hair becomes longer, thicker, and more pigmented, particularly in the scalp, axillae, pubic eminence, and the face in males. General skin pigmentation increases and acne lesions often develop. As the skin ages, it loses elasticity and exposure to the environment, particularly sun and wind, cause the skin to become dry and wrinkled.

The human skin displays remarkable regional and racial differences, for example, skin of the eyebrows is thick, coarse, and hairy; that on the eyelids is thin, smooth, and covered with almost invisible hairs. Lips are hairless, whilst males have coarse hair over the upper lip and cheeks and jaws. Freckles, also called ephelides (singular ephelis), can also be found on the skin. They are small, brownish, well-circumscribed, stainlike spots on the skin, occurring most frequently in red- or fair-haired people. Freckles do not form on surfaces that have not been exposed to the sun. The ultraviolet radiation in sunlight causes the production of melanin to increase, however, the number of melanocytes remains the same.

The skin is driest at its surface, with a water content of 10 to 25%, and a pH of between 4.2 and 5.6. The lower epidermal layers contain up to 70% water and the pH gradually increases to 7.1 to 7.3. The "acid mantle" derives from the lactic acid and carboxylic amino acids in the sweat secretions mixed with the sebaceous secretions. The lower fatty acids (propionic, butyric, caproic or caprylic) have been demonstrated to have fungistatic and bacteriostatic action, possibly due to the low pH which they produce. The isoelectric point of keratin is between 3.7 and 4.5 and hence materials applied to the skin should have a pH greater than this value.

PASSAGE OF DRUGS THROUGH THE SKIN
Model systems for skin

A number of systems are available for studying transdermal drug absorption. In humans, cadaver skin is widely used, as is breast skin from mammary reduction operations. An alternative is the porcine skin model. Pigs have a marked advantage in studies of this type since their sebaceous glands are inactive, which can be particularly useful for the study of epidermal lipids. Large areas of full thickness epidermis can be removed by applying an aluminium block heated to 60°C for 30 seconds. The hamster cheek pouch also appears to be free of follicles and may be a useful model for absorption studies[4].

There is much interest in drug absorption through the appendageal pathway, but it is hampered by a lack of reliable techniques allowing direct and appendageal absorption to be studied. Hairless rodents still possess underdeveloped follicles, and attempts to study burn scar tissue as follicle-free skin[5] have obvious weaknesses. The Syrian hamster ear is rich in follicles, and a stratification procedure may allow the various routes of absorption to be separated in this model[6].

Routes of absorption

Drug diffusion from a transdermal delivery system to the blood can be considered as passage through a series of diffusional barriers. The drug has to pass first from the delivery system through the stratum corneum, the epidermis and the dermis, each of which has different barrier properties. Differences in composition of these layers cause them to display different permeabilities to drugs, depending on molecular properties such as diffusion coefficient, hydrophobicity, and solubility.

The first limiting factor is the vehicle or device. In a transdermal device, the primary design goal is the maintenance of the desired constant drug concentration at the skin surface for a suitable length of time. This has been achieved with a wide variety of technologies. The second and major barrier for most compounds is the stratum corneum. Skin from which stratum corneum has been removed is highly permeable, while the removed stratum corneum is nearly as impermeable as the entire skin[7]. Skin from cadavers has approximately the same permeability as living skin, suggesting that the underlying tissues present little resistance to drug adsorption[8].

Absorption can occur through several possible routes on an intact normal skin. It is widely accepted that the sebum and hydrophilic secretions offer negligible diffusional resistance to drug penetration. Drug molecules may penetrate not only through the skin but also via the eccrine glands and the sebaceous apparatus; this is known as transappendageal absorption. This route is often neglected since it is difficult to study. The most useful techniques are autoradiography of labelled drugs[9] although several studies have used confocal microscopy with fluorescent drug models. As the openings of glands comprise only a fraction of a percent of the skin surface, transappendageal absorption is often considered unimportant; however it is likely that some materials do penetrate readily by this route. It has been suggested that this route is more rapid than transepidermal transport, and so provides a loading dose, which is sustained by slower diffusion through the epidermis[10].

There are two possible routes of passage of drugs through the stratum corneum; these are via the hydrophilic keratinised cells or the lipid channels organized largely in bilayers between the cells. The lipoidal nature of the lipid channels favours passage of hydrophobic molecules, and since many drugs are hydrophobic, this is their major route of entry[11]. Transdermal drug absorption is influenced considerably by the degree of hydration of the skin, probably due to a combination of several factors including improved contact or wetting, and hydration of the lipid channels of the stratum corneum. Application of oily materials can improve the skin hydration by reducing the evaporation of moisture from underlying tissues. Hydration increases the penetration of polar molecules more than non-polar ones[12] so it is possible that hydration of the lipid channels is more important than hydration of keratinised cells. It is possible to hydrate the lipids in the stratum corneum (despite their hydrophobic nature) because they contain a large fraction of surface-active 'polar lipids' which are surfactant-like in nature (for example, phospholipids), and the phase behaviour of these materials depends strongly on the hydration of their polar groups.

The stratum corneum can act as a reservoir for drugs, causing the pharmacological response to continue for a short time after the device has been removed. If the skin is then allowed to dry out, the drug will diffuse into underlying tissues more slowly, and application of an occlusive patch which rehydrates the skin can cause release of the drug at a later time.

The final barrier is the living portion of the epidermis and the dermis. Diffusion rates in these viable tissues are much higher than in the stratum corneum and consequently they offer little resistance to absorption. However, the tissues are much more hydrophilic than the stratum corneum, and so act as a barrier to extremely hydrophobic compounds which cannot partition into them. As a result transdermal absorption is optimal for compounds with intermediate polarity which can pass through both the stratum corneum and dermal tissues.

Advantages and disadvantages of transdermal delivery

Drugs applied transdermally avoid the chemically hostile gastrointestinal environment containing acid, food and enzymes. Consequently, this route is useful if there is gastrointestinal distress, disease, or surgery, and one of the first applications of this delivery method was for the treatment of travel sickness. The most attractive feature of transdermal delivery is that first-pass metabolism of the drug is avoided since the blood drains directly into the main venous return. Patient compliance is good since a single device can administer drug for several days, and so is not subject to the problems of multiple daily dosing with tablets. Transdermal devices are usually well accepted, although they can cause irritation to the skin, the degree of which depends both on the drug and the formulation. Finally, the devices have major pharmacokinetic benefits; they can provide a sustained plasma profile over several days, without severe dips occurring at night, and without the potential for dose-dumping which can be a hazard with orally administered sustained release devices. Because the drug is delivered continuously, it can have a short biological half-life. Removal of the device causes the plasma levels to fall shortly thereafter, although some drugs can be stored in the hydrophobic regions of the skin and be released slowly into the blood.

There are however several disadvantages. Drugs may be metabolised by bacteria on the skin surface. Epithelial bacteria can in fact be more prevalent under a transdermal device, since the increased hydration and uniform temperature can encourage growth. Enzymatic activity in the epithelium may be different to that in the gastrointestinal tract, leading to unexpected routes of breakdown of drugs[13]. However, once the enzyme systems are understood they have the potential to activate pro-drugs to active species. It appears that it is possible to influence the metabolism of the drug in the skin by the use of host-guest inclusion complexes; thus for example the incorporation of PGE1 into a cyclodextrin complex reduced the rate of metabolism to other prostaglandins in the epidermis, leading to more efficient delivery[14].

Maintaining contact between a drug delivery device and the skin can present problems. Application of the device occludes the skin, trapping water and sebum from the glands. This, together with the flexing of the skin, can lead to loss of contact and discomfort. The choice of adhesive is restricted since irritation must be minimised, and in early devices, for example those used for clonidine, the drug had to be transported through the adhesive. In many modern devices the adhesive is loaded with drug thus becoming an integral part of the sustained release device. Irritation is often attributed to acrylic adhesives[15]. Silicone-based adhesive disks are a good alternative in this case.

One of the primary functions of the skin is as a protective barrier to foreign agents, and hence it is not surprising that a complex relationship exists between the skin and the body's immune system. A number of cell types (e.g. Langerhans cells and keratinocytes of the epidermis, indeterminant cells, tissue macrophages, mast cells, neutrophilic granulocytes and vascular endothelial cells of the dermis) are directly involved with the immune system and the transdermal route can cause drug sensitization. If an individual becomes sensitized to drug which has been delivered transdermally, it may become impossible to administer that drug by any other route[16].

Finally, transdermal technology is often uneconomical compared to the simple oral tablet, and so is only used where specific advantages are gained.

FACTORS AFFECTING PERCUTANEOUS ABSORPTION
Individual variation

Individual variation can be as severe a problem as for other drug delivery systems, for example the absorption of hydrocortisone can show nearly a ten-fold variation between individuals[17]. Thus dosage must be titrated to achieve a therapeutic benefit and the transdermal system does have the advantage in this respect that treatment can be stopped rapidly if too great a response is observed. It is straightforward to adjust the dose rate by varying the surface area of the device, although there are obviously practical limits to this.

Age

Skin condition and structure varies with age. The stratum corneum is not fully developed in neonates and this has been used to advantage in the administration of transdermal theophylline and caffeine[18]. It can also pose a major problem since externally applied materials, such as antiseptics and disinfectants, can be absorbed easily. Pre-term infants have very little barrier function, since this does not develop until 9 months after conception. In older people the stratum corneum thickens and is less hydrated, increasing its barrier function.

Site

Drug absorption varies greatly with site of application. Hydrocortisone, for example, penetrates the scrotum 40 times more rapidly than the forearm or back, the commonly used application sites. Heavily keratinised sites, notably the arch of the foot, are several times less efficient than the forearm. This pattern appears to apply to most drugs and offers the interesting possibility of titrating the dose by varying the position of the transdermal device. Patients who experience local irritation may re-site devices, which causes a problem when areas are chosen with very different absorption characteristics. Indeed, recently, it has been suggested that the site of application of the delivery device should be varied to reduce the skin sensitivity[16].

Occlusion

Occlusion increases adsorption considerably in many cases, probably due to increased hydration of the stratum corneum, improving permeability to both polar and non-polar drugs[19]. The increased humidity under the dressing may increase the bacterial load hence potential bacterial degradation of the drug needs to be studied.

Temperature

Temperature affects drug penetration by two mechanisms. Firstly it alters the physiology of the skin, and secondly the physicochemical diffusion rates in the device increase with temperature. The skin temperature is strongly influenced by its surroundings, and may be 20°C cooler than body temperature or several degrees hotter. Fortunately many transdermal patches act as insulators and so the actual variation beneath the device is likely to be significantly lower. The external temperature is more likely to influence the diffusion rate in the controlled release system itself. In disease the body temperature may vary;

temperature-induced variations in the diffusion coefficient may alter the absorption rate by up to a factor of two over this temperature range[20].

Temperature also influences blood flow in the surface vasculature and so might be expected to influence adsorption through this route. However, this possibility has not yet been proven[21] and since the device and the stratum corneum are rate-limiting, the effects of blood flow might be expected to be minimal.

Race

Race appears to influence penetration to a small extent. Negroid stratum corneum has more layers and is generally less permeable, although there is no difference in actual thickness between negroid and European stratum corneum[22]. It is not known if the presence of melanocytes influences the penetration of drugs.

Disease

The skin is the part of the body which comes into direct contact with the environment and hence it is usually the first part of the body to sustain damage or be exposed to irritant substances. Thus, dermatitis is a fairly common complaint. The symptoms generally begin as itching, sweat retention, increased sensitivity and pain, but lead to swelling, oozing, crusting and scaling, with thickening and hyperpigmentation. Inflammation occurs in response to a number of factors e.g. mechanical, chemical, thermal stimuli, infections or imbalance in the autoregulation processes. All these processes can reduce barrier action and lead to increased permeability of the skin to drugs. Allergic contact dermatitis from drugs is a significant obstacle to the development of transdermal drug delivery systems and various animal models are being investigated to test methods for its prevention[23].

Any damaged or diseased area of the skin is likely to display compromised barrier properties and consequently higher drug absorption. Skin permeability is increased in psoriasis and ichthyosis[24][25]. This is unusual since both of these conditions result in thickening of the stratum corneum, but presumably it does not retain structural integrity.

Irritation and inflammation increase penetration even if the skin layer is unbroken[26]; ultraviolet light and sunburn also increase permeability. Burning from more conventional sources such as scalding causes greater penetration, the extent increasing with burn temperature but not apparently with burn duration[27].

VEHICLES AND DEVICES

For topical delivery of drugs, ointments, creams, lotions and gels are used. These materials have a long history but are not suitable for controlled transdermal delivery since they do not provide a protected reservoir of drug or a controlled area of application. There are at least four systems currently employed for systemic delivery of drugs (Figure 8.3). All of these have two main features; a reservoir containing the drug, and a physical mechanism to control the rate at which drug diffuses from the device. The first is the microsealed system, which is a partition-controlled delivery system containing a drug reservoir with a saturated suspension of drug in a water-miscible solvent homogeneously dispersed in a silicone elastomer matrix. A second device is the matrix-diffusion controlled system. The third and most widely used system for transdermal drug delivery is the membrane-permeation controlled system, in which diffusion across a polymer membrane controls the delivery rate. A fourth system, recently made available, is the gradient-charged system[28]. In many formulations the adhesive is spread across the entire face of the device and becomes part of the release rate control. This is considered to be a superior approach to simply using a ring of adhesive around the periphery, because it provides more reliable contact with the skin over the delivery area. The objective in designing all of these systems is to make the release

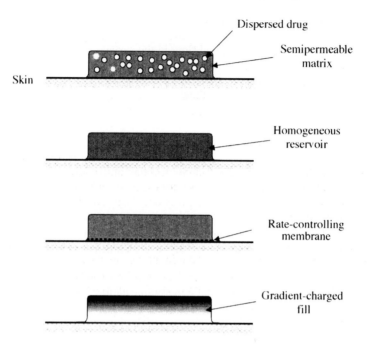

Figure 8.3 Typical devices used for transdermal drug delivery

rate from the device rate-limiting so that individual physiological variations will not affect the absorption rate. This normally means that only small amounts of drug can be delivered, so the drug must be active in small doses.

The variety of devices, and means for absorption rate control, available is well illustrated by the products available for the transdermal delivery of nicotine, which is one of the most successful applications to date[29]. The Elan ProStep™ patch uses a hydrogel reservoir and absorption is controlled by skin permeability. The Ciba Habitrol™ patch and Cygnus-Kabi Nicotrol™ patch have polymer matrices containing nicotine, and release is controlled by diffusion through the matrix, which is slower than diffusion through the skin. The Alza Nicoderm™ patch also has a matrix reservoir but also uses a polyethylene membrane to control the release rate. This type of device provides protection against the most significant concern of the membrane-controlled devices, that the membrane would become ruptured and dose-dumping would occur. If the drug reservoir is held in a matrix then the release rate of this component can be engineered to be slightly higher than that of the membrane, so that it is not rate-limiting in the intact device, but provides protection in the event of membrane damage.

In the future we can expect to see an increasing number of more sophisticated devices produced by microtechnology. Altea Technologies is currently marketing a Micropor™ system which produces tiny pores of a few micrometres diameter in the stratum corneum using hot-wire technology. Henry et al[30] have reported the use of microfabrication to produce arrays of microneedles which pierce the stratum corneum but are not long enough to trigger pain receptors. Technologies such as these have obvious extensions to delivery by iontophoresis and electroporation.

PENETRATION ENHANCERS

Because transdermal absorption is relatively slow, there has been a large amount of work concerned with finding materials which will increase the penetration rate of drugs through the skin. Such materials are called penetration enhancers. Penetration enhancers are believed to operate by increasing the permeability of the stratum corneum, either in the lipid or the keratinised protein regions. It is unlikely that many materials penetrate as far as the epidermis in sufficient concentration to increase its ability to transport hydrophobic drugs. The largest class of penetration enhancers appear to fluidise the lipid channels. These include dimethyl sulphoxide (DMSO) at high concentrations, decylmethyl sulphoxide, and azone. These materials are known to influence lipid structure[31] but are also polar and capable of swelling proteinaceous regions. Lipid fluidity appears to be the most important factor since at low concentrations substances such as DMSO swell keratin but do not appreciably improve absorption. However, it is only high surface concentrations (>60%) which affect skin lipid fluidity and cause an increase in drug penetration.

Certain penetration enhancers, such as propylene glycol, assist other enhancers to enter the skin. For example, azone is more soluble in propylene glycol than water, so propylene glycol assists its penetration. Additionally, propylene glycol may hydrate keratinised regions of the stratum corneum. Consequently, the azone/propylene glycol mixture is one of the most efficient of currently used penetration enhancers. Isopropyl palmitate combined with triethylene glycol monomethyl ether provides an excellent transdermal flux enhancer *in vitro*, but its effectiveness *in vivo* has not yet been reported[32]. A range of other enhancers of less importance, including fatty acids, esters, urea, and terpenes, have been reviewed by Walker and Smith[33].

Biodegradable enhancers like dodecyl N,N-dimethylamino acetate (DDAA) and N-(2-hydroxyethyl)-2-pyrrolidone have been synthesized to decrease duration of action and toxicity. DDAA and azone caused approximately equal transdermal penetration enhancement of model drugs *in vitro*, but DDAA was less irritant and its irritant effects lasted for only 4 days[34].

A further possibility for penetration enhancement is to influence the nature of the lipid channels by altering lipid biosynthesis in the skin. The intercellular lipid domains of the stratum corneum contain a mixture of cholesterol, free fatty acids, and ceramides. Each of these lipid classes is required for normal barrier function. Selective inhibition of either cholesterol, fatty acid, or ceramide synthesis in the epidermis delays barrier recovery rates after the barrier has been damaged. Possible enhancers using this approach are 5-(tetradecyloxy)-2-furancarboxylic acid which inhibits fatty acid synthesis, and fluvastatin which inhibits cholesterol synthesis. A study by Tsai[35] in hairless mice demonstrated that these two agents in combination could increase the absorption rate of lidocaine by a factor of 8.

Surfactants appear to assist the penetration of polar materials, and it is believed that their mode of action is on the keratinised protein regions of the stratum corneum[36]. It is possible that a combination of hydration and protein conformational change is responsible for this effect. The most powerful surfactants, such as sodium dodecyl sulphate, denature and uncoil keratin proteins, leading to a more porous hydrated structure, through which drugs can diffuse more easily. Such materials also are known to have membrane-solubilizing actions so they probably also influence lipid structure. They are however too irritant for clinical application.

The use of colloidal systems such as liposomes to enhance drug penetration is not particularly successful to date. Conventional liposomes do not appear to pass through intact stratum corneum although there is some evidence that they are phagocytosed by keratinocytes, at least *in vivo,* and so may be taken up in damaged skin where the stratum corneum is broken[37]. A number of authors have examined the possibility that liposomes may be able to enhance the absorption of drugs by the appendageal route, but these studies are complicated by the difficulty of handling model systems[38]. "Transfersomes" have been used for percutaneous delivery in animals and humans[39]. These are liposomes which are constructed from lipid mixtures which are extremely deformable, so that they can squeeze through the pores between the layers of stratum corneum lipid (typically 20-30 nm). The driving force for this penetration is the water activity gradient in the skin; if the skin is occluded so that the water concentration gradient in the stratum corneum is removed, transfersomes do not penetrate.

A number of workers have reported the use of cyclodextrins as penetration enhancers for extremely lipophilic drugs. It is difficult to assess such studies since the cyclodextrin influences the vehicle behaviour as well as that of the skin, and hydrophilic cyclodextrins would not be expected to show significant absorption through the stratum corneum. This area has been reviewed in detail by Matsuda and Arima[40].

The skin will respond to drugs and/or skin permeation enhancers by inflammatory and immune reactions. A fundamental difficulty with the development of penetration enhancers is that an attempt is being made to alter the skin structure; this is almost certain to provoke an irritant reaction. Both sodium dodecyl sulphate and DMSO are irritant; azone is probably the least irritant, partly since it is active at low (1%) concentrations. This problem is made more severe since irritation is often found in transdermal therapy even before penetration enhancers are used.

IONTOPHORESIS

Iontophoresis is the use of an electric current applied to the skin to drive drugs through the epithelium. Iontophoresis enhances transdermal drug delivery by three mechanisms: (a) the ion-electric field interaction provides a directional force which drives ions through the skin; (b) flow of electric current increases the permeability of the skin; and (c) electroosmosis produces bulk motion of the solvent itself that carries ions or neutral species, with the solvent 'stream'. Electroosmosis is the movement of the solvent which occurs when an electric field is imposed near a charged surface. The membrane attracts a predominance of counterions and the movement of these ions in the field causes the solvent to flow in the same direction to maintain the osmotic balance. As both human skin and hairless mouse skin are negatively charged above about pH 4, the adjacent solvent layer contains a predominance of positive ions and electroosmotic flow occurs from anode to cathode. Thus, delivery of positively charged drugs is assisted by electroosmosis, but delivery of negatively charged drugs is retarded[41]. There is evidence that iontophoretic delivery facilitates the deep penetration of drugs compared to direct topical application; for example a study of penetration of lidocaine[42] demonstrated a penetration depth of 10-12 mm compared to 5 mm for direct application.

The effects of electric current on the epithelium have been widely studied but are still incompletely understood[43]. The current does not pass uniformly through the skin, but is largely carried transappendageally via the pores, although some additional pathways open through the lipid channels[44 45]. A number of studies using dyes or tracers have demonstrated that drugs similarly follow these pathways[46 47]. In common with penetration enhancers, electrical enhancement of transdermal drug delivery is limited by similar side-effects, such as tissue damage and pain[43]. Studies of the interaction of penetration enhancers and electrical enhancement suggests that they operate through similar channels, since skin impedance drops substantially after several penetration enhancers are used[48].

A number of factors influence the iontophoretic transport of drugs:

a) The pH of the medium. As the ionization of drugs is controlled by pH, transport is optimum in the pH range in which the drug is fully ionized[49 50] although uncharged species can be carried by the electroosmotic solvent flow[41].

b) The nature of the other ions in the formulation, which compete for transport of the current. These can be ions in the formulation (for example buffers controlling the pH) or endogenous ions such as sodium, potassium, chloride and bicarbonate. The fraction of the total ionic current carried by the drug ion is called the transport number, and it is always less than 1 due to competition from other ions. Consequently when formulating iontophoretic systems, it is important to use a minimum amount of buffer, and choose competing ions with low mobilities (large highly hydrated ions)[51].

c) The current density. The drug flux is proportional to the current density, but the allowable density is limited by safety and patient tolerance to about 0.5 mA cm^{-2}. The working area can be increased but there are practical limits of a few square cm[52].

d) Molecular weight. Larger drugs have lower transport numbers and so are delivered less effectively. This is the major difficulty with the iontophoretic delivery of peptides, which for a time held much promise[53 54]. However, this is partly offset by the need to deliver only extremely small doses of these agents[55]. As the drug size increases, the importance of ionic transport decreases and the drugs become predominantly carried by the electro-osmotic solvent flow[56].

e) Concentration of drug in the delivery system. As the drug concentration at the donor site is increased, the flux across the skin increases[50 52]. This is probably due to the increase in transport number of the drug as its concentration increases relative to that of the competing ions in the system, and so is only significant if the drug is relatively large and has a low transport number. If the transport number is high, then the drug is already carrying the majority of the current and so increasing its concentration will have little effect.

f) Physiological variation. A major advantage of iontophoresis is that a relatively low level of variation in delivery rate is observed. This is probably due to the fact that the applied voltage is adjusted to achieve a specific current, and this will take account of much variability between the subjects due to, for example, site, age, and colour of skin.

g) Waveform of applied current. A number of authors have studied the effect of using AC voltages instead of a steady DC voltage, which can reduce efficiency due to polarization of the skin. Despite these studies there is little agreement about the optimum conditions for delivery[57 58].

ELECTROPORATION

Electroporation (electropermeabilization) is the creation of aqueous pores in lipid bilayers by the application of a short (microseconds to milliseconds) high voltage (200-1000V) electric pulse. It appears that electroporation occurs in the intercellular lipid bilayers of the stratum corneum by a mechanism involving transient structural changes[11]. Although DNA introduction is the most common use for electroporation, it has been used on isolated cells for introduction of enzymes, antibodies, and viruses, and more recently, tissue electroporation has begun to be explored, with potential applications including enhanced cancer tumour chemotherapy, gene therapy and transdermal drug delivery.

As presently understood, electroporation is an essentially universal membrane phenomenon that occurs in cell and artificial planar bilayer membranes. For short pulses (μs to ms), electroporation occurs if the transmembrane voltage reaches 0.5-1.5 V. Due to the small size of the cells it is necessary to apply a much higher voltage to a bulk sample in order to achieve this transmembrane voltage. In the case of isolated cells, the pulse magnitude is 10^3-10^4 V cm^{-1}. These pulses cause the formation of pores through the corneocyte which are initially only a few nanometres in diameter but enlarge as the current continues to flow. It is possible that electrical (Joule) heating increases the temperature in the channel sufficiently to melt the skin lipids and increase their permeability, in addition to forming aqueous pores[59]. This is accompanied by a large increase in molecular transport across the membrane. Membrane recovery can be orders of magnitude slower and cells can remain permeable for several minutes after the pulse or longer. It is likely that, in addition to forming aqueous pores in the skin epithelium, the electric field opens the appendageal route, although the relative importance of these pathways is not yet clear[60]. An associated cell stress commonly occurs, probably because of chemical influxes and effluxes leading to chemical imbalances, which may lead to cell death[61]. A detailed discussion of the electrical and structural changes involved in electroporation is given by Teissié et al[62].

Electroporation has been used to deliver a wide range of drugs with molecular weights up to several thousand daltons[63] and leads to an increase in permeability up to 4 orders of magnitude. Absorption is significantly higher if the field is in the 'forward' direction with respect to the drug being delivered, i.e. if the drug is cationic the electrode should be positive with respect to the skin, and vice versa for an anionic drug.

Combinations of electroporation with iontophoresis[64] and with ultrasound[65] have been demonstrated to provide further increases in drug flux over electroporation alone, and a number of macromolecules also appear to increase flux, possibly by stabilizing the transient pores in the skin[66].

SONOPHORESIS

Low-frequency ultrasound can significantly increase the permeability of human skin to many drugs, including high molecular weight proteins e.g. insulin, g interferon, and erythropoeitin[67]. This effect is termed sonophoresis. Several hypotheses have been proposed as the mechanism by which sonophoresis enhances transdermal drug absorption. These include thermal effects, generation of convective velocities, and mechanical effects. Confocal microscopy indicates that cavitation occurs in the keratinocytes of the stratum corneum upon ultrasound exposure[68]; Wu et al[69] also reported the formation of large (20 micrometre) pores in stratum corneum after exposure to ultrasound. As the ultrasound shock waves pass through the skin, they tear apart the tissue cohesion and create small vacuum bubbles. It is postulated that collapse of these cavitation bubbles induces disorder in the stratum corneum lipid bilayers, thereby enhancing transdermal transport. This seems to be a rather damaging way of increasing permeability, particularly since the stratum corneum is composed of dead cells and so cannot heal itself. Skin electrical resistance measurements support this model. Since transport through the skin is no longer rate limiting after ultrasound treatment, drug transport then depends directly on the diffusion coefficient, and hence molecular weight, of the drug.

Drug absorption can be enhanced by therapeutic ultrasound (frequency: 1-3 MHz and intensity: 0-2 W cm^{-2}), although typically by a factor of less than 10. Application of lower frequencies at higher powers causes much larger increases in absorption rate, up to a factor of 1000[70]. The absorption rate also depends on the formulation in which the drug is contained, since the drug must diffuse out of its formulation and there is little point in enhancing drug transport in skin if the device is rate-limiting. For example, insulin and vasopressin[71] were better absorbed from saline than from a hydrogel in the presence of an ultrasonic field.

The high powers normally used for sonophoresis may be reduced to therapeutic levels if a permeation enhancer is incorporated in the formulation. Thus Johnson et al[72] studied the penetration of a number of model drugs using combinations of therapeutic ultrasound and penetration enhancers, and were able to demonstrate increases in penetration of two orders of magnitude, depending on the drug/enhancer combination used.

CONCLUSIONS

Transdermal delivery has a number of advantages which can be of considerable value, most notably the ability to provide uniform plasma levels for considerable periods of time and avoidance of first-pass elimination. It also has disadvantages which are common to other delivery routes, such as intersubject variability and susceptibility to diseased states at the absorption site. At present, however, its main disadvantage is that only low plasma levels of drug can be maintained, and so it is limited to highly active drugs.

Despite these problems it is currently the optimal route for several compounds, and a number of commercial devices are well-established. It appears that transdermal delivery will be a valuable option in the development of future drug delivery systems.

REFERENCES

1. Moriearty PL. Transdermal delivery of cholinesterase inhibitors: Rationale and therapeutic potential. *CNS Drugs* 1995;4:323-334.
2. Scheuplein RJ, Blank IH. Permeability of the skin. *Physiol. Rev.* 1971;51:702-747.
3. Wertz PW. The nature of the epidermal barrier: Biochemical aspects. *Adv. Drug Deliv. Rev.* 1996;18:283-294.
4. Kurosaki Y, Nagahara N, Tanizawa T, Nishimura H, Nakayama T, Kimura T. Use of lipid disperse systems in transdermal drug delivery: Comparative study of flufenamic acid permeation among rat abdominal skin, silicon rubber membrane and stratum corneum sheet isoated from hamster cheek pouch. *Int. J. Pharmaceut.* 1991;67:1-9.
5. Illel B, Schaefer H. Transfollicular percutaneous absorption: Skin model for quantitative studies. *Acta Derm. Venerol.* 1988;68:427-430.
6. Matias JR, Orentreich N. The hamster ear sebaceous glands. I. Examination of the regional variation by stripped skin planimetry. *J. Invest. Dermatol.* 1983;81:43-46.
7. Monash S, Blank H. Location and reformation of the epithelial barrier to water vapour. *A.M.A. Arch. Dermatol.* 1958;78:710-714.
8. Tregear RT. *Physical Function of Skin* Vol 1. Academic Press, London. 1966.
9. Rogers AW. *Techniques of Autoradiography.* Elsevier, Amsterdam. 1979.
10. Katz M, Poulsen BJ. Absorption of drugs through the skin. In *Handbook of experimental pharmacology, New Series, 28 Part 1,* Brodie B.B. and Gilette J.R. (eds) Springer-Verlag, Berlin. 1971:103-174.
11. Prausnitz MR, Bose VG, Langer R, Weaver JC. Electroporation of mammalian skin: A mechanism to enhance transdermal drug delivery. *Proc. Nat. Acad. Sci. U. S. A.* 1993;90:10504-10508.
12. Behl CR, Flynn GL, Kurihara T, Harper N, Smith W, Higuchi WI. Hydration and percutaneous absorption 1. Influence of hydration on alkanol permeation through hairless mouse skin. *J. Invest. Dermatol.* 1980;75:346-352.
13. Steinstrasser I, Merkle HP. Dermal metabolism of topically applied drugs: Pathways and models reconsidered. *Pharmaceutica Acta Helvetiae* 1995;70:3-24.
14. Adachi H, Irie T, Uekama T, Manako T, Yano T, Saita M. Combination effects of O-carboxymethyl-O-ethyl-b-cyclodextrin and penetration enhancer HPE101 on transdermal delivery of prostaglandin E1 in hairless mice. *Europ. J. Pharmaceut. Sci* 1993;1:117-123.
15. Ancona AA, Arevalo AL, Macotela ER. Contact dermatitis in hospital patients. *Dermatol. Clin.* 1990;8:95-105.
16. Carmichael AJ. Skin sensitivity and transdermal drug delivery. A review of the problem. *Drug Safety* 1994;10:151-159.
17. Maibach HI. *In vivo* percutaneous penetration of corticoids in man and unresolved problems in their efficacy. *Dermatologica Suppl.* 1976;152:11-25.
18. Barrett DA, Rutter N. Transdermal delivery and the premature neonate. *Crit. Rev. Therapeut. Drug Carrier Syst.* 1994;11:1-30.
19. Feldmann RJ, Maibach HI. Penetration of ^{14}C cortisone through normal skin. *Arch. Dermatol.* 1965;91:661-666.

20. Roberts MS, Anderson RA, Swarbrick J, Moore DE. The percutaneous absorption of phenolic compounds: the mechanism of diffusion across the stratum corneum. *J. Pharm. Pharmacol.* 1978;30:486-490.

21. Arita T, Hori R, Anmo T, Washitake M, Akatsu M,Yajima T. Studies on percutaneous absorption of drugs. *Chem. Pharm. Bull.* 1970;18:1045-1049.

22. Weingand DA, Haygood C, Gaylor JR, Anglin JH. Racial variations in the cutaneous barrier. *in Current concepts in cutaneous toxicity,* Drill V.A. and Lazar P. (eds), Academic Press, New York 1980:221-235.

23. Kalish R, Wood JA, Wille JJ, Kydonieus A. Sensitization of mice to topically applied drugs: Albuterol, chlorpheniramine, clonidine and nadolol. *Contact Dermatitis* 1996;35:76-82.

24. Carr RD, Tarnowski WM. Percutaneous absorption of corticosteroids. *Acta Dermato-Venerol.* 1968;48:417-428.

25. Frost P, Weinstein GD, Bothwell J, Wildnauer R. Ichthyosiform dermatoses. III. Studies of transepidermal water loss. *Arch. Dermatol.* 1968;98:230-233.

26. Spruit D. Evaluation of skin function by the alkali application technique. *Curr. Probl. Dermatol.* 1970;3:148-153.

27. Behl CR, Flynn GL, Kurihara T, Smith W, Giatmaitan O, Higuchi WI, Permeability of thermally damaged skin.I. Immediate influences of 60°C scalding on hairless mouse skin. *J. Invest. Dermatol.* 1980;75:340-345.

28. Ranade VV. Drug delivery systems. 6. Transdermal drug delivery. *J. Clin. Pharmacol.* 1991;31:401-418.

29. Benowitz NL. Clinical pharmacology of transdermal nicotine. *Europ. J. Pharmaceut. Biopharmaceut.* 1995;41:168-174.

30. Henry S, McAllister DV, Allen MG, Prausnitz MR. Microfabricated microneedles: a novel approach to transdermal drug delivery. *J. Pharmaceut. Sci.* 1998;87:922-925.

31. Beastall JC, Washington C, Hadgraft J. The effect of Azone on lipid bilayer fluidity and transition temperature. *Int. J. Pharmaceut* 1988;48:207-213.

32. Hansen E, Sclafani J, Liu P, Nightingale J. The effect of water on a new binary transdermal flux enhancer (Peg³⁻ Me/IPP): An *in vitro* evaluation using estradiol. *Drug Develop. Ind. Pharm.* 1997;23:9-14.

33. Walker RB, Smith EW. The role of percutaneous penetration enhancers. *Adv. Drug Deliv. Rev.* 1996;18:295-301.

34. Hirvonen J, Sutinen R, Paronen P, Urtti A. Transdermal penetration enhancers in rabbit pinna skin: Duration of action, skin irritation, and *in vivo/in vitro* comparison. *Int. J. Pharmaceut.*1993;99:253-261.

35. Tsai JC, Guy RH, Thornfeldt CR, Wen Ni G, Feingold KR, Elias PM. Metabolic approaches to enhance transdermal drug delivery. 1. Effect of lipid synthesis inhibitors. *J. Pharmaceut. Sci.* 1996;85:643-648.

36. Scheuplein RJ, Ross L. Effect of surfactants and solvent on the permeability of epidermis. *J. Soc. Cosmet. Chem.* 1970;21:853-857.

37. Schaller M, Korting HC. Interaction of liposomes with human skin; role of the stratum corneum. *Adv. Drug Deliv. Rev.* 1996;18:303-309.

38. Lauer AC, Ramachandran C, Lieb LM, Niemiec S, Weiner ND. Targeted delivery to the psilosebaceous route using liposomes. *Adv. Drug Deliv. Rev.* 1996;18:311-324.

39. Cevc G. Transfersomes, liposomes and other lipid suspensions on the skin: Permeation enhancement, vesicle penetration, and transdermal drug delivery. *Crit. Rev. Therapeut. Drug Carrier Syst.* 1996;13:257-388.

40. Matsuda H, Arima H. Cyclodextrins in transdermal and rectal delivery. *Adv. Drug Deliv. Rev.* 1999;36:81-99.

41. Pikal MJ, Shah S. Transport mechanisms in iontophoresis. II. Electroosmotic flow and transference number measurements for hairless mouse skin. *Pharmaceut Res.* 1990;7:221-223.

42. Singh P, Roberts MS. Iontophoretic delivery of salicylic acid and lidocaine to local subcutaneous structures. *J. Pharmaceut. Sci.* 1993;82:127-131.

43. Prausnitz MR. The effects of electric current applied to skin: A review for transdermal drug delivery. *Adv. Drug Deliv. Rev.* 1996;18:395-424.

44. Grimnes S. Pathways of ionic flow through human skin *in vivo. Acta Derm. Venerol. (Stockholm)* 1984;64:93-98.

45. Burnette RR. Iontophoresis. In *Transdermal Drug Delivery.* Hadgraft J, (ed). Marcel Dekker, New York, 1988.

46. Papa CM, Kligman AM. Mechanism of eccrine anhydrosis. *J. Invest. Dermatol.* 1966;47:1-9.

47. Burnette RR, Ongpipattanakul B. Characterization of the pore transport properties and tissue alteration of excised human skin during iontophoresis. *J. Pharmaceut. Sci.* 1987;77:132-137.

48. Kalia YN, Guy RH. Interaction between penetration enhancers and iontophoresis: Effect on human skin impedance *in vivo. J. Cont. Rel.* 1997;44:33-42.

49. Siddiqui O, Roberts MS, Polack AE. The effect of iontophoresis and vehicle pH on the *in vitro* permeation of lignocaine through human stratum corneum. *J. Pharm. Pharmacol.* 1985;37:732-735.

50. Siddiqui O, Roberts MS, Polack AE. Iontophoretic transport of weak electrolytes through excised human stratum corneum. *J. Pharm. Pharmacol.* 1989;41:430-432.

51. Lelawongs P, Liu JC, Siddiqui O, Chien YW. Transdermal iontophoretic delivery of arginine-vasopressin (I) Physicochemical considerations. *Int. J. Pharmaceut.* 1989;56:13-22.

52. DelTerzo S, Behl CR, Nash RA. Iontophoretic transport of a homologous series of ionised and nonionised model compounds: influence of hydrophobicity and mechanistic interpretation. *Pharmaceut. Res.* 1989;6:85-90.

53. Chien YW, Siddiqui O, Sun Y, Shi WM, Lui JC. Transdermal iontophoretic delivery of therapeutic peptides/proteins. *Ann. New York Acad. Sci.* 1988;507:32-51.

54. Chou WL, Cheng CH, Yen SC, Jiang TS. The enhanced iontophoretic transport of TRH and its impedance study. *Drug Develop. Ind. Pharm.* 1996;22:943-950.

55. Yoshida NH, Roberts MS. Solute molecular size and transdermal iontophoresis across excised human skin. *J. Cont. Rel.* 1993;9:239-264.

56. Pikal MJ. The role of electroosmotic flow in transdermal iontophoresis. *Adv. Drug Deliv. Rev.* 1992;9:201-237.

57. Bagniefski T, Burnette RR. A comparison of pulsed and continuous current iontophoresis. *J. Cont. Rel.* 1990;11:113-122.

58. Hirvonen J, Hueber F, Guy RH. Current profile regulates iontophoretic delivery of amino acids across the skin. *J. Cont. Rel.* 1995;37:239-249.

59. Pliquett U. Mechanistic studies of molecular transdermal transport due to skin electroporation. *Adv. Drug Deliv. Rev.* 1999;35:41-60.

60. Weaver JC, Vaughan TE, Chizmadzhev Y. Theory of electrical creation of aqueous pathways across skin transport barriers. *Adv. Drug Deliv. Rev.* 1999;35:21-39.

61. Weaver JC. Electroporation: A general phenomenon for manipulating cells and tissues. *J. Cell. Biochem.* 1993;51:426-435.

62. Teissié J, Eynard N, Gabriel B, Rols MP. Electropermeabilization of cell membranes. *Adv. Drug Deliv. Rev.* 1999;35:3-19.

63. Prausnitz MR. A practical assessemnt of transdermal drug delivery by skin electroporation. *Adv. Drug Deliv. Rev.* 1999;35:61-76.

64. Bommannan DB, Tamada J, Leung L, Potts RO. Effect of electroporation on transdermal iontophoretic delivery of luteinizing hormone releasing hormone (LHRH) *in vitro. Pharmaceut. Res.* 1994;11:1809-1814.

65. Kost J, Pliquett U, Mitragotri S, Yamamoto A, Langer R, Weaver J. Synergistic effect of electric field and ultrasound on transdermal transport. *Pharmaceut. Res.* 1996;13:633-638.

66. Vanbever R, Prausnitz MR, Preat V. Macromolecules as novel transdermal transport enhancers for skin electroporation. *Pharmaceut. Res.* 1997;14:638-644.

67. Mitragotri S, Blankschtein D, Langer R. Ultrasound-mediated transdermal protein delivery. *Science* 1995;269(5225):850-853.

68. Mitragotri S, Edwards DA, Blankschtein D, Langer R. A mechanistic study of ultrasonically-enhanced transdermal drug delivery. *J. Pharmaceut. Sci.* 1995;84:697-706.

69. Wu J, Chappelow J, Yang J, Weimann L. Defects generated in human stratum corneum specimens by ultrasound. *Ultrasound Med. Biol.* 1998;24:705-710.

70. Mitragotri S, Blankschtein D, Langer R. Transdermal drug delivery using low-frequency sonophoresis. *Pharmaceut. Res.* 1996;13:411-420.

71. Zhang I, Shung KK, Edwards DA. Hydrogels with enhanced mass transfer for transdermal drug delivery. *J. Pharmaceut. Sci.* 1996;85:1312-1316.

72. Johnson ME, Mitragotri S, Patel A, Blankschtein D, Langer R. Synergistic effects of chemical enhancers and therapeutic ultrasound on transdermal drug delivery. *J. Pharmaceut. Sci.* 1996;85:670-679.

Chapter Nine

Nasal Drug Delivery

ANATOMY AND PHYSIOLOGY

The nose is a prominent structure located on the face between the eyes. The external openings are known as nares or nostrils which open at the back into the nasopharynx and lead to the trachea and oesophagus. The nose is the primary entrance to the respiratory tract, allowing air to enter the body for respiration. It conditions inspired air by filtering, warming, and moistening it. The nose also contains the olfactory organ, essential for the sense of smell.

The nasal cavity is an irregularly-shaped space in the front of the head extending from the bony palate upwards to the cranium (Figure 9.1). The bony framework of the nasal cavity is formed by the fusion of seven bones (Figure 9.2). It produces a chamber approximately 7.5 cm long by 5 cm high, subdivided into the right and left halves by a cartilaginous wall, the nasal septum. The septum consists of the anterior septal cartilage and posteriorly, the vomer and perpendicular plate of the ethmoid bone. It terminates at the nasopharynx.

The floor of the nose and the roof of the mouth are formed by the hard palatine bone and the soft palate, a flap of tissue. The soft palate extends back into the nasopharynx and during swallowing is pressed upward, so that food cannot lodge at the back of the nose, blocking the airway. The ability to breathe through the mouth as well as the nose is extremely beneficial, although the air inspired through the mouth is not humidified, heated and filtered to the same extent as the nose breathed air.

The forward section of the nasal cavity, which is within and above each nostril, is called the vestibule. Behind the vestibule and along each outer wall are three thin, scroll-shaped bony elements forming elevations, the conchae or turbinates, which generally run from front to rear. Each turbinate hangs over an air passage and they serve to increase the surface area of the cavities. The superior, middle and inferior turbinates form flues through which the air flows. The flues are quite narrow, and cause the air to flow in such a way that no part of the airstream is very far from the moist mucous blanket lining the air spaces. The turbulent airflow through this region, and the changes in direction caused by the turbinates, encourage inertial impaction of suspended particles. The width of the air spaces is adjusted by swell bodies in the septum and turbinates. Heating and humidification of inhaled air are important functions of the nose, which are facilitated by the abundant blood flow through

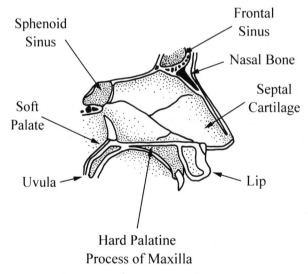

Figure 9.1 *Cross section through the nose*

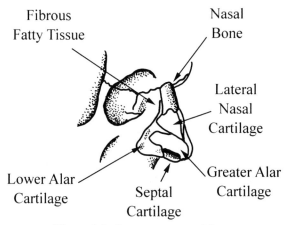

Fibrous Fatty Tissue

Nasal Bone

Lateral Nasal Cartilage

Lower Alar Cartilage

Septal Cartilage

Greater Alar Cartilage

Figure 9.2 Bony structure of the nose

the arteriovenous anastomoses in the turbinates. The rapid blood flow through the *cavernous sinusoids* matches the cross-section of the nasal cavity to meet changing demands. Humidification is produced by an abundant fluid supply from the anterior serous glands, seromucous glands, goblet cells and by transudation[1]. Air can be brought to within 97 to 98% saturation, and inspired ambient air between -20° C and +55° C can be brought to within 10 degrees of body temperature. The majority of the airflow from the nose to the pharynx passes through the middle meatus; however, up to 20% is directed vertically by the internal ostium to the olfactory region from where the airstream arches down to the nasopharynx.

Although the nose is considered by most as primarily as an organ of smell, only a relatively small region is involved in this sense, the rest of the cavity being involved in respiration. The respiratory area is lined with a moist mucous membrane with fine hairlike projections known as cilia, which serve to collect debris. Mucus from cells in the membrane wall also helps to trap particles of dust and bacteria. The olfactory region of the nasal cavity is located beside and above the uppermost turbinate. This area is mostly lined with mucous membrane, but a small segment of the lining contains the nerve cells which are the actual sensory organs. Fibres called dendrites project from the nerve cells into the nasal cavity. They are covered only by a thin layer of moisture which dissolves microscopic particles from odour-emitting substances in the air, and these chemically stimulate the olfactory nerve cells. A receptor potential in the cell is generated initiating a nerve impulse in the olfactory nerves to the brain.

The diameter of the nares is controlled by the ciliator and compressor nares muscles and the *levator labii superioris alaeque* muscle. The entrance of the nares is guarded by hairs (vibrissae) which filter particles entering the nose. The average cross-sectional area of each nostril is 0.75 cm^2. The posterior nasal apertures, the *choanae*, link the nose with the rhinopharynx and are much larger than the nares, measuring approximately 2.5 cm high by 1.2 cm wide. The nasal cavity widens in the middle and is approximately triangular in shape.

Nasal epithelia

Over 60% of the epithelial surface of the nasopharyngeal mucosa is lined by stratified squamous epithelium. In the lateral walls and roof of the nasopharynx there are alternating patches of squamous and ciliated epithelia, separated by islets of transitional epithelium, which are also present in a narrow zone between the oropharynx and the nasopharynx.

The lower area of the pharynx is lined with mucous membrane covered by stratified squamous epithelium. The posterior two-thirds of the nasal cavity is lined by pseudostratified epithelium possessing microvilli. These, along with the cilia, prevent drying of the surface and promote transport of water and other substances between the cells and the nasal secretions. The whole of the respiratory region is covered with goblet cells, which are unicellular mucous glands and supply the surface with viscid mucus.

The mucosal lining of the nasal cavity varies in thickness and vascularity. The respiratory region, which lines the majority of the cavity, is highly vascular and the surface of some of the epithelial cell types are covered in microvilli, increasing the area available for drug absorption.

Nasal lymphatic system

The nasopharyngeal region possesses a very rich lymphatic plexus, in which the lymph drains into deep cervical (neck) lymphatics. Besides capillary filtrate, some cerebrospinal fluid also drains into the nasal submucosa, which is partly absorbed by the nasal lymphatics. When the nasal mucosa is damaged by an irritant, the resulting oedema results in an increased flow of lymph.

The lymphatics of the nasopharynx play an important part in the absorption of substances which have been deposited on the nasal mucosa. It is believed that these molecules diffuse mainly through the olfactory region of the mucosa to be taken up by both the blood capillaries and lymphatics.

Nasal secretions

The composition of nasal secretion consists of a mixture of secretory materials from the goblet cells, nasal glands, lacrimal glands and a plasma transudate. In a healthy nose, the mucosa is covered by a thin layer of clear mucus which is secreted from the mucous and serous glands in the mucosa and submucosa. It is renewed approximately every 10 minutes. The mucus blanket is produced by the goblet cells, whose numbers increase with age.

Mucus consists of mucopolysaccharides complexed with sialic acid and may be partially sulphated, particularly in diseased conditions. The main component of mucus is water with 2 to 3% mucin and 1 to 2% electrolytes. Normal nasal secretions contain about 150 mEq l^{-1} sodium, 40 mEq l^{-1} potassium and 8 mEq l^{-1} calcium. Nasal mucus also contains lysozymes, enzymes, IgA, IgE, IgG, albumins, a 'kallikrein-like' substance, protease inhibitor, prostaglandins, lactoferrin, and interferon. The antibodies are present to act on bacterial particles which become trapped in the mucus lining. Many enzymes exist in nasal secretions and Table 9.1 lists the best characterized ones.

Table 9.1 Major enzymes found in nasal secretions

cytochrome P-450 dependent monooxygenases,
lactate-dehydrogenase,
oxidoreductases,
hydrolases, acid phosphotase and esterase, NAD+-dependent formaldehyde dehydrogenase, aldehyde dehydrogenase,
leucine animopeptidase,
phosphoglucomutase, glucose-6-phosphate dehydrogenase, aldolase, lactic dehydrogenase, malic enzymes, glutamic oxaloacetic transaminate, glutamic pyruvic transaminase
NAD⁻-dependent 15-hydroxyprostaglandin dehydrogenase
carboxylesterase, lysosomal proteinases and their inhibitors,
ß-glucosidase, a-fucosidase and a-galactosidase
succinic dehydrogenase,
lysozyme
steroid hydroxylases

The nasal cycle

The mucosa of each nasal passage has a separate autonomic and sensory innervation. The airflow through each nasal passage is regulated by the tumescence of the venous erectile tissue in the nasal mucosa. Engorgement of the tissue causes a constriction of the nasal passage, thus reducing airflow. This tissue exhibits cycles of constriction causing an alternation of the main airflow from one nasal passage to the other. A nasal cycle is found in about 80% of the population, yet most people are completely unaware of it since the total resistance remains relatively constant. Although the presence of the nasal cycle is well documented, its significance is still only speculated upon. One suggestion for the cycle is that each passage may rest whilst the other takes over conditioning of the inspired air.

As the nasal mucosa shrinks, droplets of secretion appear on the surface, and nasal secretion also follows the nasal cycle. The nasal cycle can be modified or overcome by a variety of endogenous and exogenous factors. Endogenous effects result from stimulation of the autonomic nervous system from fear, exercise and emotions or hormones as in pregnancy. Exogenous influences include ambient temperature, hypercapnia, allergy and infection. In addition, drugs which have sympathomimetic or parasympathomimetic action, release histamine or have antagonistic effects, will influence nasal patency by their action on the nasal vasculature. The amplitude of the nasal cycle is much more pronounced in seated or recumbent subjects compared to subjects who are standing. The nasal cycle can be overridden when recumbent. Lying on the left side will cause the right nostril to become more patent and vice versa.

Mucociliary clearance of inhaled particles

At the anterior ends of the nasal septum and turbinates, the squamous epithelium is replaced by areas of ciliated epithelium. There are approximately five ciliated to every non-ciliated cell, each ciliated cell having about 200 cilia extending from the anterior surface. Under normal conditions, these cells have a life of four to eight weeks[2]. Ciliary action clears surface fluid into the nasopharynx, where there is a transition to squamous epithelium. From here the mucus can be wiped off by the action of the soft palate and swallowed. There is also a small area in the anterior nose where ciliary action moves particles forward, from where they can then be removed by sneezing, wiping or blowing the nose. The sneeze reflex is similar to the cough reflex except that it applies to the nasal passages rather than the lower respiratory airways. During a sneeze, the uvula is depressed to channel the air through the nose and mouth to help clear the nasal passages of the irritation.

Efficient mucociliary clearance is a function of the physical properties of the mucus coupled to appropriately functioning cilia. Nasal mucus is secreted into the airway from goblet cells and mucus glands as a homogeneous gel. This floats on a 'sol' or periciliary layer that bathes the cilia, in a similar manner to the mucus lining the upper respiratory tract (Chapter 10). The mucus or gel layer acts like a conveyor belt over the 'sol' layer which is produced from serous glands and by transudation.

The cilia are approximately 6 μm long and the tip of each protrudes through the 'sol' layer into the mucus layer to propel it in an antrograde direction. The coordinated beating of the cilia moves the mucus layer along towards the pharynx. The ciliary beat frequency is estimated to be between 12 - 20Hz[3]. Intersubject variations of ciliary beat frequency are small but there is a highly significant correlation between the beat frequency and log of mucus transport time *in vivo*, indicating that this plays an important role in controlling nasal mucociliary clearance[4 5].

The filtering and deposition of airborne particles occurs predominantly by inertial impaction. The regions of highest deposition are those where the airstream bends sharply, allowing the momentum of the particles to deviate from the air path[6]. Hence, impaction points are present at the internal ostium and start of the rhinopharynx. Nearly all particles of 5-10 μm, and a significant proportion of even very small particles, are deposited, although those less than 2 μm can penetrate to the lungs. Virus-containing droplets often coalesce to exceed 5 to 6 μm in diameter and are therefore retained by the nose[7].

Nasal deposition increases with ventilation flow rate and nasal resistance. Children have much higher nasal resistances than adults but lower normal flow rates. Their nasal deposition percentages are lower than adults under similar conditions, so that despite greater nasal resistances, children have a lower particle filtering efficiency.

The average mucus flow rate is estimated to be approximately 5 mm min[-1] with a range from 0 to 20 mm min[-1]. There is some disagreement in the literature concerning the mucus flow in the anterior and posterior halves of the nasal cavity. Earlier studies reported that transit rate tended to increase in the posterior portion, possibly due to less drying of the posterior mucosal surface by the stream of inspired air[8], but others report no difference[9]. 'Slow' and 'fast' movers have been reported and there is a wide variation in mucociliary clearance rate between subjects, but within one person it is fairly consistent over moderate time spans[10]. The inter-individual and intra-individual changes in nasal clearance with time strongly suggest the important role of environmental factors. This view is supported by studies in monozygotic twins[11].

From childhood, the nose is continually challenged by pollution and upper respiratory tract infections. No affects of aging (<60 years old) on mucus flow rate are apparent and even in a group of elderly subjects (age > 60 years), 70% of subjects studied showed no significant change in flow rate. For those who did show change, age could not be proven to be the causative factor[12]. It therefore seems that the division of 'normal' healthy people into 'slow' and 'fast' movers occurs before adulthood.

Measurement of clearance

Many methods have been used to investigate nasal mucociliary clearance. Initially markers such as sky blue dye[13] and saccharin have been used to measure clearance rates[14 15]. Small amounts of powdered saccharin are placed in the nose and the time between application and detection of the taste is taken as the clearance time. Another method described is the use of aluminium discs of different colours placed on the floor and septum of the right and left nostril, used to measure transit rates in smokers and non-smokers[16]. A more quantitative method of measuring mucus flow rates is to use gamma scintigraphy to follow the distribution and clearance of radiolabelled formulations[8 14 15].

Pathological effects on mucociliary function

Environmental factors are not the sole causes responsible for changes in the efficacy of mucociliary function. There are many pathological disorders which may disrupt the nasal defence mechanism by obstruction, lesions or effects on the nasal mucus or cilia. The most usual are the common cold, closely followed by others such as hayfever, asthma and sinusitis.

Rhinitis

Rhinitis is defined as inflammation of the mucus membranes of the nasal cavity. Acute rhinitis is commonly caused by viral infections and allergic reactions. The commonest and perhaps most inconvenient are the rhinoviruses which cause the 'common cold'. It seems that bacterial infection has remarkably little capacity to disrupt ciliary clearance unless the mucosa is actually destroyed. There is a normal commensal respiratory flora in the nose. Normally, potential pathogens are phagocytosed and cleared by mucus and cilia. If organisms penetrate into the 'sol' layer, however, there is increased opportunity for further penetration and infection of host cells. Viruses are able to disrupt clearance by penetrating the mucosa and cause degeneration and shedding of epithelial cells. Once this damage has occurred, the nasal mucosa is open to bacterial infection by normal commensals.

Cold sufferers exhibit both markedly increased and decreased mucociliary clearance rates. During the hypersecretory phase (rhinorrhea) the clearance is increased and usually during recovery from a cold there is congestion which slows clearance[17]. The susceptibility to rhinoviruses in women is significantly related to the menstrual cycle, possibly due to changes in mucociliary function during the cycle[18].

Allergic rhinitis may be acute and seasonal (hayfever) or chronic (perennial rhinitis). In an allergic person, substances such as pollen or dust may more readily penetrate in and through the surface epithelium. Hayfever is the most common of all allergic diseases, affecting an estimated 10% of the population. The allergy to pollen produces rhinoconjunctivitis, for which the main symptoms are an itchy nose, sneezing and watery rhinorrhea. Mucus clearance time is decreased because nasal secretions become alkaline (pH 8) leading to increased ciliary activity[19]. There is an increase in water transport towards the epithelial surface and an altered transepithelial potential difference[20]. The same mechanisms are true for the increase in clearance seen in perennial allergic rhinitis where dust and fumes or some other allergen can provoke sneezing, rhinorrhea and nasal blockage. The physiological reaction to aerial contamination is of such a degree that it exceeds the self-cleaning capacity of the nose, impairing the nasal filter function.

Asthma

Asthmatics and bronchiectasis sufferers, both with and without allergic rhinitis, have an increased nasal mucociliary clearance time. It is therefore thought that there is some sort of mucus abnormality and ciliary malfunction working in concert[21]. Observations in asthmatics of tracheal mucus transport rates suggest that the mucociliary dysfunction observed after antigen challenge is related to airway anaphylaxis (a hypersensitivity reaction) and its chemical mediators. Pretreatment with sodium cromoglycate, a mast cell stabiliser, prevents the expected antigen induced increase in clearance time, but histamine alone is probably not the main mediator, since it stimulates mucociliary clearance. An alternative possible mediator is known as slow-reacting substance of anaphylaxis (SRS-A).

Sinusitis

Chronic sinusitis is the sequela to acute inflammation. Any condition that interferes with drainage or aeration of a paranasal sinus renders it liable to infection. If the ostium of a sinus is blocked, mucus is accumulated and pressure builds up. The nasal clearance time is increased in this condition due to the increase in quantity of mucus, which is usually highly viscous and adhesive[12]. However the inflammatory response is associated with changes in the H^+ concentration of the nasal mucus, and nasal secretions tend to be alkaline in reaction, therefore increasing ciliary activity[19].

Kartegener's syndrome

Kartegener's syndrome is an inherited disorder which comprises transposition of some or all of the major organs, bronchiectasis and sinusitis. The syndrome may also be associated with a variety of structural and functional abnormalities of cilia (the immotile cilia or ciliary dyskinesia syndrome), common due to a deficiency of the dynein arms which normally generate microtubule movement[22]. Mucociliary flow rate is therefore decreased due to ciliostasis. As well as the defects in nasal cilia associated with genetic disorders, evaluation of cilia from patients with chronic sinusitis, nasal polyposis, rhinitis and cystic fibrosis has demonstrated multiple membrane, microtubular and radial spoke alterations, although the importance of these in the pathologies is not known[2].

Sjögren's syndrome

Sjögren's syndrome is an autoimmune disorder predominantly affecting middle-aged or elderly women. The problem is a lymphocytic infiltration into the external secretory glands, which results in atrophy of the acini and consequent reduction of their secretory capacity. There is an increase in mucus transport time. Stasis in the mucus layer is due to the decreased amount of secretion. Normally, particles can become entangled in the mucus, but it seems that Sjögren's syndrome there is insufficient mucus for this to happen[12][23].

Structural dysfunction

Nasal polyps are round, soft, semi-translucent, yellow or pale glistening benign tumours usually attached to the nasal or sinus mucosa by a relatively narrow stalk or pedicle. Their presence prevents efficient humidification, temperature control and particle infiltration of inspired air. The nasal clearance is slowed down due to blockage of the nose and defects in ciliary action or mucus secretion[24]. There are two types of polyps, neutrophil and eosinophil. Eosinophil or allergic polyps are characterized by eosinophilia, seromucous secretion and steroid responsiveness, whereas neutrophil or infectious polyps demonstrate neutrophilia, purulent secretion and lack of response to steroid treatment[1].

Deviation of the nasal septum or rhinoscleroma causes obstruction which decreases clearance. People with deviated septa have longer clearance times (25 - 35 minutes) compared to normal subjects (9 - 15 minutes). Inspired air is directed onto a restricted area of mucosa and the flow rate exceeds its capacity to saturate air. This leads to an increased viscosity of the nasal mucus due to dehydration, making it unsuitable for effective ciliary action[19]. Congenital malformations such as cleft palate can also impair the function of the nose.

Laryngectomies can significantly accelerate peak transport rate in patients especially during the first sixty days after the operation, but the effect lessens with time. This could be partly due to a change in the nasal secretion[12].

Flow rates in twenty-four lepers who had differing degrees of nasal pathology indicated that, even with distortion, scarring or erosion of intranasal structures, any remaining intact mucosa which was protected from the direct impact of unmodified air, functioned normally. However heavy crusting of mucous membranes was found to inhibit or prevent mucus flow[13].

External factors affecting mucociliary clearance

There is a very wide normal range of mucociliary clearance which can be observed when particulates are introduced into the nose. Some people display the expected rapid, uninterrupted particle movement, whereas others have a slowing or even a halt in particle movement after an initial fast flow, or constantly slow movement or stasis[10]. A constitutional element in the overall control of nasal mucociliary flow may exist, but the mucus flow rate may also be influenced by many environmental factors[25].

Clearance may be altered by substances affecting, or those causing an alteration of, the physical (viscoelastic or rheological) properties of the mucus layer. Without the mucociliary and other nasal defence mechanisms, conditions such as chronic bronchitis, pneumonia and squamous metaplasia of large airways would result.

Cigarette smokers unfortunately do not inhale the smoke through their nostrils, and thus the nasal defence mechanisms are bypassed and the relatively unprotected small airways of the lung are directly accessed. Tobacco smoking is known to affect the bronchial tree but has also been shown to significantly prolong the nasal clearance. However, it does not appear to affect the ciliary beat frequency, suggesting that the defective clearance seen in smokers is due to a reduction in the number of cilia or to a change in the viscoelastic properties of mucus[26]. The effect of smoking on mucociliary transport of materials in the nose is under controversy. Some workers report that there are no differences in transit rates for smokers and non-smokers[8 16], whilst others report significantly longer nasal mucociliary clearance times in smokers (20 ± 10 minutes) compared to non-smokers (11 ± 4 minutes)[26 27]. However, the difference between the studies diminishes at relative humidities greater than 45%.

The nasal humidification system seems to be so efficient that even the driest air on entering the nasal passages is sufficiently moistened to prevent mucosal injury. However, the state of the ambient air is known to affect the mucociliary transport rate. Moderate decreases in mucus flow rate in the anterior and middle parts of the nose are observed with ambient temperatures above or below 23°C. The nasal resistance also decreases with warm air and increases with cold, as one would expect. However, none of these functional changes are sufficiently great so as to be physiologically important. There are differing opinions as to the effect of relative humidity on nasal mucociliary clearance. Some workers suggest that flow rate is correlated with relative humidity and that it increases from 6 to 9 mm min^{-1} when the relative humidity rises above 30%[8 27 28]. However, other studies have failed to find differences in either mucus flow or in nasal airway resistance, at relative humidities ranging from 10 to 70%, even though temperatures were similar to the previous studies, at around 23°C[7 9 25 29].

Other factors such as increased temperature, smog, clouds of dust and mild dehydration do not appreciably affect mucociliary clearance[13]. However nasal flushing or drinking very hot tea doubled the flow rate. The effect of irritants is greatest on the mucociliary transport in the anterior part of the nose, and for subjects with an initially slow mucus flow rate[25 29].

Chemical-induced changes

Many chemicals including nickel, chromium and aromatic hydrocarbons, have been implicated in the causation of cancer of the nose and sinuses[30]. These materials poison the nasal cilia. Occupational settings that carry an increased risk of cancer of the nose are wood-working in the furniture industry, the use of cutting oils, and employment in the shoe and leather industry. The wood dust impedes the normal mucociliary function allowing accumulation and retention of inhaled substances in the nasal cavity. The mucus transport rate decreases to less than 1 mm.min^{-1} (mucostasis). This increases the risk of developing adenocarcinoma of the nasal cavity and sinuses, especially the ethmoid[31 32]. Formaldehyde vapour also causes a slowing of clearance in the anterior nose, and exposure has been shown to precede nasal cancer in rodents[29].

Studies in rats have shown that inhalation of sulphur dioxide (SO_2) increases the thickness of the mucus blanket, and exposure to ammonia, formaldehyde and sulphur dioxide results in the cessation of ciliary movement to varying degrees[33]. Volunteers subjected to 1 ppm, 5 ppm and 25 ppm SO_2 concentrations in inspired air showed a significant decrease in mucus flow rate with the higher concentrations, the effect being greatest in the anterior part of the nose. The subjects reported discomfort proportional to the SO_2 concentration. There was also a marked decrease in cross section of the nasal airways, even at 1 ppm[25]. However, these levels are significantly higher than those normally present in the air.

Other factors which affect mucociliary clearance

An increase of mucociliary transport rate has been shown during the periovulatory phase of the menstrual cycle[18]. The mucociliary transport rate shows a diurnal cyclic pattern which is out of phase with the levels of serum IgA concentrations. The phase shift is

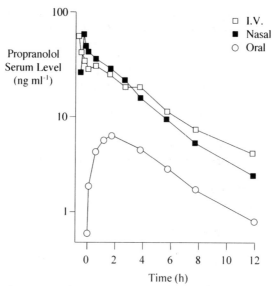

Figure 9.3 Absorption of propranolol from nasal, intravenous and oral formulations

such that the cyclic impairments of one activity will be compensated for by an improvement in the other, thus helping to preserve the nasal defence mechanism.

INTRANASAL ADMINISTRATION OF DRUGS

Currently, intranasal drug delivery is primarily employed to treat allergies and infections which cause nasal irritation, sneezing and congestion by the topical action of drugs. The observation that nasally-administered sympathomimetics and antihistamines, used for their local action, produced quite significant systemic effects, suggested that the nasal route could be used effectively to deliver drugs systemically. Much recent research has focused on delivery of large molecules via this route, particularly peptides and proteins.

The intranasal route is very useful for avoiding injections in the young and is a good way of administering drugs to the elderly. Small drugs are absorbed rapidly, at rates comparable to intravenously administered drugs (Figure 9.3). However, the physiological conditions of the nose (vascularity, speed of mucus flow, retention and atmospheric conditions) will affect the efficacy of drugs or vaccines, as will the nature of the formulations, e.g. volume, concentration, density, viscosity, pH, tonicity, and pharmacological and immunological activity. The slower the clearance of the drug, the longer the time available for drug action or absorption.

Drugs administered for local action

Topical therapy is widely used to treat allergic rhinitis. It is well known that histamine is an important mediator of allergic symptoms causing itching, sneezing and hypersecretion. Research is being directed towards discovering the relative roles of leucotrienes, prostaglandins and other arachidonic acid metabolites in the allergic process. Local eosinophilia is a characteristic feature of allergic rhinitis, some non-allergic rhinitis and nasal polyposis. Rhinitis is commonly treated with topical administration of corticosteroids, sodium cromoglycate or azelastine, an H_1-antagonist which is administered via a nasal spray.

The α-adrenergic agonist decongestant sprays containing phenylephrine, xylometazoline or tetrahydrozoline, often used in the management of allergic rhinitis, significantly increase nasal mucous velocity within ten minutes of administration. This is

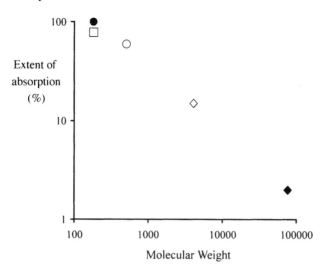

Figure 9.4 Effect of molecular weight on nasal drug absorption. ● *4-oxo-4H-1-benzopyran-2-carboxylic acid;* □ *p-aminohippuric acid;* ○ *sodium cromoglycate;* ◇ *insulin;* ◆ *dextran*

related to vasoconstriction of nasal mucosal vessels leading to a decrease in the fluid content of the mucosa[34].

Amazingly, little is known about the pathohistology and pathophysiology of the common cold. The beneficial effect of ipratropium bromide, which is a cholinoceptor antagonist, on the watery rhinorrhea in the first few days of a cold suggests that at least the early symptoms are reflexly mediated[35]. There is no convincing evidence that kinins and not histamine play a major role in symptom production[36].

Drugs administered for systemic effect

The nasal route is being actively developed as a method of delivering drugs to the systemic circulation. This route is easier and more comfortable for the patient than the parenteral route and it avoids enterohepatic recirculation and gut enzymes. This naturally makes it attractive for the delivery of peptides and recombinant DNA technology. However, absorption rates fall off sharply when the molecular weight exceeds 1000 Daltons[37] which probably explains why desmopressin[38] is delivered successfully (m. w. 1069 Daltons), whilst insulin (m. w. 6000 Daltons approx.) is not (Figure 9.4)[39].

The nasal mucosa demonstrates typical absorption mechanisms. Water soluble drugs enter via passive diffusion through aqueous channels. As the diffusion path through the nasal mucosa is short, intranasally administered drugs demonstrate a rapid rise to peak plasma concentrations, but the rapid clearance from the mucosa limits available time for absorption. Amino acids such as tyrosine and phenylalanine are absorbed by active transport, presumably by similar mechanisms to those observed in the blood brain barrier.

Currently, commercial products which utilise this route for systemic delivery exist for some gonadorelin analogues, which are hypothalmic hormones. These include buserelin for dependent prostatic cancer, oestradiol dependent endometriosis and infertility, and nafarelin also for endometriosis and infertility. A number of other hormones are being investigated at a preliminary stage, including desmopressin for diabetes insipidus and primary nocturnal enuresis and lypressin for diabetes insipidus. Anterior pituitary hormones include LHRH agonists and analogues which are used as contraceptive agents. Synthetic nasal salmon calcitonin is used in Hong Kong to treat ostoporosis[40].

A nasally delivered live attenuated influenza vaccine (FluMist™) has been developed to aid annual immunisation for influenza particularly for children and the elderly[41]. It consists of egg allantoic fluid, primarily ovalbumin and live attenuated influenza viruses types A and B.

In the US, sufentanil and midazolam are administered intranasally for sedation. Antimigraine treatments such as ergotamine tartate, sumatriptan and butorphanol are also administered intranasally to relieve the nausea and vomiting which are associated with severe migraine.

Penetration enhancers

The drive to increase the absorption of large molecular weight molecules has led to the use of penetration enhancers. Bile salts, e.g. sodium deoxycholate, sodium glycocholate and sodium taurocholate, decrease the viscosity of mucus and create transient hydrophilic pores in the membrane bilayer. EDTA, and fatty acid salts such as sodium caprate and sodium laurate, increase paracellular transport by removal of luminal calcium, thus increasing permeability of the tight junctions. Non-ionic detergents e.g. Laureth-9 alter membrane structure and permeability. It should be remembered that the penetration enhancers are generally non-specific and there remains the potential that any large molecule can enter the systemic circulation once the epithelial barrier is breached. Some penetration enhancers, e.g. Laureth-9 and bile salts, have been reported to be toxic to the nasal mucosa.

Cyclodextrins have been used as solubilizers and absorption enhancers for nasal drug delivery[42]. Methylated ß-cyclodextrins have been used to promote absorption of peptides and proteins, but mainly in animals. Limited studies show that the cyclodextrins are well tolerated in humans[43 44].

DRUG DELIVERY SYSTEMS AND DEPOSITION PATTERNS

Inhaled particles are deposited by five mechanisms; interception, electrostatic precipitation, impaction, sedimentation and diffusion. However, it is only the last three which are important in nasal drug delivery. Aerodynamic particle size is a key factor in nasal deposition. Correlation of aerodynamic particle diameter and nasal deposition efficiency at a given flow rate shows that particles of 0.5-1 μm are the least likely to impact. Above this particle size deposition increases due to inertial forces, and below it due to turbulent diffusion. Although the lung filters particles more efficiently during expiration compared to inspiration, expiratory deposition is lower than inspiratory deposition due to the loss of particles deposited in the lung[45].

There are four basic formulations which are suitable for nasal drug delivery. These are solution, suspension, emulsion and dry powders. The liquid formulations are often water based but may contain alcohol, oils or other organic solvents. Mechanical pumps and pressurised aerosol devices may be used for accurate dosing.

Liquid spray and drop preparations are most commonly used to deliver drugs intranasally. For the nasal drop to be correctly applied, some complex manoeuvres are required which include lying on a bed with the subject's head at a 90° angle and the nostrils uppermost. The drops are then applied and the head is swirled from side to side! Apart from not being very practical, the volume delivered cannot be easily controlled and contamination of the formulation can easily occur. High concentrations of preservatives cannot be used as they may damage the nasal mucosa and affect mucociliary clearance. Single use preparations may avoid the potential problems of contamination of the containers. The currently available devices are the bottle pack and a device which operates with an actuator and a chamber with a piston. This can either be a single shot or double shot device, which enables both nasal cavities to be dosed.

Liquid formulations generally clear from the nose within 30 minutes, but the exact figure is very variable and ranges of 5 to 90 minutes have been reported. Radiolabelled nasal sprays exhibit bi-phasic clearance from their initial site of deposition[46]. The first phase lasts 15-20 min in which more than 50% of the administered dose is cleared. The slower clearance is the removal of material from the non-ciliated vestibule and anterior septal area.

Dry powders are less frequently used in nasal drug delivery, even though they are preservative-free and have greatly improved stability. Powders can be administered from several devices, the most common being the insufflator. Many insufflators work with pre-dosed powder in gelatin capsules. To improve patient compliance a multi-dose powder inhaler has been developed which has been used to deliver budesonide[47].

Pressurized metered dose inhalers (pMDIs) originally developed for pulmonary delivery have been adapted for nasal use by alteration of the shape of the applicator. These have the advantage that generation of an aerosol is independent of inhalation. They are small, portable, available in a wide range of doses per actuation, provide accurate dosing and protect the contents. The disadvantages include possible irritation of the mucosa produced by the propellants and surfactants, and malfunctioning in cold conditions.

Vitamin B_{12} in a nasal gel for systemic delivery has recently been introduced into the marketplace. The gel has been used to prolong nasal retention, but the bioavailability may depend upon the mode and site of administration, since its viscosity prevents lateral spreading in the nose.

Care should be taken when studying bioadhesives for drug delivery to the nose. Any fraction of the dose which impacts on nasal hair will remain in the nose for exceptionally long periods, but it is however, not available for drug absorption[48]. Generally during studies, subjects are requested to refrain from blowing their nose, but it is this action which clears material impacted on the hair. Nasal patency will also affect the initial rate of clearance of nasal sprays from the mucosa. As would be expected, the clearance of a formulation is slower from the least patent nostril (T_{50} - least patent 39.3 ± 5.1 minutes vs most patent 24.2 ± 2.9)[48]. Vigorous breathing during inhalation of aqueous sprays does not affect nasal deposition patterns[49]. Few studies have been carried out on the pharmacokinetic inter- and intrasubject variability after nasal administration of drugs[50]. However, there appears to be a non-linear dose-response curve for some formulations[51].

The turbinates, which are covered by respiratory epithelium, are the primary sites for systemic drug absorption. Not surprisingly, drugs which are deposited posteriorly will clear faster than drugs deposited anteriorly. Nasal sprays deposit drugs more anteriorly than nasal drops and hence the type of dosing device used can affect absorption. For instance, the bioavailability of desmopressin is significantly increased when administered in a spray rather than drops. The particle size of the aerosol droplet is also very important since small particles ($< 10\mu m$) may be carried in the air into the lung whereas particles between 10 and 20 μm mainly deposit on the nasal mucosa. Aqueous sprays tend to produce droplets which are > 50 μm, with only 10% being less than 10 μm. The intensity of sniffing as the nasal spray is administered does not appear to affect the deposition pattern[52].

It should be remembered that regardless of the mechanism by which drug is administered to the nose, any drug which is not absorbed will either be blown out of the nose, or will clear to the gastrointestinal tract. When considering administering any drug to the nose, the consequence of gastrointestinal absorption should always be considered.

Mechanisms to increase nasal residence time of formulations

Two basic approaches have been used to increase the nasal residence times of drugs, and correspondingly to decrease intrasubject variation. These are firstly to use viscosity enhancers, and secondly to use a "bioadhesive" formulation to reduce the clearance rate. Two classes of bioadhesives have been used; firstly polymers which interact with the nasal mucus, and secondly microspheres. A large number of such formulations have been studied and many of them increase the residence time of the formulation, and alter the pharmacokinetics of the drug, causing increased bioavailability or duration of action. It is difficult to assess the exact physical mechanism by which these formulations operate. Many of the so-called bioadhesive polymers also act as viscosity modifiers, and many of the microsphere formulations hydrate to form glue-like gels which will adhere to the nasal tissues even in the absence of a specific particle-mucus interaction. As a result it is almost impossible to separate the importance of these effects *in vivo* and the importance of specific 'bioadhesive' interactions is questionable.

Viscosity modifiers

Spray preparations containing 0.25% methylcellulose have been reported to exhibit decreased mucociliary clearance resulting in delayed absorption of nasally administered desmopressin[53] and hydroxypropylmethylcellulose increased the residence time of spray formulations[54].

Smart hydrogel (poly(oxyethylene-b-oxypropylene-b-oxyethylene)-g-poly(acrylic acid) (GelMed Inc. USA) demonstrates great potential for nasal drug delivery. It is a thin liquid at room temperature, but it gels at body temperature. When administered as a spray to the nose, 80% cleared within 4 h, but 10% was still detectable at 20 hours post administration (Figure 9.5)[55].

Bioadhesive polymers

A number of polyelectrolyte polymers are generally considered to show specific interactions with mucus. Polyacrylic acid and polyacrylates such as Carbopol 934 were

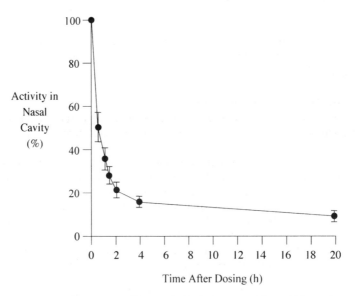

Figure 9.5 Clearance of ^{99m}Tc-labelled 'Smart Hydrogel' from the nose.

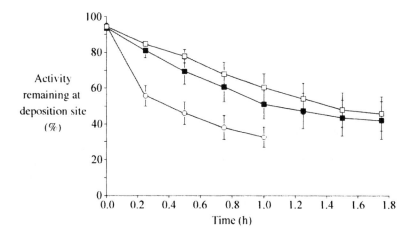

Figure 9.6 Clearance of ^{99m}Tc microspheres from the nose. □ microspheres, subject seated; ■ microspheres, subject supine; ○ DTPA solution control

shown to increase the nasal absorption and residence of insulin[56], and solutions thickened with hyaluronan showed an increased residence time[57].

Bioadhesive microspheres

Microsphere formulations studied include albumin, Sephadex, starch, dextran[58], hyaluronan[59], and chitosan[60]. The majority of these studies were intended for the delivery of peptides, particularly insulin, and caused increased absorption. Unfortunately there are conflicting reports concerning their nasal residence, and some workers have suggested that they are rapidly cleared but somehow increase nasal permeability[58]. In some cases, one is led to suspect that the isotope labelling of microspheres used for scintigraphy studies may be at fault.

The studies which demonstrate long nasal retention times for bioadhesive microspheres report that this occurs in the anterior part of the nasal cavity, which is non-ciliated and non-absorptive (Figure 9.6)[15].

Excipient and drug effects on clearance

Much interest has been shown in the ciliotoxicity of formulation excipients included in nasal sprays, although recently a differentiation is being made between ciliotoxicity and cilioinhibition[61].

In the early 1980s, it was recommended that mercury-containing preservatives, e.g. thiomersal, should not be employed in nasal preparations since these materials produced a rapid, irreversible inactivation of cilia in a chick tracheal preparation[62]. However, later studies showed that thiomersal at the concentrations used in these experiments had no effect on mucociliary transport in man[63]. Recently, the combination of topical steroids and benzalkonium chloride has produced areas of squamous cell metaplasia in rat nostrils. This was not observed in any nasal cavities exposed to the topical nasal steroid without the preservative, or to 0.9% NaCl, suggesting that benzalkonium chloride is potentially toxic[64]. It obviously does disrupt the membrane, allowing large molecules to pass through, since it enhances insulin absorption three-fold (6.31% vs 1.96%)[65]. Benzalkonium chloride is also present in many buserelin and nafarelin formulations and has also been shown to reduce ciliary beat frequency by 35% for 20 minutes *in vitro*, but it appears to have little effect *in vivo*[66]. The benzalkonium chloride story is further confused by *in vitro* studies which compared its ciliotoxicity to that of chlorobutol using concentrations of 0.005% for both compounds[67]. In commercial formulations, different concentrations of both are used i.e. 0.01% benzalkonium chloride and 0.5% chlorobutol. Hence, not surprisingly, the data generated using 0.005% chlorobutol demonstrated it to be less ciliotoxic than benzalkonium chloride, whereas studies using representative concentrations of both show that the reverse is true[68 69].

Many drugs administered in nasal preparations can also influence ciliary motility. The list of materials which are cilio-inhibitory includes anaesthetics[70], antihistamines, propranolol[71] and bile salts[72]. However, β-adrenergic and cholinergic drugs stimulate ciliary motility. Early *in vitro* studies indicated that penicillin had an inhibitory effect on ciliary function, however this was not found in subsequent studies using orally administered penicillin[73].

Dexamethasone nasal drops (used in the treatment of allergic rhinitis) may cause pathological changes leading to Cushing's syndrome[74]. Cushing's syndrome results from hypersecretion of the adrenal cortex leading to symptoms such as protein loss, fatigue, osteoporosis, amenorrhoea, impotence and oedema. The drug acts by absorption through the nasal mucosa and partly through the intestinal mucosa after a portion of the dose is swallowed. This problem does not occur with the newer intranasal steroids (e.g. beclomethasone and flunisolide) which are less readily absorbed through the nasal mucosa, and are inactivated in the liver after gastrointestinal absorption.

Care must be taken when extrapolating cilioinhibitory or toxicity data from *in vitro* to *in vivo* situations. For example, azelastine was claimed to be ciliotoxic, since it reduced *in vitro* ciliary beat frequency[75], however, this effect was not observed in animals and in long term use in allergic rhinitis patients it actually improved the nasal clearance rate[76].

Effect of formulation pH

The average baseline nasal pH is 6.4 in the anterior of the nose and 6.27 in the posterior of the nose (Figure 9.7)[77]. The ranges were 5.5 - 6.5 and 5.0 - 6.7 in adults and children respectively. Nasal pH varies with air temperature, sleep, emotions and food ingestion[37]. In acute rhinitis and sinusitis the nasal secretion is alkaline.

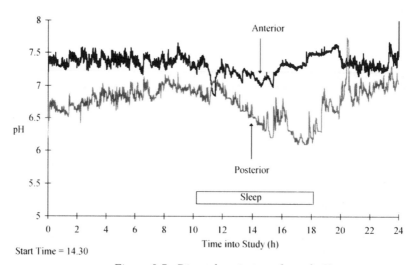

Figure 9.7. Diurnal variation of nasal pH.

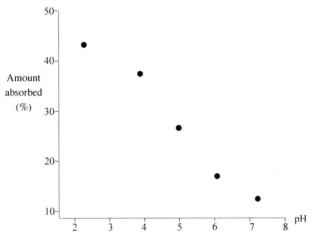

Figure 9.8 Fraction of benzoic acid absorbed in 60 minutes in the rat perfused nasal cavity model

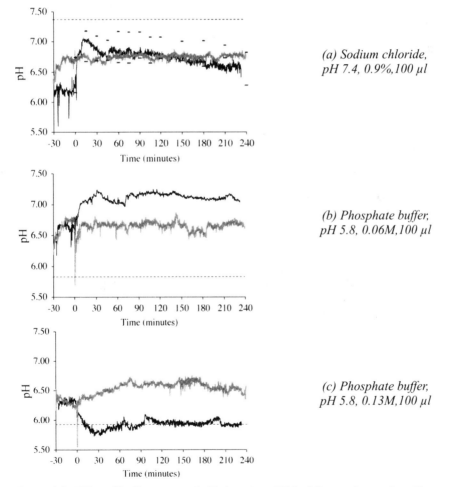

(a) Sodium chloride,
pH 7.4, 0.9%,100 µl

(b) Phosphate buffer,
pH 5.8, 0.06M,100 µl

(c) Phosphate buffer,
pH 5.8, 0.13M,100 µl

Figure 9.9 Effect of buffers on nasal pH. Anterior pH black line and posterior pH grey line

Local pH has been demonstrated *in vitro* and *ex vivo* studies to significantly affect the rate and extent of absorption of ionizable compounds (Figure 9.8)[78]. Buffering a solution to a target pH optimised for a particular drug should in theory, improve the absorption across the nasal epithelia. Reducing the pH of the mucosa enhanced the absorption of vasopressin in rats[79], but the rat tracheal cilia model shows that decreased pH has an adverse effect on ciliary beat frequency[80]. Reduction in nasal pH has also been demonstrated to result in lower blood glucose levels in dogs treated with intranasal insulin[81].

Recently, it has been demonstrated that buffers can be used to modify the pH of the human nasal cavity (Figure 9.9)[82]. Nasal anterior pH can be decreased when buffers of 0.1M and above are used. Mildly acidic solutions produce an increase in pH, presumably due to reflux bicarbonate secretion. It is more difficult to modify the pH in the posterior of the nasal cavity and stronger buffers are required to do this.

INTERSPECIES COMPARISONS

The majority of investigations published demonstrated the immense potential for nasal drug delivery. However, the majority of studies have been carried out in animals. A comparison of interspecies physiology and nasal clearance times is shown in Table 9.2. In humans, nasal drug delivery is only useful for drugs which have a low molecular weight, are active in low doses and have good aqueous solubility. It should also be borne in mind that the level of sedation used with different animals varies depending on ease of handling, and if general anaesthetics are used, these will usually reduce mucociliary transport. As a result the contribution of anaesthetics on published results can be difficult to assess.

Table 9.2 Comparison of interspecies nasal cavity characteristics[83]

Conchae complexity	Weight (kg)	Nasal volume (cm²)	Surface area (cm²)	Volume admin. per nostril (µl)	Clearance half-time (min)
Single scroll					
Man	70	20	160	150	15
Monkey	7	8	62	58	10
Double scroll					
Guinea pig	0.6	0.9	27	25	7
Mouse	0.03	0.03	2.8	3	1
Rat	0.25	0.4	14	13	5
Sheep	60	114	327	307	42
Branching					
Dog	10	20	221	207	20
Rabbit	3	6	61	58	10

CONCLUSIONS

Nasal delivery is receiving a considerable amount of attention, but there is still a lack of much fundamental physiological and biopharmaceutic information. For example, the relationship between pharmacokinetics and deposition patterns is largely unknown. Neither is it a simple route for delivery since gastrointestinal involvement will also be a contributory factor in absorption.

REFERENCES

1. Mygind N. *Nasal Allergy.* 2nd edition. Blackwell Scientific Publication, Oxford 1979.
2. Herzon FS. Nasal ciliary structural pathology. *Laryngoscope* 1983;93:63-67.
3. Satir P, Sleigh MA. The physiology of cilia and mucociliary interactions. *Ann. Rev. Physiol.* 1990;52:137-155.
4. Duchateau G, Graamans K, Zuidena J, Merkus FWHM. Correlation between nasal ciliary beat frequency and mucus transport rate in volunteers. *Laryngoscope* 1985;95:854-859.
5. Liote H. Role of mucus and cilia in nasal mucociliary clearance in healthy subjects. *Am. Rev. Respir. Dis.* 1989;140:132-136.
6. Becquemin MH. Particle deposition and resistance in the noses of aduls and children. *Europ. Res. J.* 1991;4:694-701.
7. Proctor DF, Andersen I, Lundqvuist G. Clearance of inhaled particles from the human nose. *Arch. Intern. Med.* 1973;131:132-139.
8. Quinlan MF, Salman SD, Swift DL, Wagner HN, Proctor DF. Measurement of mucociliary function in man. *Am. Rev. Resp. Dis.* 1969;99:13-23.
9. Andersen I, Lundqvist GR, Proctor DF. Human nasal function under four controlled humidities. *Am. Rev. Resp. Dis.* 1972;106:438-449.
10. Andersen I, Lundqvist GR, Proctor DF. Human nasal mucosal function in a controlled climate. *Arch. Environ. Health* 1971;23:408-420.
11. Andersen I, Camner P, Jensen P, Philipson K, Proctor DF. A comparison of nasal and tracheobronchial clearance. *Arch. Environ. Health* 1974;29:290-293.
12. Sakakura Y, Ukai R, Matima Y, Murai S, Harada T, Myoshi Y. Nasal mucociliary clearance under various conditions. *Acta Otolaryngol.* 1983;96:167-173.
13. Bang BG, Mukherjee AL, Bang FB. Human nasal mucous flow rates. *J. Johns Hopkins Med.* 1967;121:38-48.
14. Batts AH, Marriott C, Martin GP, Bond SW, Greaves JL, Wilson CG. The use of a radiolabeled saccharin solution to monitor the effect of the preservatives thiomersal, benzalkonium chloride and EDTA on human nasal clearance. *J. Pharm. Pharmacol.* 1991;43:180-185.
15. Ridley D, Wilson CG, Washington N, Perkins AC, Wastie M, Ponchel G, et al. The effect of posture on the nasal clearance of starch microspheres. *STP Pharma Sciences* 1995;5:442-446.
16. Puchelle E, Aug F, Pham QT, Bertand A. Comparison of three methods for measuring nasal mucociliary clearance in man. *Acta Otolaryngol.* 1981;91:297-303.
17. Bond SW. Intranasal administration of drugs. In *Drug Delivery to the Respiratory Tract.* Ganderton D and Jones TM (eds) Ellis Horwood, Chichester 1987;133-139
18. Armengot M, Basterra J, Marco J. Nasal mucociliary function during the menstrual cycle in healthy women. *Rev. Laryngol. Otolaryngol. Rhinol.* 1990;111:107-109.
19. Hady MR, Shehata O, Assan R. Nasal mucociliary function in different diseases of the nose. *J. Laryngol. Otol.* 1983;97:497-501
20. Suzumura E, Takeuchi K. Antigen reduces nasal transepithelial electric potential differences and alters ion transport in allergic rhinitis *in vivo. Acta Otolaryngol.* 1992;112:552-558.
21. Awotedu AA, Babalola OO, Lavani EO, Hart PD. Abnormal mucociliary action in asthma and bronchiectasis. *Afr. J. Med. Sci.* 1990;19:153-156.
22. Pederson H, Mygind N. Absence of axonemal arms in the nasal mucosa cilia in Kartagener's syndrome. *Nature (London)* 1976;262:494-495.
23. Takeuchi K. Nasal mucociliary clearance in Sjögren's syndrome. Dissociation in flow between sol and gel layers. *Acta Otolaryngol.* 1989;108:126-129.
24. Lee SW, Hardy JG, Wilson CG, Smelt GJC. Nasal sprays and polyps. *Nucl. Med. Commun.* 1984;5:697-703.
25. Andersen I, Lundqvist GR, Jensen PL, Proctor DF. Human response to controlled levels of sulphur dioxide. *Arch. Environ. Health* 1974;28:31-39.

26. Stanley PJ, Wilson R, Greenstone MA, MacWilliam L, Cole PJ. Effect of cigarette smoking on nasal mucociliary clearance and ciliary beat frequency. *Thorax* 1986;41:519-523.

27. Ewert G. On the mucus flow in the human nose. *Acta Otolaryngol.* 1965;Suppl. 200:1-62.

28. Aoki FK, Crowley JCW. Distribution and removal of human serum albumin-technetium 99m instilled intranasally. *Br. J. Clin. Pharmacol.* 1976;3: 869-878.

29. Proctor DF. Nasal mucus transport and our ambient air. *Laryngoscope* 1983;93:58-62.

30. Torjussen W, Solberg A. Histological findings in the nasal mucosa of nickel workers. *Acta Otolaryngol.* 1976;82:132-134.

31. Acheson ED, Cowdell RH, Hadfield E, Macbeth RG. Nasal cancer in woodworkers in the furniture industry. *Br. Med. J.* 1968;2:587-596.

32. Andersen HC, Solgaard J, Andersen I. Nasal cancer and nasal mucus transport in woodworkers. *Acta Otolarnygol.* 1976;52:263-265.

33. Dalhamn T. Mucus flow and ciliary activity in the trachea of healthy rats and rats exposed to respiratory irritant gases. *Acta Physiol. Scand.* 1956;36 Suppl. 123:1-15.

34. Sakethoo K, Yergin BM, Januskiewicz A, Kovitz K, Sackner MA. The effect of nasal decongestants on nasal mucus velocity. *Am. Rev. Resp. Dis.* 1978;118:251-254.

35. Borum P, Olsen L, Winther B, Mygind N. Ipratropium nasal spray: a new treatment for rhinorrhea in the common cold. *Am. Rev. Respir. Dis.* 1981;123:418-420.

36. Norman PS, Naclerio RM, Creticos PM, Togas A, Lichtenstein LM, Mediator relase after allergic and physical nasal challenge. *Int. Arch. Allergy Appl. Immunol.* 1985;77:57-63.

37. Chien YW, Su KSE, Chang S. Nasal systemic drug delivery. In *Drugs and the Pharmaceutical Sciences.* Chien, YW (ed) 1989:1-26.

38. Richardson DW, Robinson AG. Desmopressin. *Ann. Int. Med.* 1985;103:228-239.

39. Hilsted J, Madasbad S, Hvidberg A. Intranasal insulin therapy: the clinical realities. *Diabetologica* 1995;38:680-684.

40. Lee WA, Ennis RD, Longenecker JP, Bengtsson P. The bioavailability of intranasal salmon calcitonin in healthy volunteers with and without a permeation enhancer. *Pharm. Res.* 1994;11:747-750.

41. Bryant ML, Brown P, Gurevich N, McDougall IR. Comparison of the clearance of radiolabelled nose drops and nasal spray as mucosally delivered vaccine. *Nucl. Med. Commun.* 1999;20:171-174.

42. Merkus FWHM, Verhoef JC, Marttin E, Romeijn SG, van der Kuy PHM, Hermens WAJJ, et al. Cyclodextrins in nasal drug delivery. *Adv. Drug Deliv. Rev.* 1999;36:41-57.

43. Hermens WAJJ, Belder CWJ, Merkus JMWM, Hooymans PM, Verhoef J, Merkus FWHM. Intranasal estradiol administration to oophorectomized women. *Europ. J. Obstet. Gynecol. Reprod. Biol.* 1991;40:35-41.

44. Merkus FWHM, Schipper NGM, Verhoef JC. The influence of absorption enhancers on the intranasal insulin absorption in normal and diabetic subjects. *J. Cont. Rel.* 1996;41:69-75.

45. Heyder J, Rudolf G. Deposition of aerosol particles in the human nose. *Inhaled Part.* 1975;4:107-126.

46. Batts Lansley A. mucociliary clearance and drug delivery via the respiratory tract. *Adv. Drug Deliv. Rev.* 1993;11:299-327.

47. Malmberg H, Holopainen E, Simola M, Böss I, Lindquist N. A comparison between intranasal budesonide dry powder in the treatment of hay fever symptoms. *Rhinol.* 1991;29:137-141.

48. Washington N, McGlashan JA, Jackson SJ, Bush D, Pitt KG, Rawlins DA, Gill, D. The effect of nasal patency on the clearance of saline in healthy volunteers. *Pharm. Res.* 2000; In press.

49. Homer JJ, Raine CH. An endoscopic photographic comparison of nasal drug delivery by aqueous spray. *Clin. Otolaryngol.* 1998;23:560-563.

50. Lethagen S, Harris AS, Sjorin E, Nilsson IM. Intranasal and intravenous administration of desmopressin: effect of F VIII/vWF, pharmacokinetics and reproducibility. *Thromb. Haemostat.* 1987;58:1033-1036.

51. Anik ST, McRae G, Nerenberg C. Nasal absorption of nafarelin decapeptide[D-Nal(2)6] LHRH in rhesus monkey. *J. Pharm. Sci.* 1984;73:684-685.

52. Newman SP, Steed KP, Hardy JG, Wilding IR, Hooper G, Sparrow RA. The distribution of an intranasal insulin formulation in healthy volunteers: Effect of different administration techniques. *J. Pharm. Pharmacol.* 1994;46:657-660.

53. Harris AS, Svensson E, Wagner ZG, Lethagen D, Nilsson IM. Effect of viscosity on particle size, deposition and clearance of nasal delivery systems containing desmopressin. *J. Pharm. Sci.* 1988;77:405-408.

54. Pennington AK, Ratcliffe JH, Wilson CG, Hardy JG. The influence of solution viscosity on nasal spray deposition and clearance. *Int. J. Pharmaceut.* 1988;43:221-224.

55. Jackson SJ, Bush D, Washington N, Ron ES, Schiller M. Determination of the nasal retention of Smart hydrogel™ using gamma scintigraphy (abstract). *J. Pharm. Pharmacol. (suppl. 4)* 1997;49:84.

56. Nagai T, Nishimoto Y, Nambu N, Suzuki Y, Sekine K. Powder dosage form for nasal administration. *J. Cont. Rel.* 1984;1:15-22.

57. Pritchard K, Lansley AB, Martin GP, Halliwell M, Marriott C, Benedetti M. Evaluation of the bioadhesive properties of hyaluronan derivatives: detachment rate and mucociliary transport studies. *Int. J. Pharmaceut.* 1996;129:137-145.

58. Edman P, Bjork E, Ryden L. Microspheres as a nasal delivery system for peptide drugs. *J. Cont. Rel.* 1992;21:165-172.

59. Illum L, Farraj NF, Fisher AN, Gill I, Miglietta M, Benedetti LM. Hyaluronic acid ester microspheres as a nasal delivery system for insulin. *J. Cont. Rel.* 1994;29:133-141.

60. Genta I, Costantini M, Montanari L. Chitosan microspheres for nasal delivery: Effect of cross-linking agents on release characteristics. *Proc. Cont. Rel. Soc.* 1996;23:377-378.

61. Marttin E, Schipper NGM, Verhoef JC, Merkus FWHM. Nasal mucociliary clearance as a factor in nasal drug delivery. *Adv. Drug Deliv. Rev.* 1998;29:13-38.

62. Van de Donk HJM, Mercus FWHM. Nasal drops: do they damage ciliary movement? *Pharm. Int.* 1981;2:157.

63. Bond SW, Hardy JG, Wilson CG. Deposition and clearance of nasal sprays. *Proceedings of the 2nd Europ. Congr. Biopharmaceut. Pharmacokinet.* 1983:93-97.

64. Berg OH, Lie K, Steinsvag SK. The effects of topical nasal steroids on rat respiratory mucosa *in vivo*, with special reference to benzalkonium chloride. *Allergy* 1997;52:627-632.

65. Dondeti P, Zia H, Needham TE. *In vivo* evaluation of spray formulations of human insulin for nasal delivery. *International Journal of Pharmaceutics* 1995;122:91-105.

66. Braat JPM, Ainge G, Bowles JAK. The lack of effect of benzalkonium chloride on the cilia of the nasal mucosa in patients with perennial allergic rhinitis: a combined functional, light scanning and transmission electron microscopy study. *Clin. Exp. Allergy* 1995;25:957-965.

67. Joki S, Saano V, Nuutinen J, Virta P, Karttunen P, Silvasti M, et al. Effects of some preservative agents on rat and guinea pig tracheal and human ciliary beat frequency. *Am. J. Rhinol.* 1996;10:181-186.

68. Batts AH, Marriott C, Martin GP, Wood CF, Bond SW. The effect of some preservatives used in nasal preparations on the mucus and ciliary components on mucociliary clearance. *J. Pharm. Pharmacol.* 1990;42:145-151.

69. Schipper NGM, Verhoef J, Romeijn SG, Merkus FWHM. Absorption enhancers in nasal insulin delivery and their influence on nasal ciliary functioning. *J. Cont. Rel.* 1992;21:173-186.

70. Van de Donk HJM, Van Egmond ALM, Van den Huevel AGM, Zuidema J, Mercus FWHM. The effects of drugs on ciliary motility. I Decongestants. *Int. J. Pharmaceut.* 1982;12:57-65.

71. Duchateau GSMJE. Studies on nasal drug delivery. *Pharm. Weekblad* 1987;9:326-328.

72. Duchateau GSMJE, Zuidema J, Merkus FWHM. Bile salts and intranasal drug absorption. *Int. J. Pharmaceut.* 1986;31:193-199.

73. Vinther B, Elbron D. Nasal mucociliary function during penicillin treatment. *Acta Otolaryngol.* 1978;86:266-267.
74. Kimmerle R, Rolla AR. Iatrogenic Cushing's syndrome due to dexamethasone nasal drops. *Am. J. Med.* 1985;79:535-537.
75. Su XY, Po ALW. The effect of some commercially available antihistamine and decongestant intra-nasal formulations on ciliary beat frequency. *J. Clin. Pharm. Ther.* 1993;18:219-222.
76. Garay RP. Azalastaine: well known ciliotoxic agent? *Int. J. Pharm.* 1996;136:181-183.
77. Hehar SS, Mason JD, Stephen AB, Washington N, Jones NS, Jackson SJ, Bush D. twenty four hour ambulatory nasal pH monitoring. *Clin. Orolaryngol. Appl. Sci.* 1999;24:24-25.
78. Gibson RE, Olanoff LS. Physicochemical determinants of nasal drug absorption. *J. Cont. Rel.* 1987;6:361-366.
79. Morimoto K, Yamaguchi H, Iwakura Y, Morisaka K, Ohashi Y, Nakai Y. Effects of viscous hyaluronate-sodium solutions on the nasal absorption of vasopressin and an analogue. *Pharmaceut. Res.* 1991;8:471-474.
80. Su XY, Po ALW. Surface-response study of the effect of pH and tonicity on ciliary activity. *S.T.P. Pharma Sciences* 1994;4:82-85.
81. Hirai S, Ikenaga R, Matsuzawa T. Nasal absorption of insulin in dogs. *Diabetes* 1978;27:269-299.
82. Washington N, Steele RJC, Jackson SJ, Bush D, Mason J, Gill DA, Pitt K, Rawlind DA.. Determination of baseline human nasal pH and the effect of intranasally administered buffers. *Int. J. Pharmaceut.* In press.
83. Gizurarson S. The relevance of nasal physiology to the design of drug absorption studies. *Adv. Drug Deliv. Rev.* 1993;11:329-347.

Chapter Ten

Pulmonary Drug Delivery

STRUCTURE AND FUNCTION OF THE PULMONARY SYSTEM
    The lung
    Upper airway
    Structure of the tracheo-bronchial tree
    Epithelium
        Upper airways
        Bronchi and bronchioles
        Alveoli
        Alveolar-capillary membrane
    Lung permeability
    Lung mucus
    Lung defences
    Lung surfactant
    Blood supply
    Lymphatic system
    Nervous control
        Cough reflex
    Biochemical processes which occur in the lung
    Breathing
    Respiratory disease
        Asthma
        Acute bronchitis
        Chronic bronchitis
        Pulmonary emphysema
        Bronchiectasis
DOSAGE FORMS FOR PULMONARY DRUG DELIVERY
    Pressurized inhalation aerosols
    Dry powder inhalers
    Nebulizers
    Spacer devices and ancillary equipment
ASSESSMENT OF DEPOSITION BY GAMMA SCINTIGRAPHY
    Choice of radiolabel
    Labelling inhalation formulations
    Labelling dry powder inhalers
    Validation
FACTORS AFFECTING PARTICLE DEPOSITION IN THE LUNG
    Physicochemical properties
    Deposition patterns from different dose forms
    Physiological variables
    Inhaler technique
    Effects of disease
DRUG ABSORPTION
PHARMACOKINETICS

DRUGS ADMINISTERED VIA THE PULMONARY ROUTE
     Anti-allergy agents
     Beta receptor agonists
     Adrenocorticosteroids
     Leukotriene inhibitors
     Other bronchodilating agents
     Mucolytics
     Systemically-absorbed drugs
REFERENCES

STRUCTURE AND FUNCTION OF THE PULMONARY SYSTEM

The major function of the pulmonary system is the oxygenation of blood and the removal of carbon dioxide from the body. Breathing ventilates the respiratory tissue leading to gaseous exchange in the lungs. The tissue is therefore specialized to present the largest available surface area within the protection of the thoracic cavity. The large oxygen requirement is necessary to support the high metabolic rate of mammals.

The respiratory system in man is divided into the upper and lower respiratory tracts. The upper respiratory tract consists of the nose, nasal passages, paranasal passages, mouth, Eustachian tubes, the pharynx, the oesophagus and the larynx. The trachea and bronchi are sometimes included as part of the upper respiratory tract. The lower respiratory tract consists of the true respiratory tissue, i.e. the air passages and alveoli.

The lung

The organ lung comprises a left and right lung, divided in slightly unequal proportions, that occupy most of the intrathoracic space. The right lung represents 56 percent of the total lung volume and is composed of three lobes, a superior, middle, and inferior lobe, separated from each other by a deep horizontal and an oblique fissure. The left lung, smaller in volume because of the asymmetrical position of the heart, has only two lobes separated by an oblique fissure. The space between the lungs is filled by a connective tissue space containing the heart, major blood vessels, trachea with the stem bronchi, oesophagus and thymus gland. In the thorax, the two lungs rest with their bases on the diaphragm, while their apices extend above the first rib.

Upper airway

As discussed in Chapter 9, the function of the nose is to provide humidification, filtration and warming of the inspired air. Although the nose is designed as the primary route of entry for gases, most people also breathe through the mouth, particularly during stress. In this case many of the nasal defensive pathways are lost. Hence the lung also has to have mechanisms to condition the air and remove foreign particles.

The nasopharynx is primarily a passageway from the nose to the oral pharynx for air and secretions. It is also connected to the tympanic cavity of the middle ear through the auditory tubes that open on both lateral walls. The act of swallowing briefly opens the normally collapsed auditory tubes and allows the middle ears to be aerated and pressure differences to be equalized. In the posterior wall of the nasopharynx is located a lymphatic organ, the pharyngeal tonsil.

The larynx is an organ of complex structure that serves a dual function: as a controlling air canal to the lungs and as the organ of phonation. Below the larynx lies the trachea, a tube about 10 to 12 centimetres long and two centimetres wide. Its wall is stiffened by 16 to 20 characteristic horseshoe-shaped, incomplete cartilage rings that open towards the back and are embedded in a dense connective tissue. The dorsal wall contains a strong layer of transverse smooth muscle fibres that span the gap of the cartilage. In an adult, the trachea is 11 to 13 cm in length and 1.5 to 2.5 cm in diameter, and bifurcates to form the right and left main bronchi (Figure 10.1). The right bronchus divides into the upper, middle and lower branches whilst the left bronchus divides only into an upper and a lower branch. These lobar bronchi give rise to branches called 'segmental bronchi'. The branching angle of 37° appears to be optimal to ensure smooth airflow.

Structure of the tracheo-bronchial tree

The hierarchy of the dividing airways, and partly the blood vessels, in the lung largely determines the internal lung structure. Functionally the system can be subdivided into three zones, a proximal, purely conducting zone, a peripheral, purely gas-exchanging zone, and a transitional zone in between. Morphologically the relatively thick-walled, purely air-conducting tubes can be distinguished from those branches of the airway tree structurally designed to permit gas exchange.

Every branching of the tracheo-bronchial tree produces a new 'generation' of tubes, the total cross-sectional area increasing with each generation (Figure 10.2). The main bronchi are known as the first generation, the second and third generations are the lobar and segmental bronchi respectively. The fourth to ninth generations are the small bronchi and in these segmental bronchi the diameters decrease from approximately 4 to 1 mm. At a diameter of less than 1 mm they lie inside the lobules and are then correctly termed

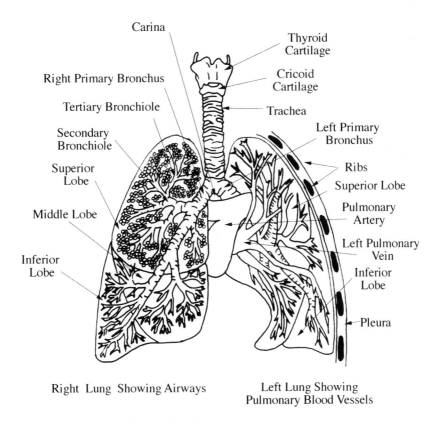

Right Lung Showing Airways   Left Lung Showing Pulmonary Blood Vessels

Figure 10.1 Structure of the lungs

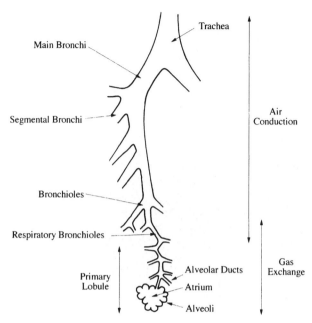

Figure 10.2 The tree structure of the lung

bronchioles. Here the function of the tissue changes from conducting airway to gas exchange. Although the decrease in diameter minimizes the deadspace, it is associated with a large increase in resistance to flow. For example, a 10% reduction in diameter is associated with an increase in airway resistance of more than 50%. Thus the airways should be as wide as possible to minimize resistance, but this will of course increase deadspace. In the body these opposing factors are balanced by finely tuned physiological control which is easily disturbed by lung pathologies such as asthma and bronchitis.

The respiratory gases diffuse from air to blood, and vice versa, through the 140 square metres of internal surface area of the tissue compartment. The gas-exchange tissue proper is called the pulmonary parenchyma, while the supplying structures, conductive airways, lymphatics, and non-capillary blood vessels belong to the non-parenchyma. The parenchyma of the lung consists of approximately 130,000 lobules, each with a diameter of about 3.5 mm and containing around 2,200 alveoli. It is believed that each lobule is supplied by a single pulmonary arteriole. The terminal bronchioles branch into approximately 14 respiratory bronchioles, each of which branches further into the alveolar ducts. The ducts carry 3 or 4 spherical atria that lead to the alveolar sacs supplying 15-20 alveoli (Figure 10.3). Additional alveoli arise directly from the walls of the alveolar ducts, and these are responsible for approximately 35% of the total gas exchange. It has been estimated that there are 300 million alveoli in an adult human lung. The volume of an alveolus changes with the degree of inflation, but assuming 75% lung inflation, the diameter of an alveolus is thought to be between 250 and 290 μm. It is estimated that each alveolus has a volume of 1.05×10^{-5} ml, with an air-tissue interface of 27×10^{-4} cm^2. For these calculations, it was assumed that the lung had a total air volume of 4.8 l, a total respiratory zone volume of 3.15 l and a total alveolar air-tissue interface of 81 m^2.

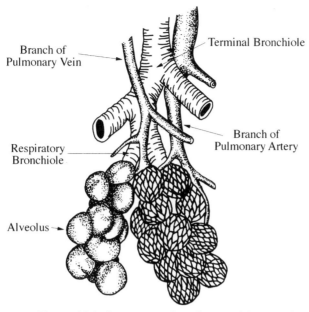

Branch of
Pulmonary Vein

Terminal Bronchiole

Respiratory
Bronchiole

Branch of
Pulmonary Artery

Alveolus

Figure 10.3 Structure and perfusion of the alveoli

Epithelium

Upper airways

The nasal cavity, the nasopharynx, larynx, trachea and bronchi are lined with pseudostratified, ciliated, columnar epithelium with many goblet cells. There are also coarse hairs in the nasal region of the respiratory tract.

Bronchi and bronchioles

The bronchi, but not the bronchioles, have mucous and serous glands present. The bronchioles, however, possess goblet cells and the wall contains a well-developed layer of smooth muscle cells, capable of narrowing the airway. The epithelium in the terminal and respiratory bronchioles consists largely of ciliated, cuboidal cells and smaller numbers of Clara cells. The ciliated epithelial cells each have about 20 cilia with an average length of 6 µm and a diameter of 0.3 µm. Each cilium is composed of a central doublet and 9 peripheral filaments which function as a structural support. Contractions result in successive beats of the cilia creating a wave which consists of a fast propulsion stroke followed by a slow recovery stroke. Clara cells become the most predominant type in the most distal part of the respiratory bronchioles. They have ultrastructural features of secretory cells but the nature and function of the secretory product is poorly understood.

Alveoli

In the alveolar ducts and alveoli the epithelium is flatter and becomes the simple, squamous type, 0.1 to 0.5 µm thick. The alveoli are packed tightly and do not have separate walls, adjacent alveoli being separated by a common alveolar septum with communication between alveoli via alveolar pores (Figure 10.4). The alveoli form a honeycomb of cells around the spiral, cylindrical surface of the alveolar duct. The exposed alveolar surface is normally covered with a surface film of lipoprotein material.

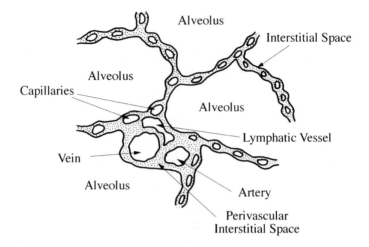

Figure 10.4 Cross-section of the alveoli

There are several types of pulmonary alveolar cells. Type I (or small type A), are non-phagocytic, membranous pneumocytes. These surface-lining epithelial cells are approximately 5 μm in thickness and possess thin squamous cytoplasmic extensions that originate from a central nucleated portion. These portions do not have any organelles and hence they are metabolically dependent on the central portion of the cell. This reduces their ability to repair themselves if damaged.

Attached to the basement membrane are the larger alveolar cells (Type II, type B or septal cells). These rounded, granular, epithelial pneumocytes are approximately 10 to 15 μm thick. There are 6 to 7 cells per alveolus and these cells possess great metabolic activity. They are believed to produce the surfactant material that lines the lung and to be essential for alveolar repair after damage from viruses or chemical agents.

Alveolar-capillary membrane

The blood and alveolar gases are separated by the alveolar capillary membrane (Figure 10.4) which is composed of a continuous epithelium of 0.1 to 0.5 μm thickness, a collagen fibre network, a ground substance, a basement membrane and the capillary endothelium. The interstitium is composed of the basement membrane of the endothelium, a ground substance, and epithelium. It forms a three dimensional skeleton to which the alveoli and capillaries are attached. Maximum absorption probably occurs in the areas where the interstitium is the thinnest (80 nm) since the surfactant is also thin in these areas (15 nm). Drainage of the interstitial fluid occurs by passage into the lymphatics, which often happens long after passage along the alveolar wall.

The thickness of the air-blood barrier varies from 0.2 μm to 10 μm. The barrier is minimal when the thickness is less than 0.5 μm since the epithelium and endothelium are present only as thin cytoplasmic extensions and the interstitium exists as a narrow gap between mostly fused membranes. When the diameter exceeds 0.5 μm additional structural elements are present. The minimal barrier thickness is nearly identical in structure and dimensions in all mammalian species that have been investigated. This is in contrast to the alveolar surface areas which increase proportionally with body weight.

Lung permeability

The alveolar epithelium and the capillary endothelium have a very high permeability to water, most gases and lipophilic substances. There is an effective barrier however for many hydrophilic substances of large molecular size and for ionic species. The alveolar type 1 cells have tight junctions, effectively limiting the penetration of molecules to those with a radius of less than 0.6 nm. Endothelial junctions are much larger, with gaps of the order of 4 to 6 nm. Clearance from the alveoli by passage across the epithelium bears an approximate inverse relationship to the molecular weight. The normal alveolar epithelium is almost totally impermeable to proteins and small solutes, for example the half-time for turnover of albumin between plasma and the alveolar compartment is of the order of 36 hours[1]. The microvascular endothelium, with its larger intercellular gaps, is far more permeable for all molecular sizes and there is normally an appreciable leak of protein into the systemic circulation.

Lung mucus

A thin fluid layer called the mucous blanket, 5 μm in depth, covers the walls of the entire respiratory tract (Figure 10.5). This barrier serves to trap foreign particles for subsequent removal and prevents dehydration of the surface epithelium by unsaturated air taken in during inspiration.

There are about 6000 tracheo-bronchial glands in man, with an average of one cell per square millimetre of surface area. The ratio of goblet cells to ciliated cells is 1 to 5 in the large airways and 1 to several hundred in the bronchioles. The mucus largely originates from the vagally innervated, submucosal glands, with a smaller contribution from goblet cells. Within the gland, distal serous cells secrete a watery fluid, whereas the mucus cells near the neck secrete a gel. It is speculated that the secretions of the serous cells help in the movement of the swollen gel to the surface. Although the mucus producing cells are under vagal control and can be regulated by cholinergically mediated drugs, goblet cells discharge mucus without physiological stimulation.

The main component of nasal mucus appears to be a mucopolysaccharide complexed with sialic acid. Mucus contains 2-3% mucin, 1-2% electrolytes, and the remainder water. Tracheo-bronchial mucus has viscoelastic properties and it averages 5% solids, including

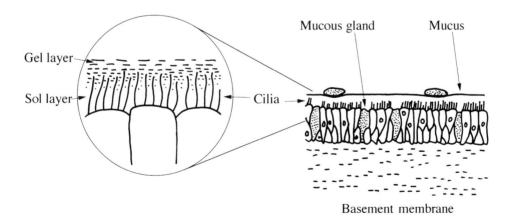

Figure 10.5 The mucociliary escalator

2% mucin, 1% carbohydrate, less than 1% lipid and 0.03% DNA. Pulmonary secretions are slightly hyperosmotic, but those secreted from the smaller bronchi and bronchioles are thought to be isosmotic, being in equilibrium with tissue and vascular fluids. The pH of rat tracheal secretions has been reported to be between 6.0 and 7.6.

Increased mucus secretion is brought about by cholinergic and a-adrenergic agonists which act directly on the mucus secreting cells of the submucosal gland. Serous secretions are stimulated by b-agonists or cholinergic stimulation, whereas the goblet cells do not appear to be innervated. The peripheral granules, in which the mucus is stored, are discharged continuously and form a reservoir which is secreted after exposure to an irritant stimulus. Disease states can drastically change the distribution of goblet cells and composition of respiratory tract fluids. Conditions such as chronic bronchitis are characterized by increased sputum and chronic irritation, leading to an increased number of glandular and goblet cells which result in a crowding of ciliated cells. Mucus transport is thus slowed and the increased viscosity of the mucus exacerbates the problem.

Lung defences

The respiratory tract possesses a complicated but comprehensive series of defences against inhaled material due to its continual exposure to the outside environment. The lung has an efficient self-cleansing mechanism referred to as the mucociliary escalator (Figure 10.5). The mucus gel layer floats above the sol layer which has been calculated to be approximately 7 μm thick. The cilia extend through this layer so that the tip of the villus protrudes into the gel. The co-ordinated movement of the cilia propels the mucous blanket and deposited foreign materials at the rate of 2-5 cm min⁻¹ towards the pharynx where they are swallowed. It has been estimated that 1 litre of mucus is cleared every 24 hours. Cigarette smokers demonstrate a considerable slowing in the clearance mechanisms of the large airways, resulting in an accumulation at the hilius, the junction between the lymph node and efferent lymphatic vessel.

The alveolar phagocytes or "dust cells" remove inhaled particles which reach the alveoli since this region is not ciliated. These cells can ingest and destroy bacteria and viruses and engulf inhaled particulates, migrating to the ciliated areas of the bronchial tree, where they are transported up the mucociliary escalator. Some macrophages with engulfed particles slowly penetrate the alveolar wall, especially in the region of the alveolar duct, pass into the tissue fluid and lymphatics. They also secrete chemicals that attract white blood cells to the site, and hence they can initiate an inflammatory response in the lung. Particles picked up by macrophages are removed by them into the lymphatic system of the lung and stored in adjacent lymph glands. Soluble particles are removed into the bloodstream, to be finally excreted by the kidney.

The composition of expectorated liquid and sputum varies, but consists of tracheobronchial, salivary, nasal and lacrimal gland secretions plus entrapped foreign material, dead tissue cells, phagocytes, leucocytes, alveolar lining and products of microbial infections.

Lung surfactant

The elastic fibres of the lung and the wall tension of the alveoli would cause the lung to collapse if this were not counterbalanced by the presence of the lung surfactant system. This covers the alveolar surface to the thickness of 10 to 20 nm. The surfactant has a liquid crystalline or gel structure which consists of phospholipids (74%), mucopolysaccharides and possibly proteins. It forms a continuous covering over the alveoli and is constantly renewed from below. Fifty percent of the surfactant comprises dipalmitoyl lecithin, replacement of which is rapid with a half-life of 14 hours. Enzymes, lipids and detergents can destroy the surfactant. If the surfactant is removed by irrigation of the lung with saline, no harm appears to result since it is rapidly replaced. Generation of surfactant in neonates does not occur until the time of birth, so preterm infants often suffer from respiratory problems. Replacement surfactants, such as Exosurf® (GlaxoWellcome) can be administered to alleviate this problem.

Blood supply

The pulmonary artery arises from the right ventricle of the heart and thus supplies the lung with de-oxygenated blood. The lung tissue itself receives a supply of oxygenated blood from the bronchial arteries. Smaller capillaries branch from the main arteries to supply the terminal bronchioles, respiratory bronchioles, alveolar ducts, air sacs and alveoli. The average internal diameter of the alveolar capillary is only 8 μm with an estimated total surface area of 60 to 80 square metres and a capillary blood volume of 100 to 200 ml. The large surface area allows rapid absorption and removal of any substance which may penetrate the alveoli-capillary membrane thereby producing good sink conditions for drug absorption. Blood takes only a few seconds to pass through the lungs and it has been estimated that the time for passage through the alveolar capillaries of males at rest to be about 0.7 s, falling to 0.3 s on exercise.

Lymphatic system

In the adult lung, the lymphatic channels surround the bronchi, pulmonary arteries and veins. A deep system of lymphatics has been identified which lie adjacent to the alveoli. Movement of fluid from the alveolar lumen to the lymphatics has been described as a two-stage process. The first step is the passage across the epithelial lining through the intercellular clefts and/or through the cytoplasmic layer by diffusion or pinocytosis. The second step is the movement of fluid along the alveolar wall into the lymphatic area.

Nervous control

Both sympathetic and parasympathetic nerves supply the tracheo-bronchial tree. The primary role of these nerves is the control of ventilation of the lungs under varying physiological demand and the protection of the lung by the cough reflex, bronchoconstriction and the secretion of mucus. The lung is heavily innervated, as are the smooth muscle sheets that surround the airways, the intercostal muscles and the diaphragm.

Stimulation of the sympathetic nerves via the ß₂ adrenergic receptors primarily results in active relaxation of bronchial smooth muscle. Stimulation of parasympathetic nerves via the nicotinic and muscarinic receptors results in increased glandular activity and constriction of bronchial smooth muscle.

Cough reflex

Cough is accomplished by suddenly opening the larynx during a brief Valsalva manoeuvre which is a forceful contraction of the chest and abdominal muscles against a closed glottis. The resultant high-speed jet of air is an effective means of clearing the airways of excessive secretions or foreign particles. Cough receptors are found at the carina (the point at which the trachea divides into the bronchi) and bifurcations of the larger bronchi. They are much more sensitive to mechanical stimulation, and inhalation of dust produces bronchoconstriction at low concentration and elicits the cough reflex with larger amounts. Lung irritant receptors, located in the epithelial layers of the trachea and larger airways, are much more sensitive to chemical stimulation and produce a reflex bronchoconstriction and hyperpnoea (over respiration) on stimulation by irritant gases or histamine. The constriction is relieved by isoprenaline or atropine which suggests that the effect is due to contraction of smooth muscle, mediated through post-ganglionic cholinergic pathways.

Biochemical processes which occur in the lung

Almost all of the drug-metabolizing enzymes found in the liver are also present in the lung, although in much smaller amounts. The lung has been observed to be responsible for the release of 5-hydroxytryptamine, synthesis of prostaglandins, conversion of angiotensin I to angiotensin II, histamine release, and inactivation of bradykinin. The mast cells located around the small blood vessels and in the alveolar walls are rich in histamine, heparin, 5-hydroxytryptamine and hyaluronic acid. Histamine release accounts for many of the symptoms of bronchial asthma and allergies. It causes capillary dilatation, increased capillary permeability, contraction and spasm of smooth muscle, skin swelling, hypotension and increased secretion of saliva, mucus, tears and nasal fluids.

The mammalian lung can actively synthesize fatty acids, particularly palmitic and linoleic, and incorporate these into phospholipids which are predominantly saturated lecithins. The active synthesis of proteins by the alveolar cells has also been reported.

Breathing

Breathing is an automatic and rhythmic act produced by networks of neurons in the hindbrain (the pons and medulla). The respiratory rhythm and the length of each phase of respiration are set by reciprocal stimulatory and inhibitory interconnection of these brainstem neurons.

The forces that normally cause changes in volume of the chest and lungs stem not only from muscle contraction but also from the elastic properties of both the lung and the chest. A lung is similar to a balloon, it resists stretch, tending to collapse almost totally unless held inflated by a pressure difference between its inside and outside. Air moves in and out of the lungs in response to differences in pressure. When the air pressure within the alveolar spaces falls below atmospheric pressure, air enters the lungs (inspiration), provided the larynx is open; when the air pressure within the alveoli exceeds atmospheric pressure, air is blown from the lungs (expiration). The flow of air is rapid or slow in proportion to the magnitude of the pressure difference. Atmospheric pressure remains relatively constant, hence flow is determined by how much above or below atmospheric pressure the pressure within the lungs rises or falls.

The respiratory pump is versatile, capable of increasing its output 25 times, from a normal resting level of about 6 L min^{-1} to 150 L min^{-1} in adults.

Respiratory disease

The respiratory tract is the site of an exceptionally large range of disorders since it is exposed to the environment and therefore dust or gases in the air may cause damage to the lung tissue or produce hypersensitivity reactions. Secondly, the entire output of the heart has to pass through its large network of capillaries, hence diseases that affect the small blood vessels are likely to reach the remainder of the lung. Cough is a particularly important sign of all diseases that affect any part of the bronchial tree. The presence of blood in the sputum is an important indication of disease. It may result simply from an exacerbation of an existing infection, it may also indicate the presence of inflammation, capillary damage, tumour or tuberculosis.

Asthma

Particles of foreign protein may be deposited directly in the lung and hence it is not surprising that allergic reactions are very common. The most common and most important of these is asthma. The most common triggers are pollens, mould spores, animal proteins of different kinds, and proteins from a variety of insects, particularly cockroaches and mites that occur in house dust. Spasmodic asthma is characterized by contraction of the smooth muscle of the airways and, in severe attacks, by airway obstruction from mucus that has accumulated in the bronchial tree resulting in difficulty in breathing.

Extrinsic asthma is caused by an identifiable allergen, in which antigens affect tissue cells sensitized by a specific antibody. Intrinsic asthma occurs without an identifiable antigen or specific antibody. Extrinsic asthma commonly manifests in childhood because of a genetic predisposition or "atopic" characteristic. Hayfever and asthma are common atopic conditions. Exacerbation of extrinsic asthma is precipitated by contact with any of the proteins to which sensitization has occurred; airway obstruction is often worse in the early hours of the morning, for reasons not yet entirely elucidated. Intrinsic asthma may develop at any age, and there may be no evidence of specific antigens. Persons with intrinsic asthma experience attacks of airway obstruction unrelated to seasonal changes, although it seems likely that the airway obstruction may be triggered by infections, which are assumed to be viral in many cases.

Acute bronchitis

Acute bronchitis most commonly occurs as a consequence of viral infection. It may also be precipitated by acute exposure to irritant gases, such as chlorine, sulphur dioxide and ammonia. The bronchial tree in acute bronchitis is reddened and congested and minor blood streaking of the sputum may occur. Most cases of acute bronchitis resolve over a few days and the mucosa repairs itself.

Chronic bronchitis

This is a common condition and is generally produced by cigarette smoking and characterized by chronic cough and excess sputum production. The mortality rate from chronic bronchitis and emphysema soared after World War II in all western countries. The number and size of mucous glands lining the large airways increase after a number of years of smoking. The speed at which this occurs may be enhanced by breathing polluted air and by a damp climate. The changes are not confined to large airways, though these produce the dominant symptom of chronic sputum production. Changes in smaller bronchioles lead to obliteration and inflammation around their walls. All of these changes together, if severe enough, can lead to disturbances in the distribution of ventilation and perfusion in the lung, causing a fall in arterial oxygen tension and a rise in carbon dioxide tension. By the time this occurs, the ventilatory ability of the patient, as measured by the velocity of a single forced expiration, is severely compromised. It is not clear what determines the severity of these changes, since many people can smoke for decades without evidence of significant airway changes, while others may experience severe respiratory compromise after 15 years or less of exposure.

Pulmonary emphysema

This irreversible disease consists of destruction of alveolar walls and the consequent increase in size of the air spaces distal to the terminal bronchiole. It occurs in two forms, centrilobular emphysema, in which the destruction begins at the centre of the lobule, and panlobular (or panacinar) emphysema, in which alveolar destruction occurs in all alveoli within the lobule simultaneously. In advanced cases, the destruction is so great, that the two forms cannot be distinguished. Centrilobular emphysema is the form most commonly seen in cigarette smokers, and some observers believe it is confined to smokers. It is more common in the upper lobes of the lung (for unknown reasons) and probably causes abnormalities in blood gases out of proportion to the area of the lung involved by it. By the time the disease has developed, some impairment of ventilatory ability has occurred. Panacinar emphysema may also occur in smokers, but it is the type of emphysema characteristically found in the lower lobes of patients with a deficiency in the antiproteolytic enzyme known as alpha1-antitrypsin. Like centrilobular emphysema, panacinar emphysema causes ventilatory limitation and eventually blood gas changes. Other types of emphysema, of less importance than the two major varieties, may develop along the dividing walls of the lung (septal emphysema) or in association with scars from other lesions.

Bronchiectasis

Bronchiectasis consists of a dilatation of major bronchi. It is believed usually to begin in childhood, possibly after a severe attack of whooping cough or pneumonia. The bronchi become chronically infected, and excess sputum production and episodes of chest infection are common. The disease may develop as a consequence of airway obstruction or of undetected (and therefore untreated) aspiration into the airway of small foreign bodies such as plastic toys.

DOSAGE FORMS FOR PULMONARY DRUG DELIVERY

Direct delivery of a drug to the lung has a number of advantages over oral administration, including the use of less drug to achieve the same therapeutic benefit, a reduction in the likelihood of systemic side effects, and a more rapid onset of action. There are two possible mechanisms for delivery of drugs to the lung, either via an aerosol or direct instillation. The most commonly used is the aerosol, which consists of finely divided liquid droplets or solid particles in a gaseous suspension. An atomizer is the general term for a device which generates an aerosol and may be electrically, pneumatically or mechanically powered. Unfortunately today, the term aerosol, in general usage, has become synonymous with a pressurized package.

Pharmaceutical aerosols may be divided into two types. Space sprays disperse the drug as a finely divided spray with particles not exceeding 50 μm. Surface-coating aerosols produce a coarse or wet spray and are used to coat surfaces with a residual film. Only space sprays are used for pulmonary drug delivery. The main types of device used at present to produce aerosols are nebulizers, metered dose inhalers (MDI) and dry powder inhalers (DPI), although development of the technology is causing the distinctions between these devices to become blurred.

Pressurized inhalation aerosols

Pressurized metered dose inhalers for delivery of medications have been available since the mid 1950s. In these systems, the drug is usually a polar solid which has been dissolved or suspended in a non-polar liquefied propellant. If the preparation is a suspension, as is most commonly the case, the powder is normally micronised by fluid energy milling and the suspension is stabilized by the addition of a surfactant. Lecithin, oleic acid, and the Span and Tween series surfactants have been widely used for this type of formulation. Oleic acid is particularly favoured and is added in some excess over the amount required for suspension stabilization, since it also functions as a lubricant for the metering valve.

Metered dose inhalers (MDIs) are the most commonly used drug delivery system for inhalation (Figure 10.6). The propellants have a high vapour pressure of around 400 kPa at room temperature, but since the device is sealed, only a small fraction of the propellant exists as a gas. The canister consists of a metering valve crimped on to an aluminum can.

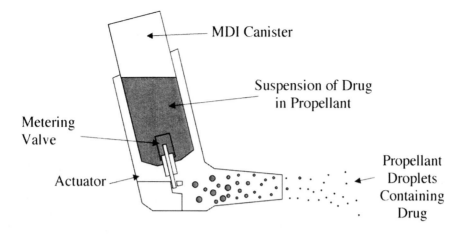

MDI Canister

Suspension of Drug
in Propellant

Metering
Valve

Propellant

Actuator

Droplets
Containing
Drug

Figure 10.6 The metered dose inhaler

Individual doses are measured volumetrically by a metering chamber within the valve. Each MDI canister can hold between 100 and 200 doses of between 20 μg and 5 mg of drug, which is released within the first 0.1 s after actuation.

The valve stem is fitted into an actuator incorporating a mouthpiece. The aerosol, consisting of propellant droplets containing drug, is delivered from the actuator mouthpiece at very high velocity, probably about 30 ms[-1]. There is partial (15 - 20%) evaporation of propellant prior to exit from the atomizing nozzle ("flashing"), and further break up of droplets beyond this point caused by the violent evaporation of the propellant. This results in a wide droplet size distribution from 1 to 5 μm. Only 10% of the particulates delivered in a single dose released by a metered-dose inhaler actually reach the lungs, since the bulk of it impacts in the oropharynx and the mouthpiece. Reduction of the plume velocity, for example in the Gentlehaler[®] device[2] causes a significant reduction in oropharyngeal deposition.

A flurry of activity in aerosol formulation and technique of administration occurred following the adoption of the Montreal Protocol in 1987. This banned the manufacture of certain chlorofluorocarbon (CFC) propellants[3] by developed countries for environmental reasons. The temporary exception was for those used in the treatment of asthma and chronic obstructive lung disease. In many inhalers CFC propellants have now been replaced with hydrofluoroalkanes (HFAs). These compounds do not deplete the atmospheric ozone layer, but unfortunately are still considered "greenhouse gases," and may contribute to global warming[4].

With drugs which can be dissolved in the propellant, delivery to lungs can be increased to 40% of the ejected dose[5] since the particle size of the drug remaining after propellant vaporization can be very small. Altering the vapour pressure of these systems can also improve deposition. Lung depositions of 51 and 65% were reported with low and high vapour pressures respectively[6]. The changeover of propellant from CFCs to HFAs has had a notable effect on the delivery of some drugs, notably beclomethasone dipropionate. This has a 51% delivery to the lungs in HFA, in which it is soluble, compared to 4% in CFC, in which it is a suspension[7]. Unfortunately both HFAs and CFCs are relatively poor solvents and so it not often possible to take advantage of this type of formulation, even with the addition of cosolvents such as ethanol.

In order to be effective, metered dose aerosols must be triggered as the patient is inhaling. Some patients have difficulty with this feat of coordination, and breath actuated inhalers such as the Autohaler® have been designed to overcome this by triggering the valve as the patient breathes in[8]. The Mist-Assist® inspiratory flow control device (IFCD, Ballard Medical, Draper, UT) is a compact device (similar in size to a spacer) through which both an MDI or medication from a nebulizer can be administered. By use of a floating ball within the inspiratory chamber, it provides visual and auditory (clicking sound) feedback to optimize timing of medication delivery and rate of inspiratory flow. Most important, the inspiratory flow rate (and therefore inspiratory resistance) can be adjusted on the device. This inspiratory flow control enhances laminar flow of particles and gas and increases the lung deposition.

Dry powder inhalers

The environmental concerns surrounding the use of chlorofluorocarbons have led to a resurgence of interest in dry powder inhaler devices. Early dry powder inhalers such as the Rotahaler® used individual capsules of micronized drug which were difficult to handle. Modern devices use blister packs (e.g. Diskus®) or reservoirs (e.g. Turbuhaler®) (Figure 10.7). The dry powder inhalers rely on inspiration to withdraw drug from the inhaler to the lung and hence the effect of inhalation flow rate through various devices has been extensively studied. The major problem to be overcome with these devices is to ensure that the finely micronized drug is thoroughly dispersed in the airstream. It has been recommended that patients inhale as rapidly as possible from these devices in order to provide the maximum force to disperse the powder[9]. The quantity of drug and deposition pattern varies enormously depending on the device[10], for example the Turbuhaler® produces significantly greater lung delivery of salbutamol than the Diskus®. Vidgren and coworkers[11] demonstrated by gamma scintigraphy that a typical dry powder formulation of sodium cromoglycate suffers losses of 44% in the mouth and 40% in the actuator nozzle itself.

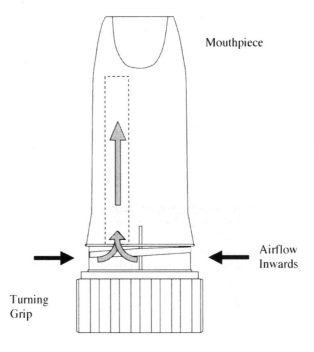

Mouthpiece

Airflow
Inwards

Turning
Grip

Figure 10.7 A simplified view of the Turbuhaler, a typical dry powder device

Nebulizers

Medical nebulizers can be divided into two main groups, pneumatic and electric. A pneumatic generator operates from a pressurized gas source, while an electric generator derives its power from an electric source. There are two types of pneumatic nebulizers (jet and hydrodynamic) and one electric generator (ultrasonic) presently used for medical purposes.

The jet nebulizer is a system in which a high-velocity gas flow is directed over a tube that is immersed in a water reservoir (Figure 10.8). The expansion of the driver gas decreases the pressure over the tube, which draws the formulation into the gas stream. The high shear rate in the jet stream then nebulizes it. The hydrodynamic nebulizer uses a system that prepares a film of water for aerosol formation by flowing it over a hollow sphere. A small orifice in the sphere expels gas at supersonic velocity. This high-velocity gas ruptures the thin film of water and produces a continuous dispersion of fine, liquid particles. A gas cylinder or compressor supplies the gas pressure. The ultrasonic nebulizer consists of a piezo-electric crystal which produces high frequency sound waves in the liquid in the nebulizing unit. The surface waves produce small droplets (Faraday crispations) which are conducted away by an airstream for inhalation. All these devices produce relatively broad droplet size distributions in which a large fraction of coarse droplets are present. Consequently most use some sort of baffle system in the airstream; coarse droplets impact on this and are returned to the reservoir for re-nebulization, while the smaller particles avoid the baffle and are passed to the patient.

The properties of nebulizers vary widely; while all produce droplets with sizes in the range 1-10 μm, they vary significantly in droplet size distribution and pulmonary deposition[12 13]. Despite this they have a number of advantages that is causing a renewal of interest in their use. Because MDIs and DPIs have a relatively high gas flow rate, they show high oropharyngeal impaction. This problem is reduced in nebulizers since the airflow can be adjusted to suit the patient's inhalation rate. Continuous nebulization can deliver very large quantities of drugs if necessary, from aqueous solutions without major formulation prob-

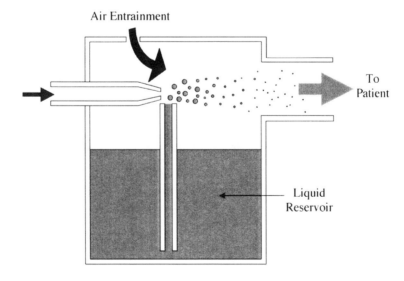

Figure 10.8 An air-driven nebulizer

lems. Unfortunately most nebulizers are bulky and require a fixed power source, which limits their use severely.

In order to combine these advantages of nebulizers with the portability of MDIs, Boehringer Ingelheim have developed the Respimat®, a spring-driven spray with a similar outward appearance to a conventional MDI. Unlike an MDI, the Respimat® delivers its spray in a slow low-velocity cloud. This leads to increased central pulmonary deposition[14], which is probably due to the increased time available for droplet evaporation before inhalation, and the reduced plume velocity, which reduces oropharyngeal impaction. Since these two factors are the main reasons for the success of spacer devices (see below), the addition of a spacer to a Respimat® caused no significant improvement in deposition.

Spacer devices and ancillary equipment

A number of techniques have been used in an attempt to improve the deposition of inhaled drug particles. The best known of these are the various kinds of spacers, chambers which are placed between the inhaler device and the patient's mouth (Figure 10.9). These devices cause considerable improvements in the fraction of dose deposited in the lungs and operate through a number of mechanisms. Firstly they provide a delay time before inhalation to allow full evaporation of propellant, so that the particles have reached their minimum size. Secondly they slow down the particle cloud so that the impaction velocity on the oropharynx is reduced, thus reducing impaction in this region. Finally they have a reservoir function which makes the timing of inhalation by the patient less critical. A typical example of such a device is the Nebuhaler®, which was studied by Kenyon et al. for the delivery of Budenoside[15]. The Nebuhaler® caused a significant increase (from 12% to 38%) in pulmonary deposition, and an improvement in peripheral deposition. When assessing studies of such devices, it is important to realize that the spacer itself acts as an impaction filter and a proportion of the larger droplets are removed by it. In addition plastic devices accumulate wall charges and act as electrostatic precipitators, causing significant drug losses which vary with handling, humidity and cleaning or priming history[15].

Several methods have been developed to fire the aerosol device when the patient's breathing is correctly timed. We have already mentioned the Autohaler® which is fired by a pressure switch. More recent devices such as the SmartMist® and AERx® add the sophistication of microprocessor control so that usage can be logged and the device can be controlled with a degree of sophistication [16] [17].

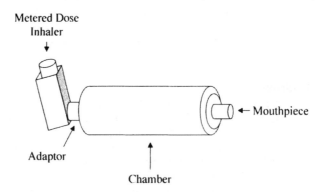

Figure 10.9 A typical spacer device

ASSESSMENT OF DEPOSITION BY GAMMA SCINTIGRAPHY

One of the most convenient methods to assess the pattern of distribution of therapeutic aerosols in the lung is by the use of gamma scintigraphy [18]. This can measure deposition in the lung, oropharynx and stomach. A critical feature for the success of gamma scintigraphy is a meticulously validated radiolabelling process to give confidence that the radiolabel is behaving in a manner which is representative of the system under study. Conventional planar gamma scintigraphy does not allow clear distinction between central and peripheral deposition since there is an overlay of structures e.g. alveoli, small and large airways, which is most marked centrally. Single photon emission computed tomography (SPECT)[19] and positron emission tomography, (PET) have the potential to give more detailed data on regional lung deposition as the image they provide is three-dimensional. Currently these techniques are more expensive and employ higher radiation doses, so are less widely used than planar imaging.

The procedures used for planar scintigraphic assessment of deposition are straightforward. The patient is given the appropriate number of doses of labelled formulation containing 1-2 MBq of activity, usually with a specified inhalation technique, and is then imaged with anterior and posterior views for 30 seconds to 1 minute. There is little point in performing kinetic studies of activity decay over longer periods since it is extremely difficult to ensure that the movement of the label *in vivo* represents a measurement of any useful physiological or formulation behaviour. If simultaneous pharmacokinetic studies are to be performed, the 'charcoal block' technique can be used, in which the subject is given a charcoal suspension drink prior to administration of the formulation. The object of this is to absorb any drug which may be swallowed and absorbed by the normal gastrointestinal route.

In order to facilitate the construction of regions of interest in the images, krypton 81m gas is commonly used to show the total ventilated area of the lungs. This radioactive gas has a half-life of 13 seconds and therefore the subject is imaged while breathing in the gas from a generator. This area can then be compared to the deposition of radiolabel from a test system. The region of interest can be drawn around the whole lung volume, but it is more common to divide the lung into central and peripheral areas, despite the fact that some peripheral areas must overlie the central area due to the viewing projection. The ratio of peripheral to central deposition is usually termed a 'penetration index'.

Studies based on 3-dimensional acquisition such as SPECT are performed in a similar manner but using a much higher (>100 MBq) activity level. Perring and coworkers[19] combined this technique with CT imaging of the lungs and used computer-based methods to transform the data to a concentric-shell lung model, and were thus able to provide a much more rigorous analysis of lung penetration. At present however the technique is considerably more specialized than planar imaging, which is used for the majority of routine studies.

Choice of radiolabel

Aqueous phases can be followed using technetium-99m labelled diethylenetriaminepentaacetic acid (DTPA). It is absorbed from the lungs with a half time of about 1 h and rapidly cleared from the body via the kidneys. If prolonged imaging is needed, then a label that clears more slowly from the lung such as ^{99m}Tc-labelled albumin should be used. Materials such as ^{99m}Tc stannous phytate show better alveolar deposition than pertechnetate or ^{111}In-DTPA with a slow clearance[20]. It has been hypothesized that phytate bears a strong structural resemblance to triphosphoinositide, a component of the lung surfactant material, and that it binds to alveolar wall receptors competing for inositol receptors. ^{99m}Tc Hexakis (t-butyl isonitrile) TBIN has been used to label the lipid phase of an aerosol[21].

Some attempts have been made to label the drug itself. A bronchodilator, the anti-cholinergic compound ipratropium bromide, has been labelled using a cyclotron-produced radionuclide ^{77}Br. This radionuclide has a half-life of 58 hours with peak gamma-ray energies, 239 and 521 KeV which are not ideal but are usable for scintigraphic studies. The powder produced was incorporated into pressurized canisters and it was shown that upon actuation, radioactivity was lost from the canisters at a rate equal to that of the drug[22].

Labelling inhalation formulations

Significant effort has been expended in attempts to radiolabel particles in aerosol formulations. All have significant problems and require validation prior to use, since it is possible that the label may not become associated with the drug particle.

1. In many early studies, the label in solution was added to the dry canister, and the solvent evaporated prior to adding the MDI propellants and solids. Some workers extract the ^{99m}Tc into butanone prior to adding it to the canister[23]. The whole is then sonicated in an attempt to redistribute the label. This is one of the least satisfactory methods, since it normally uses a water-soluble label such as ^{99m}Tc-DTPA. This forms a dry film on evaporation, which is later broken up into an ill-defined population of particles in the water-immiscible propellant. It has been suggested that the label associates with the surfactant layer around the particles, but since some of the surfactant will be present in solution, the validity of this ill-characterized technique seems unclear.

2. The drug is labelled by co-crystallizing or co-precipitating with added label prior to micronizing and formulation. This is extremely difficult since the levels of activity required to label a micronizable batch of drug (1-10 g minimum) are extremely high if a useful activity (e.g. 1 MBq in 100 µg) is to be obtained in the final doses. Extensive radiation protection is required and the apparatus requires a significant decay time. In addition there may be no guarantee of success since the label may crystallize or precipitate separately from the drug and form its own population of particles.

3. Addition of labelled particles (e.g. Teflon) to the formulation. These can be made to specific sizes, e.g. by spinning disc generator. The main problem here is that is difficult to ensure that the size distribution of the test particles is representative of that of the drug, and thus it becomes extremely difficult to ensure that the labelled particles behave *in vivo* in the same way as the drug particles. In addition the preparation of very small labeled model particles is problematic.

4. Addition of a propellant-soluble label such as ^{99m}Tc hexamethylpropyleneamine oxidase (HMPAO) to the pMDI. This label then evaporates down on to the surface of the drug particle when the pMDI is actuated. This is probably the most interesting technique but makes a number of assumptions; firstly that propellant evaporation is complete by the time the plume enters the upper airways (which is widely contested), and secondly that each propellant droplet contains at least one drug particle. Droplets which contain no drug particles will evaporate down to a very small size which is determined by the concentration of label and soluble components (surfactants and lubricants) and may thus suggest a deposition pattern which does not match that of the drug.

5. Spray-drying of the label on to the particle surface prior to formulation[24]. This method can be used for powders intended for both MDI and DPI administration. It has the advantage that the label is specifically associated with the particle, but validation is required in the case of MDI formulations to ensure that the label does not redissolve into the propellant.

Labelling dry powder inhalers

Dry powder inhalers contain usually pure drug and a carrier. Usually the diameter of the carrier substance particles is greater that the pure drug. In order to ensure that only the drug is labelled, it has to be labelled prior to mixing with the carrier. To achieve this the drug has to be suspended in a solvent which dissolves the label but not the drug. The radiolabel is added to the drug suspension, which is then evaporated. The drug particles are disaggregated, blended with carrier and loaded into the inhaler.

Validation

Whichever of these techniques is chosen, it is necessary to ensure that the label behaves in an aerodynamic manner in the same way as the drug particles. The most rigorous way to do this is to fire the device into a multistage classifier (normally an Andersen sampler with 8-10 stages) and verify that the distribution of radiolabel activity in the various stages is the same as the distribution of drug measured by direct chemical assay. If the label distributes similarly to the drug in the classifier, it is a reasonable assumption that it will do so *in vivo*, although it is not impossible that differences may still exist. For example, while the classifier operates in normal air, the air in the lung has nearly 100% humidity. This can lead to differences in particle growth rates that are not seen *in vivo*.

Generally, it is not necessary to perform a measure of label binding, as is the case in oral formulations, since it must be assumed that the micronized drug particle will dissolve instantaneously on contact with the pulmonary mucosa, and absorption of the drug and label will be rapid. Thus in most cases anything other than an immediate measure of drug/label distribution is of little value. The exception is for formulations such as liposomes and microparticles, in which the delivery agent is postulated to remain intact in the lung for a period of time and hence clearance can be measured[17].

FACTORS AFFECTING PARTICLE DEPOSITION IN THE LUNG

Aerosols used by patients should reach the desired location in sufficient quantity to be effective, and hence it is important to consider the factors which influence the amount and distribution of retained aerosols. The physical characteristics of the aerosol cloud such as particle size, velocity, charge, density and hygroscopicity will affect its penetration and deposition. Deposition is also affected by physiological variables, including respiration rate, airway diameter, presence of excessive mucus and respiratory volume.

Physicochemical properties

The three main mechanisms of deposition are inertial impaction, sedimentation and Brownian diffusion, the particle diameter determining the relative importance of these mechanisms.

Inertial impaction is the most important mechanism of deposition for particles greater than 5 μm in diameter[25]. If particles are large or are travelling at high velocities they may be unable to follow a change in direction in the airstream, for example in the upper airways at bifurcations, and hence they will impact on the airway walls. Impacted deposition is also enhanced where airways are partially obstructed at high flow rates, and by a turbulent airflow in the trachea and major bronchi. Sedimentation occurs when particles settle under gravity. The rate of settling is proportional to the square of the particle diameter (Stokes' law) and so becomes less important for small particles. Brownian diffusion is an important mechanism of deposition only for particles less than about 0.5 μm in diameter. The particles are displaced by random bombardment of gas molecules and collide with airway walls.

As a consequence of these diameter-sensitive processes, the deposition of particulates in the lung is highly dependent on their size (Figure 10.10). Droplets larger than 10 μm

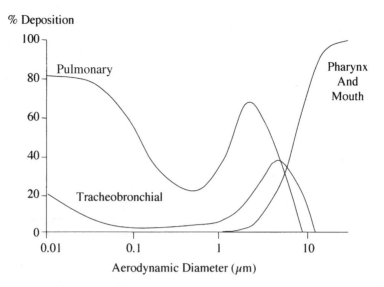

Figure 10.10 Dependence of deposition of particulates on particle size

impact in the upper airways and are rapidly removed by mucociliary clearance. Smaller droplets which escape impaction in the upper airways, in the range 0.5 to 5 μm, are sufficiently large to deposit by sedimentation, while those below 0.5 μm are too small to sediment efficiently and migrate to the vessel walls by Brownian motion. The optimum diameter for pulmonary penetration has been determined by studies of the deposition of monodisperse aerosols to be 2 to 3 μm[26]. Smaller particles are exhaled before sedimentation can occur, although breath-holding can improve deposition in these cases. Extremely small aerosols, below 0.1 μm, appear to deposit very efficiently through Brownian diffusion to the vessel walls, but such fine aerosols are extremely difficult to produce.

Often the particle size does not remain constant as an aerosol moves from the delivery system into the respiratory tract. Volatile aerosols may become smaller through evaporation whereas hygroscopic aerosols may grow dramatically. The exact relative humidity within airways is not known, but particles produced from dry atmospheric aerosols have been found to double in diameter when the relative humidity is increased to 98%. Particle growth due to absorption of moisture does not appear to affect total drug deposition in the respiratory tract[27].

Air in the deep branches of the lung has been estimated to contain around 40 g water per cubic metre. Most aerosol particles will absorb moisture to a degree that depends on temperature, relative humidity and the nature of the aerosol particle. The degree of saturation is also device dependent since aerosols formed by jet nebulizers may have a very low humidity, while ultrasonic nebulizers produce an aerosol with a much higher humidity.

Thermophoresis of particles has been reported to occur in the lung. This is a movement of droplets towards the cooler areas due to the more rapid Brownian motion in the warm areas. It is thought that this effect is small and short-lived in the lung, since the air in the deeper airways is rapidly brought to thermal equilibrium. Finally, electrostatic effects, in which the droplets are attracted to the vessel walls by virtue of a surface charge interaction, are thought to be unimportant in pulmonary delivery, due to the high humidity.

Deposition patterns from different dose forms

The delivery device largely influences the deposition of drug via the emitted particle size and velocity of the aerosol, as described above. Consequently it is important that the device emits a plume of particles in the 2-5µm size band. A number of formulation factors may conspire to prevent this; for example the particles suspended in MDI propellants are generally aggregated, and it is assumed that they are disaggregated efficiently by the shear forces in the actuator. Poor formulation, for example a poor choice of surfactant in the suspension, may cause the particles to be irreversibly aggregated. A similar problem occurs in dry powder devices, in which the fine drug powder is often cohesive and may not readily disperse. In the Turbuhaler® (AstraZeneca) the particles are broken up by a spiral in the mouthpiece producing a high resistance to the patient's inspiratory flow[28]. The Turbuhaler® produces twice as many particles with diameters less than 4.7 micrometres than does the MDI with spacer. The Diskus® (GlaxoWellcome) is also a dry powder inhaler, but this device has a low resistance to inspiratory flow. Thus, it is a less efficient producer of respirable particles under 4.7 micrometres than an MDI plus a metal spacer device, or the Turbuhaler®. As a consequence, the Turbuhaler® DPI delivers 20% to 30% of drug to the lung, approximately twice as much drug as the equivalent dose in the corresponding MDI.

Physiological variables

The average respiratory rate is approximately 15 breaths per minute with a tidal volume of about 500 ml and a residence time for tidal air of 3 seconds. A slowing of the respiratory rate increases the dwell time and retention of aerosol particles in the lung. Increasing the respiratory rate decreases dwell time, increases the turbulent flow and particle velocity. Severe turbulence retards the flow of gases into and out of the lung and results in premature deposition of the aerosol particles high into the respiratory tract since the collision rate with the walls is increased. Slowing inspiration and expiration minimizes turbulent flow. As a result deposition to the deep lung can be improved if the breath is held after actuation[17].

The resting pressure within the trachea is equal to atmospheric pressure, but during inspiration the pressure may drop to 60 to 100 mm Hg below atmospheric pressure, creating the gradient responsible for the inward flow of the aerosol cloud. The flow into each segment of the lung may vary considerably according to the pressure differential across each passageway and its resistance. Increasing the pressure differential increases the flow and penetration by aerosols. Aerosol delivery with children is problematic due to compliance issues and smaller airways and lung volumes.

Inhaler technique

Inhaler technique is a common problem, particularly in the elderly. Pressurized metered-dose inhalers in particular can be difficult to administer properly. There are significant variables of inhaler technique, such as timing of actuation and inspiratory flow rate. In a study which assessed the use of seven common inhaler devices in 20 patients with chronic obstructive pulmonary disease, fourteen patients had a fault that would result in no drug delivery at some time during the study. The fault occurred at some point for each inhaler device[29]. These faults were most common with the Diskhaler®. Patients ranked the metered dose inhaler and Accuhaler highest for ease of use and preference. Even when the correct method of using an inhaler is taught to the patients, their technique declines within 1 hour after instruction.

Although a large volume of inhalation is desirable, a fast inspiratory flow rate is not. Marked differences in bronchodilator response occur in patients with known airway reactivity following inhalation of beta-adrenergic bronchodilators at a slow rate[30].

Bronchodilation was significantly reduced when the inhaled flow rate was increased to 80 l.min^{-1} from 25 l.min^{-1}. The slow inhalation flow rate most likely allows the aerosol to penetrate more readily to the target receptor sites in the small, peripheral airways. Most asthmatic patients, however, tend to inhale too rapidly and pressurized inhalers in this group were used at peak inspiratory flow rates ranging from 50 l.min^{-1} to 400 l.min^{-1} [31]. A period of breath-holding increases the number of particles deposited in the lungs at their furthest point of penetration by the process of sedimentation. A new strategy to improve aerosol delivery to the lung involves devices that limit the inspiratory flow rate and increase inspiratory resistance. Examples of these devices are the Turbuhaler® or an inspiratory flow control device (IFCD) plus a metered-dose inhaler. Each is superior to drug delivery via a metered-dose inhaler plus the more common spacer device.

Effects of disease

The inhalation of aerosols, their penetration and deposition into the lungs, their absorption and activity is affected by the severity of pulmonary disease. Bronchoconstriction or obstruction of airways will lead to diversion of flow to non-obstructed airways. In advanced disease the remaining airways and alveoli may be increasingly exposed to inspired particles. Disease-induced structural changes, such as the increased resistance to airflow seen in patients with obstructive airway disease, leads to a more central deposition of aerosol. Asymptomatic smokers also tend to deposit aerosol particles centrally, possibly due to airway goblet cell hypertrophy.

Narrowing of airways by mucus, inflammation or bronchial constriction can increase linear velocities of airflow, enhance inertial deposition and cause more deposition in the central airways. In adult respiratory distress syndrome, characterized by acute inflammatory oedema, the lung permeability to proteins increases and accumulation of fluid occurs. Lung deposition from MDIs was not found to be significantly different in asthmatics when compared to normals[7,32], however a greater proportion of the dose was located more centrally in asthmatic subjects. This resulted in faster clearance of the drug as penetration into the lung is lessened[33].

A large number of other diseases and conditions can lead to altered respiratory flow. These include microbial infections, pneumoconiosis, carcinoma and obstructive pulmonary disease. In the majority of cases these lead to increasing lung rigidity, a decrease in tidal volume and an increase in respiratory rate, together with mechanical obstruction of parts of the airway. It is unfortunate that all these factors reduce deposition in exactly the region in which treatment is needed, so that the dose may target only the healthy regions of the lung.

DRUG ABSORPTION

Inhaled drugs can be absorbed from their deposition site in various parts of the respiratory tract, including the upper airways, mouth, pharynx and lower airways. Due to the large surface area and blood supply, there is considerable interest in delivering drugs systemically via the lung, particularly for drugs such as peptides which are degraded in the gastrointestinal tract. Since the blood from the pulmonary circulation is returned to the heart and is pumped to the tissues, no first-pass metabolism occurs in the liver. The rate-limiting portion of the barrier is thought to be the alveolar membrane itself[34]. It is believed that this barrier exhibits passive transport characteristics similar to other organs lined with epithelial cells. Lipid soluble drugs are usually absorbed by passive diffusion at rates that correlate with their lipid/water partition coefficients. Anaesthetics and respiratory gases cross the alveolar-capillary membrane quite readily, water crosses easily and in large quantities, but isotonic sodium chloride is only slowly absorbed. The membrane is only slightly permeable to aqueous solutes. Hydrophilic compounds are absorbed by diffusion through aqueous membrane pores, their absorption rate being inversely related to their molecular size.

Compounds such as disodium cromoglycate are at least partly absorbed by a saturable, carrier-type transport mechanism[35]. Interestingly, high molecular weight amides and alkyl amines pass more readily than their low molecular weight homologues, suggesting that a number of specific transport systems may be present.

PHARMACOKINETICS

Pharmacokinetic studies of drug absorption have been hindered by the need to separate pulmonary absorption from that occurring in the gastrointestinal tract. Drug will be swallowed following oropharyngeal deposition when the aerosol is fired, and the dose administered by this route may be greater than that entering the lungs. In addition drug impacting on the upper airways may be cleared by the mucociliary escalator and swallowed at a later time. Pulmonary absorption is expected to be fast since the drug arrives rapidly at the target site, compared to the delay involved in transit through the gastrointestinal tract. Studies involving salbutamol administered from a pressurized aerosol showed that peak plasma levels were reached 3-5 hours after dosing, but in this case the peak plasma level was probably related to the gastrointestinal absorption of the swallowed part of the dose[36]. Another study involving terbutaline indicated that after inhalation, the peak plasma level was reached within 30 to 60 minutes[37]. In this experiment ingested charcoal was used to prevent absorption from the gastrointestinal tract; without charcoal the peak plasma level was reached at 1-6 hours. This confirms that absorption from the airways is more rapid than from the gut. However, it may be possible that the peak plasma concentration results from absorption from the oral and pharyngeal mucosa for some drugs.

DRUGS ADMINISTERED VIA THE PULMONARY ROUTE

Anti-allergy agents

When the asthmatic response is triggered by an external allergen such as pollen, a major part of the primary immune response consists of the release of histamine from mast cells, a process termed 'degranulation'. Histamine has a wide range of actions in tissues, but in the bronchial tissues it causes constriction of smooth muscle via the H_1 receptors. This action can be prevented by sodium cromoglycate, which inhibits mast cell degranulation. As a result it has a powerful prophylactic action in asthma, but is of little use for relief of an acute attack. It is valuable for the management of extrinsic asthma and exercise-induced asthma. Cromoglycate is now thought to have an additional actions such as inhibition of pulmonary sensory C-fibre discharge[38 39]. A new drug in the category of anti-allergics is nedocromil sodium, which is equipotent with sodium cromoglycate[40].

Beta receptor agonists

When an asthmatic attack has been triggered by histamine at H_1 receptors, the objective is to redilate the bronchi with a β_2 receptor agonist in the upper and mid airways. These cause relaxation of bronchial smooth muscle and thus allow the airway to dilate. These materials are mainstays of the treatment of asthma, as well as a variety of other pulmonary diseases in which it is desired to decrease airway resistance. They provide rapid symptomatic relief where the predominant cause of reduced airway calibre is bronchial smooth muscle contraction, or they may be used as regular maintenance therapy to avert symptoms. Their preventative effect is particularly seen in the suppression of exercise-induced asthma[41]. Beta receptor agonists also increase the rate of mucociliary clearance, known to be abnormally slow in patients with obstructive airways disease. Inhaled β_2 receptor agonists are less effective if airway inflammation is a major factor in the disease. The oldest member of the class is salbutamol (called albuterol in the USA), and a range of other materials are available, including metaproterenol, fenoterol and terbutaline.

Adrenocorticosteroids

Adrenocorticosteroids (generally simply termed 'steroids') inhibit the inflammatory process by mechanisms which are poorly understood. It is possible that they may include interference with prostanoid formation and the inhibition of the cellular signalling between cells involved in the immune response. They prevent not only the early inflammatory phenomena such as oedema and increased blood flow, but also later effects such as phagocyte activity and capillary proliferation. The drugs used, e.g. beclomethasone dipropionate, betamethasone and budesonide, exert a topical effect in the lungs but are generally inactivated when swallowed. The doses required are low (400 - 800 µg daily), resulting in low plasma concentrations thereby minimizing systemic side effects. Modern treatment of asthma in childhood favours the use of small doses of steroid to keep inflammatory processes suppressed.

Leukotriene inhibitors

The cysteinyl leukotrienes (LTC_4, LTD_4, LTE_4) are products of arachidonic acid metabolism and are released from various cells, including mast cells and eosinophils. These eicosanoids bind to cysteinyl leukotriene receptors (CysLT) found in the human airway. Cysteinyl leukotrienes and leukotriene receptor occupation have been correlated with the pathophysiology of asthma, including airway edema, smooth muscle contraction, and altered cellular activity associated with the inflammatory process, which contribute to the signs and symptoms of asthma. Singulair (Montelukast sodium) is an orally active compound that binds with high affinity and selectivity to the $CysLT_1$ receptor (in preference to other pharmacologically important airway receptors, such as the prostanoid, cholinergic, or ß-adrenergic receptor). Montelukast sodium inhibits physiologic actions of LTD_4 at the $CysLT_1$ receptor without any agonist activity.

Other bronchodilating agents

Other bronchodilators include anticholinergic drugs which act by blocking the muscarinic action of acetylcholine, and thus preventing bronchial muscles from being constricted via innervation. Since reflex bronchoconstriction may be mediated through the stimulation of pulmonary sensory fibres, there is much interest in inhibition of this pathway as a method of controlling asthma. A quaternary derivative of atropine, ipratropium bromide, is commonly delivered by nebulizer and has been successful in the control of acute asthma. Methyl-xanthines (for example theophylline and aminophylline) have been used for many years in the USA as a first line treatment for asthma, but theophylline cannot be inhaled and must be injected, as it is an irritant to the lung. Methyl-xanthines are however less effective than $ß_2$-receptor agonists administered by aerosol[41].

Mucolytics

Various pharmacological agents alter the rheological function of mucus, which has been exploited particularly to thin mucus to aid in its clearance from the bronchi. Water, saline and mucolytic aerosols are important as aids in the removal of the bronchial secretions which accumulate in chronic bronchitis, bronchiectasis, cystic fibrosis and asthma. Inorganic and organic iodides act directly on mucus and are used therapeutically. Addition of potassium iodide reduces the apparent viscosity, presumably due to an effect of the halide on the configuration of the glycoprotein[42].

Traditionally aerosols have been used in an attempt to liquefy secretions and induce sputum clearance, either by mucociliary action or coughing. Inhalation of aerosolized water does liquefy and clear secretions[43]. It can however be an irritant and cause bronchoconstriction in asthmatics[44]. Saline aerosol is bland and may well improve mucociliary clearance, particularly in a hypertonic concentration where it facilitates expectoration[41]. It may liquefy sputum by enhancing chloride (and water) flux across the bronchial mucosa[45]. Mucolytic aerosols are also widely used; N-acetyl-cysteine (Airbron) being best known in Britain, and 2 mercapto-ethane ethane sulphonate (Mistabron) in Europe. Mistabron appears to enhance mucociliary clearance in patients with chronic bronchitis[46]. Other molecules such as DL-penicillamine and dithiothreitol act on the sulphhydryl bonds in mucus causing thinning, though nebulization of dithiothreitol causes intense irritation and is therefore unsuitable for clinical exploitation[47].

On rare occasions antihistamines and antibiotics may by given as aerosols. Antibiotics are given because in asthmatics the mucus thickens and "plugs" the bronchiole. This plug may then become a focus for infection. Some antibiotics, notably the tetracyclines[48], interact with mucus glycoprotein causing thickening. The exudates formed during inflammation and disease probably cause a mucus thickening by physical entrapment of mucus with biopolymers such as albumin, IgG, or IgA leading to changes in mucus viscoelasticity.

Systemically-absorbed drugs

As has been mentioned, the pulmonary route has been used to achieve systemic delivery. A product containing ergotamine tartrate is available as an aerosolized dosage inhaler (360 µg per dose) and has the advantage of avoiding the delay in drug absorption due to gastric stasis associated with migraine. In vaccine delivery, aerosol administration of para-influenza Type 2 vaccine has been found to be more effective than subcutaneous injection[49]). Penicillin reaches the bloodstream in therapeutic quantities after pulmonary delivery, but kanamycin is poorly absorbed from the lung so can only be used for local drug delivery.

The deep lung has been investigated as a site for delivering large molecule proteins and peptides as it is believed that the morphology of the alveolar epithelium predisposes it to absorb large molecule compounds. The pulmonary route has been explored for the delivery of insulin and human growth hormone, and absorption was found to be greatest in those subjects with the highest penetration index, implying that deep central deposition is a prerequisite for absorption[50 51]. The pharmacokinetics of these materials, which have extremely short intravenous half-lives of 3 and 40 minutes respectively, were dominated by the slower limiting pulmonary absorption rate.

REFERENCES

1. Straub NC. Pulmonary edema due to increased microvascular permeability to fluid and protein. *Circ. Res.* 1978;43:143-151.

2. Newman SP. Scintigraphic assessment of therapeutic aerosols. *Crit. Rev. Therapeut. Drug Carrier Syst.* 1993;10:65-109.

3. DíSousa S. The Montreal protocol and essential use exemptions. *J. Aerosol Med.* 1995;8:S13-17.

4. Bisgaard H. Delivery of inhaled medication to children. *J. Asthma* 1997;34:443-467.

5. Ashworth HL, Wilson CG, Sims EE, Wooton PK, Hardy JG. Delivery of propellant soluble drug from a metered dose inhaler. *Thorax* 1991;46:245-247.

6. Harnor KJ, Perkins AC, Wastie ML, Wilson CG, Sims EE, Feely LC, Farr SJ.. Effect of vapour pressure on the deposition pattern from solution phase metered dose inhalers. *Int. J. Pharmaceut.* 1993;95:111-116.

7. Leach C. Enhanced drug delivery through reformulating MDIs with HFA propellants - drug deposition and its effect on preclinical and clinical programs. In *Respiratory drug delivery V* Dalby, RN, Byron, PR and Farr, SJ (eds). Buffalo Grove, Interpharm Press 1996:133-144.

8. Newman SP, Weisz AWB, Talaee N, Clarke SW. Improvement of drug delivery with a breath actuated pressurised aerosol for patients with poor inhaler technique. *Thorax* 1991;46:712-716.
9. Pitcairn GR, Hunt HMA, Dewberry H, Pavia D, Newman SP. A comparison of *in vitro* drug delivery from two dry powder inhalers, the Aerohaler and the Rotohaler. *STP Pharma Sciences* 1994;4:33-37.
10. Lipworth BJ, Clark DJ. Comparative lung delivery of salbutamol given via Turbuhaler and Diskus dry powder inhaler devices. *Europ. J. Clin. Pharmacol.* 1997;53:47-49.
11. Vidgren MT, Kärkkäinen A, Paronen TP, Karjalainen P. Respiratory tract deposition of ^{99m}Tc-labelled drug particles administered via a drug powder inhaler. *Int. J. Pharmaceut.* 1987;39:101-105.
12. Hardy JG, Newman SP, Knock M. Lung deposition from four nebulizers. *Resp. Med.* 1993;87:461-465.
13. Farr SJ, Ho KKL, Kellaway IW. A gamma scintigraphic study of tracheo-bronchial deposition and clearance of nebulised aerosols. *STP Pharma Sci.* 1994;4:23-28.
14. Newman SJ, Brown J, Steed KP, Reader SJ, Kladders H. Lung deposition of fenoterol and flunisolide delivered using a novel device for inhaled medicines. *Chest* 1998;113:957-963.
15. Kenyon CJ, Thorsson L, Borgstrom L, Newman SP. The effects of static charge in spacer devices on glucocorticosteroid aerosol deposition in asthmatic patients. *Europ. Respir. J.* 1998;11:606-610.
16. Gonda I, Schuster JA, Rubsamen RM, Lloyd P, Cipolla D, Farr SJ. Inhalation delivery systems with compliance and disease management capabilities. *J. Cont. Rel.* 1998;53:269-274.
17. Farr SJ, Rowe AM, Rubsamen R, Taylor G. Aerosol deposition in the human lung following administration from a microprocessor controlled pressurised metered dose inhaler. *Thorax* 1995;50:639-644.
18. Newman SP, Wilding IR. Gamma scintigraphy: an *in vivo* technique for assessing the equivalence of inhaled products. *Int. J. Pharmaceut.* 1998;170:1-9.
19. Perring S, Summers Q, Fleming JS, Nassim MA, Holgate ST. A new method of quantification of the pulmonary regional distribution of aerosols using combined CT and SPECT and its application to nedocromil sodium administered by metered dose inhaler. *Br. J. Radiol.* 1994;67:46-53.
20. Isitman AT, Manoli R, Schmidt GH, Holmes RA. An assessment of alveolar deposition and pulmonary clearance of radiopharmaceuticals after nebulization. *Am. J. Roentgenol. Radium Ther. Nucl. Med.* 1974;120:776-781.
21. Wilson CG, Washington N, Washington C, Frier M, Poole S, Yeadon M. Investigation into the disposition and clearance of an artificial lung surfactant when delivered by aerosol or intratracheal instillation. *Pharmaceut. Sci.* 1995;1:271-275.
22. Short MD, Singh CA, Few JD, Studdy PT, Heaf PJD, Spiro SG. The labelling and monitoring of an inhaled, synthetic, anticholinergic bronchodilating agent. *Chest* 1981;80:918-921.
23. Borgstrom L, Newman S. Total and regional lung deposition of terbutaline sulphate inhaled via a pressurised MDI or via a Turbuhaler. *Int. J. Pharmaceut.* 1993;97:47-53.
24. Arppe J, Vidgren M. Practical gamma labelling method for metered-dose inhalers and inhalation powders. *STP Pharma Sciences* 1994;4:19-22.
25. Raabe OG, Howard RS, Cross CE. *In Bronchial Asthma* Gershwin M.E. (ed), Grune and Stratton, London and New York. 1986:495-514.
26. Gonda I. A semi-empirical model of aerosol deposition in the human respiratory tract for mouth inhalation. *J. Pharm. Pharmacol.* 1981;33:692-696.
27. Moren F, Andersson J. Fraction of dose exhaled after administration of pressurised inhalation aerosols. *Int. J. Pharmaceut.* 1980;6:295-300.
28. Newman SP, Moren F, Trofast E, N. T, Clarke SW. Deposition and clinical efficacy of terbutaline sulphate from Turbuhaler, a new multi-dose powder inhaler. *Europ. Respir. J.* 1989;2:247-252.
29. Oliver S, Rees PJ. Use in chronic obstructive pulmonary disease. *Int. J. Clin. Pract.* 1997;51:443-445.

30. Newman SP, Pavia D, Clarke SW. Simple instructions for using pressurized aerosol bronchodilators. *J. Royal Soc. Med.* 1980;73:776-779.

31. Coady TJ, Davies HJ, Barnes P. Evaluation of a breath actuated pressurized aerosol. *Clin. Allergy* 1976;6:1-6.

32. Melchor R, Biddiscombe MF, Mak VHF, Short MD, Spiro SG. Lung deposition patterns of directly labelled salbutamol in normal subjects and patients with reversible airflow obstruction. *Thirax* 1993;48:506-511.

33. Saari SM, Vidgren MT, Koskinen MO, Turjanmaa VM, Waldrep JC, Nieminen MM. Regional lung deposition and clearance of ^{99m}Tc-labeled beclomethasone-DLPC liposomes in mild and severe asthma. *Chest* 1998;113:1573-1579.

34. Taylor AE, Guyton AC, Bishop VS. Permeability of the alveolar membrane to solutes. *Circ. Res.* 1965;16:352-362.

35. Pauwels R. Pharmacokinetics of inhaled drugs. *In Aerosols in Medicine. Principles, Diagnosis and Therapy,* Moren S, Newhouse MT, Elsevier, Biomedical Sciences Division 1985.

36. Walker SR, Evans ME, Richards AJ, Paterson JW. The clinical pharmacology of oral and inhaled salbutamol. *Clin. Pharmacol. Ther.* 1972;13:861-867.

37. Nilson HT, Simonsson BG, Strom B. The fate of 3H-terbutaline sulphate administered to man as an aerosol. *Eur. J. Clin. Pharmacol.* 1976;10:1-7.

38. Church MK. Is inhibition of mast cell mediator release relevant to the clinical activity of anti-allergenic drugs? *Agents and Actions* 1986;18:288-293.

39. Richards IM, Dixon M, Jackson DM, Vendy K. Alternative modes of action of sodium cromoglycate. *Agents and Actions* 1986;18:294-300.

40. Riley PA, Mather ME, Keogh RW, Eady RP. Activity of neocromil sodium in mast cell dependent reactions in the rat. *Int. Arch. Allergy Appl. Immunol.* 1987;82:108-110.

41. Clarke SW, Newman SP. Therapeutic aerosols 2- Drugs available by the inhaled route. *Thorax* 1984;39:1-7.

42. Martin R, Litt M, Marriott C. The effect of mucolytic agents on the rheological and transport properties of canine tracheal mucus. *Am. Rev. Resp. Dis.* 1980;121:495-500.

43. Palmer KNV. Reduction of sputum viscosity by a water aerosol in bronchitis. *Lancet* 1960;1:91.

44. Shoeffel RE, Anderson SA, Attounyan REC. Bronchial hyper-reactivity in response to inhalation of ultrasonically nebulized solutions of distilled water and saline. *Br. Med. J.* 1981;283:1285-1287.

45. Nadel JA. New approaches on regulation of fluid secretions in airways. *Chest* 1981;80:849-851.

46. Clarke SW, Lopez-Vidriero MT, Pavia D, Thomson ML. The effect of sodium-2-mercaptoethane sulphonate and hypertonic saline aerosols on bronchial clearance in chronic bronchitis. *Br. J. Clin. Pharmacol.* 1979;7:39-44.

47. Lightowler JE, Lightowler NM. Comparative mucolytic studies on dithiothreitol, N-acetylcysteine and L-cysteine on human respiratory mucus *in vitro* and their effects on the role of flow of mucus in the exposed trachea of the rat on topical administration. *Arch. Int. Pharmacodyn. Ther.* 1971;189:53-58.

48. Marriott C, Kellaway IW. The effect of tetracyclines on the viscoelastic properties of bronchial mucus. *Biorheol.* 1975;12:391-395.

49. Wigley FM, Fruchtman MH, Waldman RH. Aerosol immunisation of humans with inactivated parainfluenza type 2 vaccine. *N. Engl. J. Med.* 1970;283:1250-1253.

50. Colthorpe P, Farr SJ, Taylor G, Smith IJ, Wyatt D. The pharmacokinetics of pulmonary-delivered insulin: a comparison of intratracheal and aerosol administration to the rabbit. *Pharmaceut. Res.* 1992;9:764-768.

51. Colthorpe P, Farr SJ, Smith IJ, Wyatt D, Taylor G. The influence of regional deposition on the pharmacokinetics of pulmonary-delivered human growth hormone in rabbits. *Pharmaceut. Res.* 1995;12:356-359.

Chapter Eleven

Ocular Drug Delivery

INTRODUCTION

The external eye is readily accessible for drug administration. As a consequence of its function as the visual apparatus, mechanisms are strongly developed for the clearance of foreign materials from the cornea to preserve visual acuity. This presents problems in the development of formulations for ophthalmic therapy.

Topical administration is direct, but conventional preparations of ophthalmic drugs, such as ointments, suspensions, or solutions, are relatively inefficient as therapeutic systems. Following administration, a large proportion of the topically applied drug is immediately diluted in the tear film and excess fluid spills over the lid margin and the remainder is rapidly drained into the nasolacrimal duct. A proportion of the drug is not available for immediate therapeutic action since it binds to the surrounding extraorbital tissues. In view of these losses, frequent topical administration is necessary to maintain adequate drug levels. Systemic administration of a drug to treat ocular disease would require a high concentrations of circulating drug in the plasma to achieve therapeutic quantities in the aqueous humor, with the increased risk of side effects.

Three important factors have to be considered when attempting drug delivery to the eye-

1. how the blood-eye barrier (systemic to ocular) or cornea (external to ocular) is crossed to reach the site of action,

2. how to localize the pharmacodynamic action at the eye and minimise drug action on other tissues

3. how to prolong the duration of drug action such that the frequency of drug administration can be reduced.

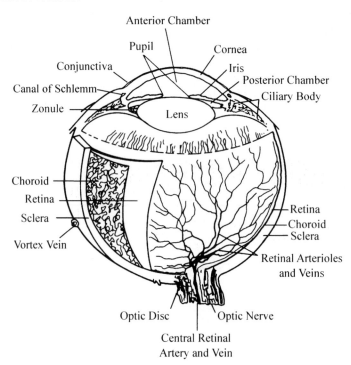

Figure 11.1 Vertical section through the human eye

STRUCTURE OF THE EYE

The outer shape of the eye comprises two spheres of different radii, one set into the other (Figure 11.1). The anterior sphere, the cornea, is the smaller and more curved of the two and is completely transparent. The posterior sphere or sclera is a white, opaque, fibrous shell which encloses the ocular structures. Both tissues are relatively non-distensible and protect the eye from physical damage. The ring where the two areas join is called the limbus.

The outer tissues of the eye consist of three layers

1. the outermost layers, the sclera and cornea, provide protection for the delicate structures within

2. the middle layer, the uveal tract, has a nutritive function, being mainly vascular and consisting of the choroid, ciliary body and the iris

3. the innermost layer is the retina containing photoreceptors and is concerned with the reception of visual stimuli. The inner eye is divided by the lens that separates the aqueous and vitreous humors. The iris separates the aqueous humor into the anterior and posterior chambers.

The cornea

The cornea is made up of the stroma (up to 90% of its thickness) which is bounded externally by epithelium and the Bowman's membrane and internally by Descemet's membrane and the endothelium (Figure 11.2). The mean thickness of the cornea in man is just over 0.5 mm in the central region and is composed of five to six layers of cells. It becomes 50% thicker towards the periphery as the epithelium increases to eight to ten cell layers. The cells at the base are columnar, but as they are squeezed forward by new cells, they become flatter. These cells can be classified into three groups: basal cells, an intermediate zone of 2 - 3 layers of polygonal cells (wing shaped) and squamous cells. The permeability of the intact corneal epithelium is low until the outermost layer is damaged, suggesting that tight junctions exist between the cells in this layer. The outer layer of the surface cells possesses microvilli, which presumably help to anchor the precorneal tear film. The cells of the basal layer show extensive interdigitation of plasma membranes and are therefore relatively permeable.

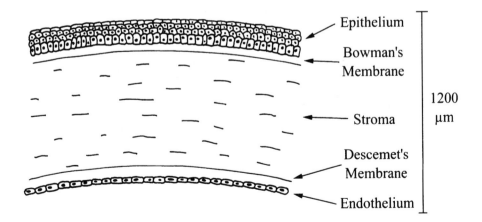

Figure 11.2 The five layers of the cornea

Immediately adjacent to the epithelium is a less ordered region of the stroma or Bowman's membrane. It is not sharply differentiated from the stroma beneath it and could be described as Bowman's layer rather than a membrane.

The stroma substantia propria consists of a set of lamellae, or plates, running parallel with the surface and superimposed on each other like the leaves of a book. Between the lamellae lie the corneal corpuscles, cells that synthesize new collagen essential for the repair and maintenance of this layer.

The stroma can be considered to have a comparatively open structure that normally allows diffusion of solutes having molecular weight below 500,000 Daltons. It can act as a barrier for very lipophilic substances that pass freely through the epithelium, while it is easily penetrated by hydrophilic solutes.

Descemet's membrane is located on the interior surface of the stroma and it is secreted by the endothelium. It is made up of a different type of collagen from that in the stroma. The endothelium consists of a single layer of flattened cells 5 μm high and 20 μm wide. These cells form a regular mosaic, each with close contact with its neighbours. The endothelium is about 200 times more permeable than the epithelium and thus represents a weak barrier. The endothelium is in contact with the aqueous humor of the anterior chamber. The endothelial layer is crossed by a passive flux of water towards the stroma, which has a tendency to swell. An active pump mechanism generates a flux in the opposite direction that controls corneal tumescence.

Although the cornea covers only one-sixth of the total surface area of the eyeball, it is considered the main pathway for the permeation of drugs into the intraocular tissues.

The conjunctiva and sclera

The conjunctiva lines the posterior surface of the eyelids and covers the exterior surface of the cornea. The portion that lines the lids is called the palpebral conjunctiva; the portion covering the white of the eyeball is called the bulbar conjunctiva. The palpebral conjunctiva is vascular and the bulbar conjunctiva is transparent. The area between the lids and the globe is termed the conjunctival sac that is open at the front at the palpebral fissure and only complete when the eyes are closed.

The sclera is composed primarily of collagen and mucopolysaccharide and forms the posterior five sixths of the protective coat of the eye. Its anterior portion is visible and constitutes the white of the eye. Attached to the sclera are the extraocular muscles. Through the sclera pass the nerves and the blood vessels that penetrate into the interior of the eye. At its posterior portion, the site of attachment of the optic nerve, the sclera becomes a thin sieve like structure, the lamina cribrosa, through which the retinal fibres leave the eye to form the optic nerve. The episcleral tissue is a loose connective and elastic tissue that covers the sclera and unites it with the conjunctiva above.

The choroid and retina

The choroid is the middle pigmented vascular coat of the posterior five-sixth of the eyeball. It is continuous with the iris in the front. It lies between the retina and the sclera and prevents the passage of light rays.

The retina is the light sensitive inner lining to the eyeball. It consists of seven nervous layers and one pigmented layer.

The aqueous humor

The aqueous humor is a clear colourless fluid with a chemical composition rather similar to that of blood plasma, but with a lower protein content. Its main function is to keep the globe reasonably firm and it is secreted continuously by the ciliary body into the posterior chamber. It flows as a gentle stream through the pupil into the anterior chamber, from which it is drained by he canal of Schlemm.

The vitreous body is a jelly made up of a form of collagen, vitrosin, and the muco-polysaccharide, hyaluronic acid. Its composition is similar to that of the cornea, but the proportion of water is much greater, about 98 percent or more, compared with about 75 percent for the cornea. The vitreous body serves to keep the underlying retina pressed against the choroid.

The eyelids

The eyelids are movable folds of modified fleshy skin consisting of orbital and palpe-bral portions positioned in front of the eyeball (Figure 11.3). They have an obvious protec-tive function and play an important role in the maintenance of the tear film and lacrimal drainage. Fibrous tarsal plates provide the framework for the lids.

Between the bulbar and the palpebral conjunctiva there are two loose, redundant portions forming recesses that project back. These recesses are called the upper and lower fornices, or conjunctival sacs. The looseness of the conjunctiva in this region makes move-ments of lids and eyeball possible.

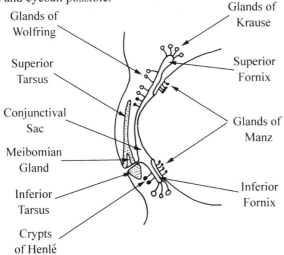

Figure 11.3 Vertical section through the eyelids and conjunctiva

The precorneal tear film

The maintenance of a clear, healthy cornea requires that the anterior surface of its epithelial layer be kept moist. The precorneal tear film is a very thin fluid layer continu-ously bathing the corneal epithelium, the conjunctiva and walls of the conjunctival cul-de-sac. Normal secretion of tears by the lacrimal system is necessary for:

1. nutrition of the cornea,
2. protection against bacterial infection,
3. removal of cellular debris and foreign matter
4. formation of a stable, continuous fluid film over the cornea producing a high quality optical surface.
5. lubrication for the movement of the eyelids.

The average tear volume in a human is 7 μl, 1 μl of which is contained in the precorneal tear film, and 3 μl in each of the tear margins. Prior to blinking, the tear volume can

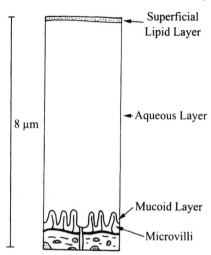

Figure 11.4 The structure of the tear film according to Wolff

increase to about 30 μl. The maximum amount of fluid that can be held in the conjunctival sac is only about 10 μl. As the tear layer is so thin, evaporation and lipid contamination of the mucin component of the tear fluids quickly destroys its continuity. This results in dry spots that appear usually within 15 to 30 seconds after a blink, at scattered locations on the corneal surface. The blinking action of the eyelids, which usually occurs before the actual formation of dry spots, is required to re-form the tear film layer. The blink interval should therefore, be shorter than the tear break-up time.

The precorneal tear film was first thought to be a three layered structure consisting of a superficial oily layer, a middle aqueous layer, and an adsorbed mucus layer (Figure 11.4), secreted by several glands (Figure 11.5)[1]. Recent research suggests that the mucus fraction extends through the tear film[2].

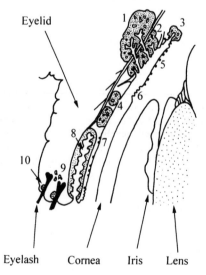

Main lacrimal glands
1. Orbital lobe
2. Palpebral lobe

Accessory lacrimal glands
3. Glands of Krause
4. Glands of Wolfring

Mucin secretors
5. Goblet cells
6. Glands of Manz
7. Crypts of Henle

Oil secretors
8. Meiomian gland
9. Glands of Moll
10. Glands of Zeis

Figure 11.5 The glands secreting the components of the precorneal tear film

The superficial oily layer is approximately 0.1 μm thick and consists of wax and cholesterol esters secreted by the Meibomian glands, the glands of Zeis at the palpebral margin of each eyelid, and the glands of Moll situated at the root of each lash. This layer reduces the evaporation from the underlying aqueous phase by a factor of 10 to 20, preventing the cornea from drying.

The aqueous layer lies below the oily layer and is the largest component of the tear film (6-10 μm thick), consisting of watery lacrimal secretions provided by the numerous accessory lacrimal glands of Kraus and Wolfring, most of which are situated in the upper conjunctival fornix.

The mucoid layer is secreted by conjunctival goblet cells, the crypts of Henlé, which are situated on the conjunctival surface of the upper and lower tarsus, and the glands of Manz positioned in a circular ring on the limbal conjunctiva. Mucin is involved in adhesion of the aqueous phase to the underlying cornea, and thus keeps the cornea wettable.

Physical properties of tears

The normal pH of tears varies between 7.0 and 7.4. The pH of the tear film is influenced by any dissolved substances, particularly by the bicarbonate-carbon dioxide buffer system. When the eyelids are open, the pH of the precorneal tear film increases through loss of carbon dioxide. Solutions instilled into the lower fornix with pH below 6.6 and above 9.0 are associated with irritation, reflex tears and rapid blinking.

The surface tension of tear fluid at 33°C, the surface temperature of the eye, has been measured as between 44 and 50 mN.m^{-1} [3]. The instillation of a solution containing drugs or adjuvants that lower the surface tension may disrupt the outermost lipid layer of the tear film. The lubricant and protective effect of the oily film disappears and dry spots may be formed due to tear film evaporation. The dry spots cause irritation and reflex blinking is elicited to eliminate the sensation of a foreign body in the eye. In many cases, the sensation may be delayed for 30 minutes to 1 hour following the application, dependent on the concentration and nature of the instillate.

The evaporation process influences the tonicity of human tears when the eye is open. The osmolarity after prolonged eye closure or during sleep is 293 to 288 mOsm. After the eye is opened, the osmolarity progressively rises at a rate of 1.43 mOsm.kg^{-1}.h^{-1} to 302 to 318 mOsm.kg^{-1}. Due to their molecular weight and low concentrations, proteins contribute only slightly to the total osmotic pressure, but they do influence tear viscosity. The viscosity of human tears ranges from 1.3 to 5.9 mPa.s with a mean value of 2.9 mPa.s.

Lacrimal drainage system

An efficient drainage system exists to remove excess lacrimal fluid and cell debris from the precorneal area of the eye (Figure 11.6). Tears initially drain through the lacrimal puncta, which are small circular openings of the lacrimal canalculi, situated on the medial aspect of both the upper and lower lid margins. They then pass through the mucous membrane lined lacrimal passages. The superior and inferior canalculi (approximately 8 mm in length and 1 mm in diameter) unite in the region of the medial canthus to form the common canalculus. This opens into the lacrimal sac about 3 mm below its apex. At its lower end, it is continuous with the nasolacrimal duct that passes downwards to open into the inferior meatus of the nose with a valvular mechanism at its opening. The tears finally pass into the nasopharynx.

The drainage of tears is an active process involving the lacrimal pump that is dependent on the integrity of the orbicularis muscle of the eyelids. Closure of the eyelids draws the lacrimal fluid from the puncta and canalculi into the sac by a suction effect. Opening the

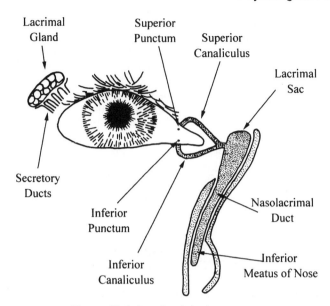

Figure 11.6 Lacrimal drainage system

lids forces the lacrimal fluid from the sac into the nasolacrimal duct and then into the nose through the lower end of the sac. The valvular mechanism opens during this movement.

Blood-eye barriers

Several barriers prevent material entering the ocular circulation. The vessels of the iris have thick walls that prevent leakage of materials into the aqueous humor. The epithelium in the ciliary processes is a unique membrane that prevents the passage of most molecules, including antibiotics and proteins. However, molecules may enter the posterior chamber of the eye during the active secretion process that forms aqueous humor. Topically applied fluorescein is seen to leak across the choroidal circulation, without passing into the retinal pigment layer. Injury or inflammation can damage the blood-eye barriers, since the capillary endothelial and epithelial cells separate, resulting in destruction of the intercellular barrier and leakage of material.

The external eye is readily accessible for drug administration; however, as a consequence of its function as the visual apparatus, mechanisms are strongly developed for the clearance of foreign materials from the cornea to preserve visual acuity. This presents problems in the development of formulations for ophthalmic therapy.

Systemic administration of a drug to treat ocular disease would require a high concentration of circulating drug in the plasma to achieve therapeutic quantities in the aqueous humour, with the increased risk of side effects. Topical administration is more direct, but conventional preparations of ophthalmic drugs, such as ointments, suspensions, or solutions, are relatively inefficient as therapeutic systems. A large proportion of the topically applied drug is immediately diluted in the tear film and excess fluid spills over the lid margin and the remainder is rapidly drained into the nasolacrimal duct. A proportion of the drug is not available for therapeutic action since it binds to the surrounding extraorbital tissues. In view of these losses frequent topical administration is necessary to maintain adequate drug levels. This results in transient periods of over- and under-dosing (Figure 11.7).

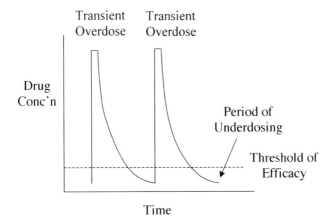

*Figure 11.7 Sawtooth pattern of therapy following administration
of ophthalmic drugs as eye drops*

Three factors have to be considered when drug delivery to the eye is attempted. Firstly, how to cross the blood-eye barrier (systemic to ocular) or cornea (external to ocular) to reach the site of action; secondly, how to localise the pharmacodynamic action at the eye and minimise drug action on other tissues and finally, how to prolong the duration of drug action such that the frequency of drug administration can be reduced.

FACTORS AFFECTING DRUG PERMEATION

The sequential barriers of epithelium, stroma and, to a lesser extent, the endothelium pose difficulties for drug absorption through the cornea (Figure 11.2). The epithelial and endothelial cells are rich in lipids and are mostly permeable to fat soluble substances. The stroma is acellular with a high water content, making it permeable to water soluble substances. In order for drugs to be well absorbed, they need to have a mixed hydrophilic/hydrophobic nature with an intermediate partition coefficient in the range of 10 to 100.

The stroma can be considered as a single compartment with the aqueous humor since the endothelium separating them is only a weak barrier and hence is not rate limiting. Both the epithelium and the aqueous tissues can act as drug reservoirs. The hydrophilic stroma serves as a depot for water-soluble compounds such as catecholamines and their metabolites, whereas the epithelium is the main depot for lipophilic molecules such as chloramphenicol.

Ionization and pH

The majority of drugs are ionizable, but for a drug to pass the lipid barriers of the epithelium and endothelium, it needs to be hydrophobic, which generally means unionized. The ionized form prefers the trans-stromal route since this is primarily hydrophilic. After an ophthalmic formulation is instilled into the eye, it is mixed with the tears present in the conjunctival sac and with the precorneal tear film. The pH of the mixture is mainly determined by the pH of the instilled solution as the tear film is of small volume with low buffering capacity. Since the pH can so easily be influenced by the delivery vehicle, it can be exploited to optimize absorption. For example, pilocarpine, a weak base, is administered in a vehicle of low pH, in which it is ionized. In this form it can be absorbed before the tear film secretion returns the local pH to physiological levels. Adjustment of the vehicle buffer capacity allows some measure of control over the duration of the pH disturbance.

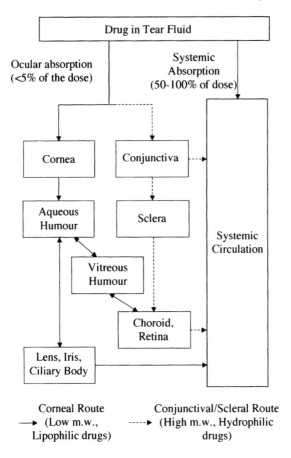

Figure 11.8 Transcorneal penetration into the aqueous humour. The losses are significant and it usual for less than 5% of the instilled dose to penetrate into the intraocular tissues following a 25 μl drop

Protein binding

Estimates of the total protein content of tears range from 0.6 to 2% w/v, the major fractions consisting of albumin, globulin and lysozyme. Drugs bound to the protein in the tear fluid may not permeate the cornea due to the additional bulk of the protein molecule; also binding of drugs to protein in conjunctival tissues competes for the drug available for corneal absorption (Figure 11.8). Binding increases in certain disease states, particularly inflammatory conditions, due to higher secretion of proteins in tissue exudate.

If two drugs have to be applied to the same eye, an interval of five to ten minutes should elapse between administration of each drug. If the second drug is applied too soon after the first, it may displace the first drug, which will then be rapidly cleared, thereby reducing its effect.

Pigmentation and drug effects

There have been only a limited number of studies carried out in this area, but these suggest that the intraocular distribution of drugs vary with levels of eye pigmentation. For example, a ten-fold increase in pilocarpine deposition in the iris-ciliary body of the pigmented

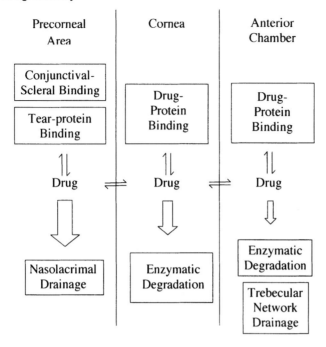

Figure 11.9 Losses during disposition into the eye. The precorneal losses are significant; binding and clearance processes further reduce the concentration of applied drug to the interior tissues

rabbit eye is found when compared with albinos, although the pilocarpine concentration in the aqueous humor was indistinguishable between the two[4]. Pilocarpine is metabolised by tissue esterases and esterase activity is highest in the iris and ciliary body, followed by the cornea and aqueous humor[5]. In the pigmented eyes, the phamacological effect was reduced owing to a higher amount of esterase activity in the cornea and iris-ciliary body.

Drug distribution in the eye

The amount of drug reaching the anterior chamber of the eye is determined by the net result of two competing processes:

1. the rate of drug loss from the precorneal area.
2. the rate of drug uptake by the cornea

Once the drug penetrates the cornea and enters the aqueous humor, it is distributed to all the internal tissues of the eye. The anterior chamber is in contact with the cornea, iris, ciliary body, lens and vitreous humor. The drug is rapidly distributed to these tissues and concentrations mirror those of the aqueous humor. Deeper into the intraocular tissues, the concentration is reduced by aqueous humor turnover and non-specific binding as illustrated in Figure 11.9.

Drug penetration through the sclera and conjunctiva

The sclera could constitute an important penetration route for some drugs, particularly those with low corneal permeation. Drugs may diffuse across the sclera by three possible pathways:

1. through perivascular spaces

2. through the aqueous media of gel-like mucopolysaccharides
3. across the scleral collagen fibrils.

An *in vitro* study using isolated corneal and scleral membranes of the rabbit has shown that scleral permeability was significantly higher than the respective corneal permeability for many hydrophilic compounds[6]. The ratio of permeability coefficient of sclera to that of cornea was reported 1.2 - 5.7 for some blockers and 4.6 for inulin. The permeability coefficients were in the order propranolol > penbutolol > timolol > nadolol for the cornea and penbutolol > propranolol > timolol > nadolol for the sclera. It was suggested that the mechanism for scleral permeation was diffusion across the intercellular aqueous media, as in the case of the structurally similar corneal stroma. This mechanism alone however, cannot explain the substantially higher permeability of penbutolol and propranolol compared with the other compounds of similar molecular weight. A partitioning mechanism may account for these observations. The conjunctival/scleral route has also been reported to be the predominant pathway for the delivery of p-aminoclonidine to the ciliary body[7].

FACTORS INFLUENCING DRUG RETENTION
Proper placement of the eyedrops

Accurate and proper placement of an eye drop may considerably improve the efficacy of drug delivery, as the capacity of the conjunctival sac is dependent on the position of the head and technique of instillation. A drop is placed in the inferior cul-de-sac by gently pulling the lower lid away from the globe and creating a pouch to receive the drop. After gently lifting the lid to touch the globe, a small amount of liquid is entrapped in the inferior conjunctival sac, where it may be retained up to twice as long as when it is simply dropped over the superior sclera. Drainage from the cul-de-sac may be further reduced by punctual occlusion or simple eyelid closure, which prolongs the contact time of the drug with the external eye. This serves two purposes; first it maximises the contact of drug with the periocular tissues increasing absorption through the cornea and secondly, the systemic absorption is reduced (Figure 11.10).

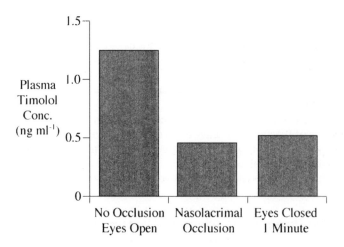

Figure 11.10 Effect of eyelid closure or nasolacrimal occlusion on systemic absorption of timolol

Influence of instilled volume

When an ophthalmic formulation is instilled into the eye, it is mixed with the precorneal tear film. The osmotic pressure of the mixture depends upon the osmolarity of the tears and of the ophthalmic formulation. If the osmotic pressure obtained is within defined limits, no discomfort is experienced, but if the osmotic pressure is outside these limits the patient experiences irritation eliciting reflex tears and blinking. The original osmolarity of the precorneal tear film is regained two minutes after the non-isotonic solution is administered, mainly due to a rapid flow of water across the cornea. The instillation of a hypotonic drug solution creates an osmotic gradient between the tear film and the surrounding tissues. This induces a flow of water from the eye surface to the cornea, hence the drug concentration on the eye surface is temporarily increased.

The rapid rate of tear turnover and efficient drainage in the eye profoundly affects the bioavailability of topically applied ophthalmic drugs. Increasing the tear volume suddenly, such as following the instillation of an eyedrop, produces rapid reflex blinking which quickly re-establishes the normal tear pool. Typically, the volume of an ophthalmic solution will be 30-50 μl, which is instilled into the lower fornix. The reflex blink can cause as much as 20 μl to spill over the lid margin onto the skin. Most of the remainder is pumped into the nasolacrimal duct until the total tear volume returns to its normal value of 7 μl. As the precorneal volume of fluid (lacrimal and instilled) becomes smaller, the turnover rate of lacrimal fluid will have a greater influence on the residual drug concentration. Therefore, a larger instilled volume will maximize the penetration of ophthalmic drugs, but a larger proportion will be wasted through drainage.

Significant drug absorption can occur through the mucous membrane of the nasolacrimal duct, with as much as 80% of the instilled volume draining into the gastrointestinal tract from where it can be absorbed into the systemic circulation. Severe systemic side-effects can arise which can lead to toxicity problems, particularly in geriatric and paediatric patients. To minimise loss to other absorptive pathways, the volume of the eyedrop should be sufficiently small that the tear film is not significantly perturbed. Volumes of 5-10 μl have been found to minimize side effects due to systemic absorption via the drainage apparatus, and special eyedrop tips which are capable of delivering this volume have been developed[8 9]. The extent of drug loss due to administration of volumes too large for the eye to retain has been shown in a number of cases. A 10 μl drop of 10% phenylephrine is as potent as the normal 30 μl drop of drug of the same concentration[10]. Ten and 20 μl drops of tropicamide produce more pupillary dilation compared to 40 and 80 μl drops; moreover, local irritation was seen with the larger drop size[11]. Unfortunately, although smaller drop sizes may be retained for even longer periods in the conjunctival sac and reduce systemic side effects still further, volumes less than 8 μl require high drug concentrations with consequent problems in formulation.

Preservatives

The vast majority of ophthalmic formulations contain preservatives, most commonly benzalkonium chloride. At high concentrations, preservatives can cause irritation and damage to the ocular surface. In strengths greater than 0.01%, benzalkonium chloride can damage the corneal epithelium by desquamation. Disruption of the corneal barrier increases the non-selective absorption of several compounds of differing water solubility and molecular weight. There is currently considerable interest in developing preservative free formulations to overcome these problems.

Effect of systemically administered drugs

Tear film dynamics can be affected by systemically administered pharmacological agents and locally applied adjuvants. Timolol applied topically reduces tear flow whereas pilocarpine stimulates tear flow. The adjuvant benzalkonium chloride disrupts the tear film whereas methylcellulose increases the stability of the tear film. Certain drugs can influence blink rate as well as tear secretion; for example, general anaesthetics may completely inhibit lid movements.

Drugs that are used to treat common conditions such as hypertension and allergic conditions can also influence tear film dynamics. If a patient presents with a complaint involving the tear film, it is important to rule out whether this is a side effect of other medication. Antihypertensives administered systemically (e.g. reserpine, diazoxide) stimulate tear flow whilst antihistamines reduce tear flow.

ROUTES OF DRUG ADMINISTRATION

There are three main routes commonly used for administering drugs to the eye:
1. Topical - drops or ointment
2. Systemic - oral or injection
3. Intra-ocular injection

Topical administration

Drops

The most common form of topical administration is the eye drop. It is apparently easy to use, relatively inexpensive and does not impair vision. The major problems with these types of formulation are their inability to sustain high local concentrations of drug and they only have a short contact time with the eye.

Most eye-drops consist of an aqueous medium, to which can be added buffers (phosphate, borate, acetate and glucuronate), organic and inorganic excipients, emulsifiers, and wetting agents in order to accommodate a wide range of drugs with varying degrees of polarity. Vehicles may include water, aqueous mixtures of lower alkanols, vegetable oils, polyalkylene glycols, or petrolatum based jelly. Other excipients include ethylcellulose, ethyl oleate, carboxymethylcellulose and polyvinylpyrrolidone.

Contact time between the vehicle and the eye can be increased by the addition of polymers such as polyvinyl alcohol and methylcellulose, although generally the effects on drug absorption are not dramatic. Drainage from the cul-de-sac may also be reduced by punctual occlusion or simple eyelid closure, which prolongs the contact time of the drug with the external eye. This serves two purposes - first it maximises the contact of drug with the periocular tissues increasing absorption through the cornea and second, the systemic absorption is reduced.

Perfusion

Continuous and constant perfusion of the eye with drug solutions can be achieved by the use of ambulatory motor driven syringes that deliver drug solutions through fine polyethylene tubing positioned in the conjunctival sac. The flow rate of the perfusate through a minipump can be adjusted to produce continuous irrigation of the eye surface (3-6 ml. min^{-1}) or slow delivery 0.2 ml.min^{-1}) to avoid overflow. This system allows the use of a lower drug concentration than used in conventional eye-drops, yet will produce the same potency. Side effects are reduced and constant therapeutic action is maintained. This system is not used very often due to the inconvenience and the cost involved, but may find application for irritant drugs or for sight-threatening situations.

Sprays

Spray systems produce similar results to eye-drops in terms of duration of drug action and side effects. Sprays have several advantages over eye-drops:
1. a more uniform spread of drug can be achieved
2. precise instillation requiring less manual dexterity than for eye-drop administration and is particularly useful for treating patients with unsteady hand movements
3. contamination and eye injury due to eye-drop application are avoided
4. spray delivery causes less reflex lacrimation
5. can be used by patients who have difficulty bending their neck back to administer drops.

The only disadvantage is that sprays are more expensive to produce than eye-drops so they are not widely used; however, several manufacturers have advanced spray systems at a pre-production stage. Prototype devices that force small volumes through a valving system look promising as delivery devices of the future. Recently, it has been demonstrated that one sixth of the conventional dose of pilocarpine hydrochloride delivered in this manner produces an equivalent miosis to the standard dose[12].

Use of polymers to increase viscosity

The viscosity of ophthalmic solutions is often increased to improve retention times of a drug on the corneal surface and hence bioavailability. Soluble polymers in aqueous solution are often used to extend the drug residence time in the cul-de-sac. The more commonly used viscolyzing agents include polyvinyl alcohol (PVA) and derivatives of cellulose. Cellulosic polymers, such as methylcellulose, hydroxyethylcellulose (HEC), hydroxypropyl-methylcellulose (HPMC) and hydroxypropylcellulose (HPC), are widely used as viscolyzers showing Newtonian properties. They have common properties: i) a wide range of viscosity (400 to 15000 cps); ii) compatibility with many topically applied drugs and iii) increased stability of the lacrimal film. There is a general relationship between increasing viscosity and improving bioavailability which would be expected since contact with the absorbing surface is prolonged; however, solutions that are so thick they require a force of more than 0.9 N to shear them markedly interfere with blinking.

Of the many naturally occurring polymers, sodium hyaluronate and chondroitin sulphate have been extensively investigated as potential ophthalmic drug delivery vehicles. Sodium hyaluronate is a high molecular weight polymer extracted by a patented process from sources including rooster coxcombs. The molecule consists of a linear, unbranched, non-sulphated, polyanionic glycosaminoglycan, composed of a repeating disaccharide unit (D-sodium glucuronate and N-acetyl-D-glucosamine). Sodium hyaluronate has an unusual rheological behaviour, undergoing a rapid transformation from a gel to a liquid on application of shear stress (pseudoplasticity). Hence, the viscosity is higher at the resting phase, so it provides a thickened tear film, with slow drainage and an improved distribution on the cornea during blinking. Furthermore, the carboxyl groups of hyaluronate form hydrogen bonds with hydroxyl groups of mucin in the eye, producing an intimate contact with the cornea. They demonstrate a considerably prolonged residence time when compared to saline ($T^{1/}_2$ = 11.1 minutes at 0.2% concentration and 23.5 minutes at 0.3% compared to a $T^{1/}_2$ of 50 seconds for the saline[13]).

Products based on hyaluronates are widely used in intraocular surgery as a substitute for vitreous humor and as an adjuvant to promote tissue repair. Hyaluronates protect the corneal endothelium and other delicate tissues from mechanical damage by providing a stabilised hydrogel. These unique properties give hyaluronates great potential in the ocular drug delivery.

Chondroitin sulphate is a glycosaminoglycan with a repeat unit containing ß-D-glucoronic acid and ß-D-N-acetyl galactosamine. It is similar to hyaluronic acid except for modification of the position of a hydroxyl group and the addition of sulphate groups to the galactosamine residue. Chondroitin sulphate has a good affinity to the corneal surface, preventing premature break-up of the tear film between blinks[14]. Thus, formulations containing chondroitin have been used for the treatment of dry eye and they are superior to hyaluronic acid particularly in severe cases.

Carbomers (carbopols) are polyacrylic acid polymers widely used in pharmaceutical and cosmetic industries. They have several advantages, including high viscosities at low concentrations, strong adhesion to mucosa without irritation, thickening properties, compatibility with many active ingredients, good patient acceptability and low toxicity profiles. These properties have made carbomers very valuable in the field of ophthalmic formulations, particularly for the treatment of dry eye since they have long ocular residence times.

Gelling polymers

At high concentrations, carbomers form acidic, low viscosity, aqueous solutions that transform into stiff gels when the pH is raised. Although these materials gel in the conjunctival sac upon instillation, at this concentration they can cause irritation to the eye due to their high acidity which cannot always be neutralized by the buffering action of the tear fluid. At low concentrations, the carbopol gels show long retention increasing the contact time of solutes and suspended solids.

Gelling systems that make the transition from a liquid phase to a gel or solid phase in response to a specific trigger, such as pH, temperature or concentration of ions, have been used to deliver drugs to the eye. They have the advantage over viscous solutions in that the material can be dispensed from the bottle or tube easily, and only thickens on contact with the tear film gelling *in situ*, usually in the eye cul-de-sac. The polymers used are natural (such as gellan gum) or synthetic such as cellulose acetate phthalate or a pluronic.

Gellan gum is an anionic polysaccharide formulated in aqueous solution, which forms clear gels, the strength of which increases proportionally to the amount of either monovalent or divalent cations present. Gelation occurs in the eye due to the concentration of sodium present in human tears (~2.6 $\mu g.\mu l^{-1}$). The reflex tearing, which usually leads to a dilution of ophthalmic solutions, in this case further enhances the viscosity of the gellan gum by providing cations needed for gelation. Gellan gum based formulations (0.6% w/v) do demonstrate prolonged ocular retention in man[16 17].

Other gels that form *in situ* are characterised by a high polymer concentration, such as 25% pluronics and 30% cellulose acetophthalate (CAP) which were found to cause discomfort. To reduce the total polymer content in the system, polymers were combined to improve gelling properties. A system was explored which contained carbopol, which demonstrates pH-mediated phase transitions, and methylcellulose, which exhibits thermal gelation. Such a system could be formulated as a liquid at a specific pH and room temperature but would gel on exposure to the physiological conditions of the surface of the eye i.e. pH 7.4 and 34°C[18].

Ointments

Ointments are not as popular as eye drops since vision is blurred by the oil base, making ointments impractical for daytime use. They are usually applied for overnight use or if the eye is to be bandaged. They are especially useful for paediatric use since small children often wash out drugs by crying. Ointments are generally non-toxic and safe to use on the exterior of the surface of the eye. However, ointment bases such as lanolin, petrolatum and vegetable oil are toxic to the interior of the eye, causing corneal oedema, vascularization, scarring and endothelial damage. Intraocular contamination with these vehicles should therefore be avoided. Formulations based on white petrolatum-mineral oil have a residence half-time of over an hour in man[19].

Antibiotics such as tetracyclines are used in the form of an ointment, producing effective antibacterial concentrations in the anterior chamber for several hours, whereas an aqueous solution of tetracycline is ineffective for intraocular infections. A problem with extremely lipophilic drugs, including corticosteroids, is that the therapeutic agent may not be released as it partitions into the oil base. For these drugs, alternative systems such as water-soluble inserts may be preferable.

Particulates

Poorly soluble drugs for ophthalmic administration are frequently formulated as micronised suspensions. Larger particles theoretically provide prolongation of effect due to the increased size of the reservoir; however, an increase in particle size is associated with irritation giving rise to an increased rate of removal, assisted by agglomeration of particles and ejection. The relationship between particle size and retention is poorly understood and size is probably not the only determining factor, with parameters such as zeta potential and surface chemistry also being important. Increasing the size of particles to 25 μm in diameter will increase retention time to around 12 hours in a rabbit, compared to 3 μm particles which disappear almost as fast as aqueous solutions[20]. However, increasing the particle size of 0.1% 3H-dexamethasone suspension, from 5.75, to 22 μm demonstrated that clearance of the larger particle size from the eye is faster than complete dissolution[21]. Similarly, increasing the concentration of fluorometholone solids in a suspension did not increase the aqueous humour drug concentration-time profile[22]. Hence, small particle sizes generally improve patient comfort and acceptability of suspension formulations.

Interestingly, submicron or nanosphere formulations demonstrate therapeutic advantages over aqueous solutions, although one would expect rapid clearance from the eye. For example, pilocarpine (2% w/v) adsorbed onto a biocompatible latex of average size 0.3 μm will maintain a constant miosis in the rabbit for up to 10 hours compared to 4 hours with pilocarpine eye drops[23]. Other nanoparticle systems have been investigated for the prolongation of contact time in order to increase the ocular absorption. Betaxolol-poly-e-caprolactone nanoparticles produce a significantly greater reduction in intra-ocular pressure compared to the commercial eyedrops[24]. Similar improvements were obtained with carteolol (a ß-blocker) which caused a better penetration of the drug in the nanosphere formulation.

Sustained release devices

Although some particulate systems could be classified as sustained release devices, the term is applied here only to macroscopic devices such as inserts. Provision of a matrix to sustain drug release in the eye can be achieved in several ways. For example, a hydrophilic (soft) contact lens can serve as a drug reservoir. The drug is incorporated into the lens by either instilling drops on the lens when in the eye, or pre-soaking the lens in a solution of the drug. Other systems are not placed on the cornea, but are inserted under the eyelid, such as insoluble inserts of polyvinyl alcohol or soluble collagen which dissolve in lacrimal fluid or disintegrate while releasing the drug. Soluble inserts are made of such substances as gelatin, alginates, agar and hydroxypropylmethylcellulose. These systems have been developed as a method for delivering larger amounts of drugs to the eye over a long period.

Ocuserts® (Alza Corporation, U.S.A.) are insoluble inserts containing pilocarpine used in the treatment of glaucoma, and have a one-week duration of action. The major

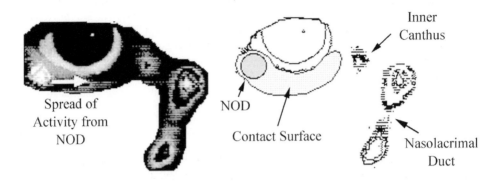

*Figure 11.11 Combined photographic and scintigraphic image of the eye (left);
illustration of contact area (right)*

advantages of this system include longer duration of drug action, avoidance of accommoda-
tive spasms in younger patients and better patient compliance. However, 20% of all patients treated with the Ocusert® lose the device without being aware of the loss. For this
reason, patients fitted with the device should be checked regularly.

Collagen shields have proven useful as the basis of a drug delivery device. The
shield is made from porcine scleral collagen that is moulded into a contact lens-like shape.
This is hardened and crosslinked by exposure to ultraviolet light. The shield conforms to
the shape of the eye and lubricates the cornea as it dissolves. The dissolution time depends
on the degree of crosslinking which can be controlled to release drug over a period from
approximately 12 to 72 hours. Drugs can be incorporated into the collagen matrix during
manufacture, adsorbed into the shield during rehydration, or topically applied over the shield
in the eye. As the shield dissolves, the drug is released gradually into the tear film, maintaining high concentrations on the corneal surface and increasing drug permeation through
the cornea[25]. Studies suggest that drug delivery by collagen shields may be helpful in the
early management of bacterial keratitis, in preference to frequent administration of topical
antibiotics, subconjunctival injection, or topical administration over a soft contact lens band-
age.

A PVA gel which hydrates on contact with the eye clears with a mean half-life of 8
minutes in normal subjects[26] but it increases the bioavailability of pilocarpine by 16 times
compared to conventional formulations. This is due to presentation of the drug in the nonionised form; and to sustained high concentration in the lower marginal tear film. Presentation of drug was confined to the sclera with little spread to cornea (Figure 11.11). As the
diffusion path from sclera to ciliary body is relatively short, this should result in high concentrations of drug in the lower hemisphere interior with much lower concentrations in the
upper segment.

Intraocular drug delivery

Over the last two decades, treatment of intraocular conditions and diseases, such as
endophthalmitis, has been attempted mainly by intravenous, topical or subconjunctival administration of suitable drugs. Sub-therapeutic intravitreal concentrations of the drugs following each of these routes frequently resulted in poor recovery of vision. Topical application of drugs for the treatment of posterior segment disorders is severely limited by the
highly efficient clearance mechanisms. Improving the precorneal residence time of topi-

cally applied drugs by viscosity enhancing agents, gelling agents, or mucoadhesive polymers has failed to provide sufficient concentrations in the vitreous humor. Similarly, subconjunctival injection of antibiotics and antivirals is also unsuccessful in achieving therapeutic concentrations in the vitreous humor. The intraocular penetration of drugs following intravenous administration is hampered by the presence of tight junctional complexes of the retinal pigment epithelium and the retinal blood vessels forming the blood-retinal barrier.

Most diseases affecting the posterior segment are chronic in nature and require prolonged drug administration. Intravitreal injections remain the main route of delivery in order to avoid the concomitant side effects seen with systemic administration. An intravitreal injection provides therapeutic concentrations of the drug adjacent to the intended site of activity and only a small dose of drug is required. However, possible retinal toxicity of the injected dose must be taken into account. Usually an intravitreal injection is restricted to a volume of 0.1-0.2 ml administered following both anterior chamber and vitreal taps. Following injection, the drug diffuses through the vitreous gel with little restriction. For most drugs the diffusion coefficient through the vitreous humor is close to that through water.

Once distributed throughout the vitreous humor, rapid elimination of the drug is observed via two routes:

1. anteriorly by simple diffusion to the posterior chamber, followed by removal to the systemic circulation along with the aqueous humor drainage

2. posteriorly across the retina where it is removed by active secretion.

Drugs lost primarily by anterior chamber diffusion have a half life in the vitreous humor of 20-30 hours, while drugs lost via the trans-retinal route, such as the penicillins, have typically much shorter half lives of 5-10 hours. Unfortunately, these time scales are still shorter than required and depot devices which deliver over days to weeks are being developed. Ocular inflammation results in the breakdown of the blood-retinal barrier and increases the elimination of non-transported drugs from the vitreous humor. In contrast, drugs that are removed by the active transport systems reside longer in the vitreous following ocular inflammation due the failure in the transport mechanism. Rate of drug loss is also enhanced in vitrectomised and lensectomised eyes.

Liposomes

Liposomal encapsulation has the potential not only to increase the activity and prolong the residence of the drug in the eye, but also to reduce the intraocular toxicity of certain drugs. For example, liposome-encapsulated amphotericin B produces less toxicity than the commercial solubilized amphotericin B formulation when injected intravitreally. The main drawbacks associated with liposomes are their short shelf life and difficulty in storage, limited drug loading capacity and instability on sterilization and finally, transient blurring of vision after an intravitreal injection. Despite these disadvantages, they have potential as drug delivery systems as they are composed of substances that are non-toxic and totally biodegradable.

Microparticulates and nanoparticles

Microspheres and nanoparticles are retained for extended periods within the eye and can provide slow, sustained release of drugs. The delivery systems are especially attractive because of the ease of manufacturing and improved stability compared to liposomes. The polymers used in the manufacture can be *erodible*, in which case the drug release is due to the polymer degradation, or *non-erodible*, where the drug is released is by diffusion through the polymer.

Intraocular devices

The administration of medications by implants or depot devices is a very rapidly developing technology in ocular therapeutics. These overcome the potential hazards associated with repeated intravitreal injection such as clouding of the vitreous humor, retinal detachment and endophthalmitis.

Implantable devices have been developed that serve two major purposes. First, to release of drug at zero order rates, thus improving the predictability of drug action, and second, to release of the drug over several months, reducing dramatically the frequency of administration.

Depot devices have been developed to treat proliferative vitreoretinopathy and retinitis associated with cytomegalovirus. Various implantable devices, such as a gentamicin osmotic minipump, a polyvinyl alcohol/ethylene vinyl acetate cup containing ganciclovir, a polysulfone capillary fibre with daunomycin in tristearin and ganciclovir intraocular implant have been suggested.

Vitrasert® is a commercially available sustained release intraocular device for ganciclovir approved for use in-patients suffering from cytomegalovirus. Apart from the anticipated problems of endophthalmitis and retinal detachment, dislocation of implant and poor intravitreal drug levels due to its placement into the suprachoroidal space have been observed.

Iontophoresis

Iontophoresis (see transdermal chapter) facilitates drug penetration through the intact corneal epithelium. The solution of the drug is kept in contact with the cornea in an eye-cup bearing an electrode. A potential difference is applied with the electrode in the cup having the same charge as the ionized drug, so that the drug flux is into the tissue. This method of administration is very rarely used, except under carefully controlled conditions. Iontophoresis allows penetration of antibiotics that are ionised and therefore do not penetrate by other methods, for example, polymyxin B used in the local treatment of infections. Although the technique is found to be suitable for a range of compounds like NSAIDS, antivirals, antibiotics, anaesthetics and glucocorticoids, its acceptability as a routine drug delivery system is limited by the lack of information on side effects from repeated or multiple applications on the same or a different site.

Commonly reported toxic effects include slight retinal and choroidal burns and retinal pigment epithelial and choroidal necrosis, corneal epithelial oedema, persistent corneal opacities and polymorphonuclear cell infiltration. Other disadvantages of iontophoresis include side effects such as itching, erythema and general irritation.

Systemic administration

Drugs are usually administered systemically for the treatment of diseases involving the optic nerve, retina and uveal tract. The blood/aqueous barrier only allows drugs to pass into the anterior chamber of the eye by one of two processes, both of which are very slow:

(1) secretion from the ciliary body
(2) diffusion from the capillaries of the iris.

Most drugs are unable to reach the anterior chamber in therapeutically active concentrations because they are either not sufficiently lipid soluble or they are bound to plasma proteins and hence cannot pass through the blood vessel wall.

Some drugs such as acetazolamide are ineffective when given topically and although it can be administered parenterally this is impractical for chronic administration. A sustained-release oral preparation of acetazolamide is valuable for patients with glaucoma since it produces consistent and sustained levels of drug. Better carbonic anhydrase inhibitors such as dorzolamide may decrease enthusiasm for acetazolamide. Recently, the sublingual route has been explored for the delivery of timolol to decrease intraocular pressure in patients with ocular hypotension.

CONCLUSIONS

Increasing the residence time of an ophthalmic formulation on the corneal surface increases the drug bioavailability and therefore reduces frequency of administration. Although recent advances have been made in ocular drug delivery systems, eye drops are still the most commonly used formulations as they are the least expensive preparations, are easy to use, and do not interfere with vision. However, frequent administration is necessary.

The retention of a drug on the corneal surface is determined by the amount of tear flow and by the blink frequency, which can be stimulated by different factors. The most important factor influencing the retention of a drug on the corneal surface appears to be the properties of the drug itself. If a drug irritates the eye, it is difficult to obtain a long retention. If the drug is non-irritant, retention time can be increased by instillation of small drops, by adjustment of the osmolarity, tonicity, pH and by choosing the appropriate preservatives and adjuvants.

REFERENCES

1. Wolff E. Mucocutaneous junction of lid-margin and distribution of tear fluid. *Trans. Opthal. Soc. UK* 1946;66:291-308.
2. Prydal JI, Kerr-Muir MG, Dilly PN. Comparison of tear film thickness in three species determined by the glass fibre method and confocal microscopy. *Eye* 1993;7:472-475.
3. Tiffany JM, Winter N, Bliss G. Tear film stability and tear surface tension. 1989;8:507-515.
4. Lee VHL, Robinson JR. Disposition of pilocarpine in the pigmented rabbit eye. *Int. J. Pharmaceut.* 1982;11:155-165.
5. Lee VHL. Esterase activities in adult rabbit eyes. *J. Pharmaceut. Sci.* 1983;72:239-244.
6. Ahmed I, Gokhale RD, Shah MV, Patton TF. Physicochemical determinants of drug diffusion across the conjunctiva, sclera and cornea. *J. Pharmaceut. Sci.* 1987;76:583-586.
7. Chien DS, Homsy JJ, Gluchowski C, TangLiu DS. Corneal and conjunctival/scleral penetration of p-aminoclonidine, AGN190342, and clonidine in rabbit eyes. *Cur. Eye Res.* 1990;9:1051-1059.
8. Brown RH, Lynch MG. Drop size of commericial glaucoma medications. *Am. J. Ophthalmol.* 1986;102:673-674.
9. Reducing the size and toxicity of eyedrops. 10th National science writers seminar in ophthalmology; 1988; Arlington.
10. Whitson JT, Love R, Brown RH, Lynch MG, Schoenwald RD. The effect of reduced eyedrop size and eyelid closure on the therapeutic index of phenylephrine. *Am. J. Ophthalmol.* 1993;115:357-359.
11. Lal A, Kumar V. The therapeutic response to topical instillation of different drop volume of tropicamide in humans. *Afro-Asian J. Opthalmol.* 1995;14:15-18.
12. Martini LG, Embleton JK, Malcolmson RJ, Richard J, Wilson CG. The use of small volume ocular sprays to improve the bioavailability of topically applied ophthalmic drugs. *Europ. J. Pharmaceut. Biopharm.* 1997;44:121-126.
13. Snibson GR, Greaves JL, Soper NDW, Prydal JI, Wilson CG, Bron AJ. Precorneal residence times of sodium hyaluronate solutions studied by quantitative gamma scintigraphy. *Eye* 1990;4:594-602.
14. Silver FH. Biomaterials used in ophthalmology. *Biomaterials, Medical Devices and Tissue Engineering.* London: Chapman and Hall, 1993:120-152.

15. Wilson CG, Zhu YP, Frier M, Rao LS, Gilchrist P, Perkins AC. Ocular contact time of a carbomer gel, Geltears®, in human. *Br. J. Ophthalmol.* 1998;82:1131-1134.
16. Greaves JL, Wilson CG, Rozier A, Grove J, Plazonnet B. Scintigraphic Assessment of an Ophthalmic Gelling Vehicle in Man and Rabbit. *Curr. Eye Res.* 1990;9:415-420.
17. Meseguer G, Buri P, Plazonnet B, Rozier A, Gurny R. Gamma scintigraphic comparison of eyedrops containing pilocarpine in healthy volunteers. *J. Ocular Pharmacol. Therapeut.* 1996;12:481-488.
18. Joshi A, Ding S, Himmelstein KJ. U.S. Patent 5 252 318. 1993.
19. Greaves JL, Wilson CG, Birmingham AT. Assessment of the precorneal residence of an ophthalmic ointment in healthy subjects. *Br. J. Clin. Pharmacol.* 1993;35:188-192.
20. Sieg JW, Triplett JW. Precorneal retention of topically instilled micronized particles. *J. Pharmaceut. Sci.* 1980;69:863-864.
21. Schoenwald RD, Stewart P. Effect of particle size on ophthalmic bioavailability of dexamethasone suspensions in rabbits. *J. Pharmaceut. Sci.* 1980;69:391-394.
22. Olejnik O, Weisbecker CA. Ocular bioavailability of topical prednisolone preparations. *Clin. Therapeut.* 1990;12:2-11.
23. Gurny R. Preliminary study of prolonged acting "drug" delivery system for the treatment of glaucoma. *Pharm. Acta. Helv.* 1981;56:130-132.
24. Marcha-Heussler L, Sirbat D, Hoffman M, Maincent P. Poly(epsilon-caprolactone) nanocapsules in carteolol ophthalmic delivery. *Pharmaceut. Res.* 1993;10:386-390.
25. Shofner RS, Kaufman HE, Hill JM. New Horizons in ocular drug delivery. In: *Ophthalmol. Clin. N. Am.* Kooner TJ (ed) Philadelphia. W.B. Saunders Co., 1989.
26. Greaves JL, Wilson CG, Birmingham AT, Richardson MC, Bentley PH. Scintigraphic studies on the corneal residence of a New Ophthalmic Delivery System (NODS): Rate of clearance of a soluble marker in relation to duration of pharmacological action of pilocarpine. *Br. J. Clin. Pharmacol.* 1992;33:603-609.

Chapter Twelve

Vaginal and Intrauterine Drug Delivery

ANATOMY AND PHYSIOLOGY

The word vagina means sheath and it is a fibromuscular tube between 6 and 10 cm long in a adult female extending from the cervix (outer end) of the uterus (Figure 12.1). The vagina lies obliquely upward and backward behind the bladder and urethra and in front of the rectum and anal canal. The axis of the vagina forms an angle of over 90° with that of the uterus, but this can vary considerably depending on the fullness of the bladder and rectum, and during pregnancy. The cervix of the uterus extends for a short distance into the vagina. It is normally pressed against its posterior wall creating recesses in the vagina at the back, on each side, and at the front of the cervix. These are known as the anterior and posterior fornices located to the front and back of the cervix. The posterior fornix is the largest of the fornices and the lateral fornices found to the sides. The upper part of the posterior wall of the vagina is covered by peritoneum which is folded back onto the rectum to form the recto-uterine pouch. The lower part of the posterior vaginal wall is separated from the anal canal by tissue known as the perineal body.

In female mammals the function of the vagina is to receive the male reproductive cells, or sperm, and is part of the birth canal. In humans, it also functions as an excretory canal for the products of menstruation.

The uterus or womb is a hollow, inverted pear-shaped fibro-muscular organ. Its shape and weight varies enormously depending on menstrual cycle and previous pregnancies. In a young female, with no previous pregnancies, the uterus is approximately 8 cm long, 5 cm wide and 2.5 cm thick and weighs approximately 30-40 g but it enlarges to four to five times this size in pregnancy.

The narrower, lower end is called the cervix; this projects into the vagina. The cervix is made of fibrous connective tissue and is of a firmer consistency than the body of the uterus. The two uterine tubes enter the uterus at opposite sides, near its top. The part of the uterus above the entrances of the tubes is called the fundus; that below is termed the body.

Between birth and puberty, the uterus gradually descends into the true pelvis from the abdomen. After puberty, the uterus is located behind the symphysis pubis and bladder and in front of the rectum. The uterus is supported and held in position by the other pelvic

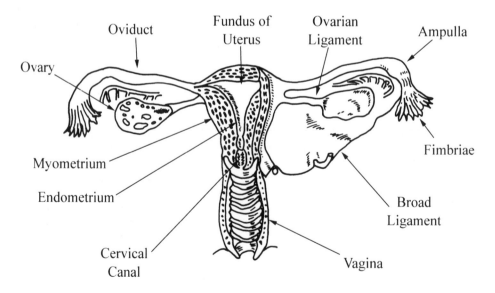

Figure 12.1 The female reproductive system

organs, the muscular floor or diaphragm of the pelvis, certain fibrous ligaments, and by folds of peritoneum. Among the supporting ligaments are two double-layered broad ligaments, each of which contains a uterine tube along its upper free border and a round ligament. Two ligaments at each side of the cervix are also important in maintaining the position of the uterus.

The triangular cavity of the uterus is remarkably flat and small in comparison with the size of the organ, except during pregnancy. The function of the uterus is to protect and nourish the embryo and foetus. At term, its thick muscular walls contract powerfully to expel the infant through the vagina.

Mucosa

The vagina has a mucous membrane comprised of stratified squamous epithelium. This has longitudinal ridges, known as the columns of the vagina, in the midline of both the anterior and posterior walls. Folds or rugae extend from them to each side. The furrows between the rugae are more marked on the posterior wall and become especially pronounced before birth of a child.

The vaginal epithelium consists of 5 layers, basal, parabasal, intermediate, transitional and superficial, however the changes between layers are gradual (Figure 12.2). Attachment of the cells is primarily by desmosomes with some tight junctions.

Attached to the mucous membrane is an outer smooth muscle coat consisting of an outer longitudinal layer and a less developed inner circular layer (Figure 12.3). The lower part of the vagina is surrounded by the bulbospongiosus muscle, a striped muscle attached to the perineal body. Covering the muscle tissue is a sheath of connective tissue which consists of blood vessels, lymphatic ducts, and nerve fibres. This layer joins those of the urinary bladder, rectum, and other pelvic structures.

The cervical canal is lined with columnar mucus secreting epithelium which is thrown into a series of V-shaped folds. Its wall, composed mainly of dense fibrous connective tissue, only has a small amount of smooth muscle.

The uterus is composed of three layers of tissue. On the outside is a serous coat of peritoneum which partially covers the organ, exudes a fluid like blood minus its cells and

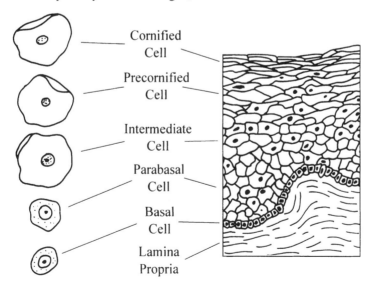

Cornified Cell

Precornified Cell

Intermediate Cell

Parabasal Cell

Basal Cell

Lamina Propria

Figure 12.2 Cross section through the vaginal mucosa

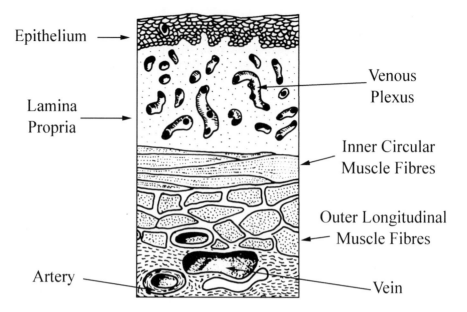

Epithelium

Lamina
Propria

Artery

Venous
Plexus

Inner Circular
Muscle Fibres

Outer Longitudinal
Muscle Fibres

Vein

Figure 12.3 Cross section through the vaginal wall

the clotting factor fibrinogen. In front it covers only the body of the cervix; behind it covers the body and the part of the cervix that is above the vagina and is prolonged onto the posterior vaginal wall; from there it is folded back to the rectum. The middle layer of tissue, the myometrium, is muscular and makes up the majority of the organ. It is very firm and consists of densely packed, unstriped, smooth muscle fibres with blood vessels, lymphatics, and nerves. The muscle is arranged in three layers of fibres running in different directions. The outermost fibres are arranged longitudinally. Those of the middle layer, which is the thickest, run in all directions without any orderly arrangement. The innermost fibres are longitudinal and circular in their arrangement.

The innermost layer of tissue in the uterus is the mucous membrane, or endometrium. It lines the uterine cavity as far as the internal os, where it becomes continuous with the lining of the cervical canal. The endometrium contains numerous uterine glands that open into the uterine cavity and that are embedded in the cellular framework or stroma of the endometrium. Numerous blood vessels and lymphatic spaces are also present. The appearance of the endometrium varies considerably at the different stages in reproductive life. It begins to reach full development at puberty and thereafter exhibits dramatic changes during each menstrual cycle. It undergoes further changes before, during, and after pregnancy; during the menopause; and in old age. These changes are for the most part hormonally induced and controlled by the activity of the ovaries. The endometrium is divided into three layers, the stratum compactum, the stratum spongiosum, and the stratum basale, which are functionally distinct, but blend together. The stratum compactum is nearest to the uterine cavity and contains the lining cells and the necks of the uterine glands; its stroma is relatively dense. Superficial blood vessels lie beneath the lining cells. The stratum spongiosum is the large middle layer and it contains the main portions of uterine glands and accompanying blood vessels; the stromal cells are more loosely arranged and larger than in the stratum compactum. The stratum basale lies against the uterine muscle; it contains blood vessels and the bases of the uterine glands. Its stroma remains relatively unaltered during the menstrual cycle.

Blood and nerve supply

The blood supply to the vagina is derived from several adjacent vessels, a vaginal artery extends from the internal iliac artery, uterine, middle rectal, and internal pudendal arteries. As the vagina is not structurally related to the gastrointestinal system, the drainage avoids the liver and hence is not subject to first pass metabolism. The blood vessels are located close to the basal epithelial layer, but pores are present in the endothelial cells lining the capillaries through which an interchange of blood and vaginal fluid constiuents can occur. The channels in the basal, parabasal and intermediate levels change width depending upon hormonal levels, expanding to their maximum width during ovulatory and luteal phases. Molecules as large as albumin and immunoglobulins are able to pass from the blood to the lumen.

The nerve supply to the lower part of the vagina is from the pudendal nerve and from the inferior hypogastric and uterovaginal plexuses.

The uterus is supplied with blood by the two uterine arteries, which are branches of the internal iliac arteries, and by ovarian arteries, which connect with the ends of the uterine arteries and send branches to supply the uterus. The nerves to the uterus include the sympathetic nerve fibres, which produce contraction of uterine muscle and constriction of vessels, and parasympathetic (sacral) fibres, which inhibit muscle activity and cause dilation of blood vessels.

Uterine and vaginal fluid

The vagina does not possess any glands except Bartholin's and Skene's glands, but these are not believed to contribute significantly to the vaginal fluid. The fluid consists mainly of cervical secretions and transudation from the blood vessels with desquamated vaginal cells and leucocytes. The fluid will also contain secretions from the endometrium and fallopian tubes. The amount and composition of fluid will vary with the menstrual cycle, but women of reproductive age produce about 1 g.h^{-1}, but post-menopausal women produce only about half this much.

Cervical secretions originate both in the uterine cavity and the cervix and they flow constantly towards the vagina. During ovulation, the secretions are watery to facilitate the movement of spermatozoa. In response to increased levels of progesterone during the luteal phase of the menstrual cycle, or during pregnancy, the secretions become more viscous to prevent the passage of microorganisms and sperm into the body of the uterus.

pH

The *Lactobacillus acidophilus* present within the vagina produces lactic acid from glycogen to maintain the pH at between 4.9 and 3.5 which has a bacteriostatic action. The anterior fornix has the lowest pH, which gradually rises towards the vestibule.

At birth, there is a passive transfer of maternal hormones and lactobacilli which are present for the first 4 weeks of life. Consequently vaginal pH is low and after the concentration of hormones has receded, the pH rises to 7 where it remains until puberty. This high pH is associated with an increased risk of infection[1].

In post-puberty women, the pH can be raised during menstruation, but also it can increase after periods of frequent acts of coitus because both vaginal transudate and ejaculate are alkaline. Acidity can also be decreased by alkaline secretion of the cervical glands. During pregnancy the mean vaginal pH is approximately 4.2[2].

Cervical bacterial flora in sexually active healthy women using oral contraceptives or intrauterine contraceptive devices is rich in anaerobes, however, barrier contraception with a condom prevents this anaerobic shift and maintains a lactobacilli-dominated flora in the cervix[3].

Enzymatic activity

The outer cell layers of the vagina contain ß-glucuronidase, acid phosphatase, with smaller amounts of α-naphthylesterase, DPNH diaphorase, phosphoamidase and succinic dehydrogenase. Basal cell layers contain ß-glucuronidase, succinic dehydrogenase, DPNH diaphorase, small amounts of acid phosphatase and a-naphthylesterase.

Alkaline phosphatase, lactate dehydrogenase, aminopeptidase and esterase activity are all markedly elevated in the follicular phase of the menstrual cycle, but fall immediately prior to ovulation[4]. Their activity begins to rise again one day after ovulation.

Mucus

Mucus is secreted by endocervical glands and its production is oestrogen dependent. It is minimal immediately after menstruation, but during the pre-ovulation stage, the raised oestrogen increases mucus production. The mucus also becomes more transparent, viscous and elastic reaching a maximum just before ovulation which lasts approximately 2 days post-ovulation.

Menstruation

The menstrual cycle lasts approximately 28 days and it can be divided into 4 phases: the follicular, ovulatory, luteal and menstrual phases. The phases equate to repair, prolifera-tion, secretion and menstruation. Repair begins even before menstruation has completely ceased. During the follicular or proliferative phase, the oestradiol levels increase, resulting in the uterine epithelium increasing in thickness from 20 layers or 0.2 mm to over 40 layers during the ovulatory phase (Figure 12.4). The major feature of the proliferative phase is the increase in ciliated and microvillus cells. The ciliogenesis begins on day 7-8 of the cycle. The stroma becomes becomes vascular and oedematous and a large number of cells includ-ing lymphocytes and macrophages derived from bone marrow are present in the endometrium. Secretion takes place from days 16-28. In this phase the oestrogen levels drop and the

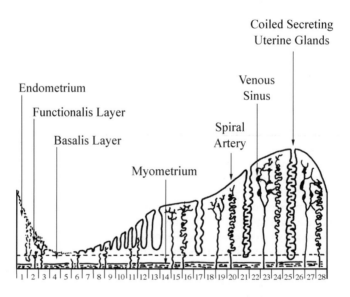

Figure 12.4 Effect of the menstrual cycle on the uterine epithelium

levels of progesterone increase and hence the effects become dominant. The drop in oestrogen can lead to the thickening of the endometrium being reduced and intermenstrual bleeding occurring. The endometrial glands produce a thick glycogen-rich mucoid secretion. There is an increase in vascularisation and the uterus is ready to receive an embryo. If implantation does not occur, the corpus luteum begins to degenerate, progesterone levels drop which causes the endometrium to breakdown. The coiled arterioles of the superficial layers of the outer endometrium contract thus depriving the superficial layers of oxygen, resulting in menstruation. Menstruation can last for anything up to about a week.

Menopause

The menopause is associated with a gradual change in the vagina which can take up to 5 to 8 years to stabilise. The length and the diameter decrease with age and the pH can rise to between 6 and 8, increasing the risk of infection. Elasticity and blood supply decrease with age and the upper vagina may atrophy. The epithelium becomes thinner which is an important consideration in intravaginal drug delivery since this would lead to an increased permeability. Vaginal secretions and hence lubrication decrease and become more watery. The levels of several enzymes, such as β-glucuronidase, acid phosphate and non-specific esterases, increase in postmenopausal women.

Disorders of the vagina

These include bacterial infections e.g. leukorrhea, vaginitis, ulcerated sores, prolapse in which the internal portions of the vagina protrude out of the vaginal orifice, and occasionally cancerous tumours. Rectocele is caused when the muscles and connective tissues supporting the rectum and back wall of the vagina are weakened, usually due to repeated childbirth or aging, and the rectum sags until it bulges into the back wall of the vagina. A rectocele often occurs together with enterocele, which is a bulge of the small intestine into the vagina. Women with small rectoceles or enteroceles may not feel much distress; a larger and more serious rectocele can cause discomfort and a sagging sensation in the pelvic area and difficulty in emptying the lower bowel. Both conditions can be corrected by surgery in which the small intestine and rectum are pushed back into place and held there by reconstructed pelvic muscles.

DRUG ABSORPTION THROUGH THE VAGINA/UTERUS

A wide range of drugs have been studied for vaginal absoprtion. These include steroid hormones such as progesterone and oestrogen, prostaglandins, iodides and salicylates[5], peanut proteins, bacterial antigens and polyvinyl alcohol (m. w. 25,000 Daltons)[6]. Insulin, hydrocyanic acid, iodides, strychnine, pilocarpine, atropine, quinine and oxyquinolone are rapidly absorbed from cat and dog vaginas[5]. Quinine and phenol red are absorbed slowly and methylene blue only in very small quantities.

A recently reported observation is that drugs administered intravaginally accumulate in uterine tissue. This has been reported for danazol, terbutaline and progesterone[7-9]. These findings have led to the hypothesis that there is a direct transport mechanism from vagina to uterus or a "uterine–first pass effect"[9].

DRUG DELIVERY
Vaginal

Traditionally, vaginally drug delivery was only used for contraceptive agents and also for treatment of local infections. Recently its potential for delivering peptides has been explored since it is vascular, permeable to many drugs[5] and drugs absorbed via this route avoid first-pass metabolism.

A major problem with using the vagina as a route for systemic drug delivery is that as the epithelium is highly sensitive to oestradiol and its thickness changes throughout the menstrual cycle, so the extent and rate of drug absorption will also vary. This has been reported for vaginal absorption of steroids[10] and vidarabine has been shown to have a 5-100 times higher permeability coefficient during the early dioestrus stage than during the oestrus stage in guinea pigs[11]. Other problems are gender specificity, personal hygiene and the influence of sexual intercourse.

The thick cervical mucosa may aid bioadhesion of drug delivery systems, but it will also act as a diffusional barrier to the drug. The distribution and coverage of materials within the vagina varies considerably with the nature of the delivery system, disintegrating tablets spread the least, whilst solutions, suspensions and foams spread the best. The rupture time of soft jelly capsules containing nonoxynol-9 after their vaginal insertion was found to rely on local pH and acidity and level of infection present. Capsules did not rupture when the vaginal pH was alkaline or if the vagina was dry[12].

Creams and gels

Creams and gels have been the usual methods for delivering contraceptives and drugs for topical delivery. These are generally considered to be messy to apply and uncomfortable when they leak into undergarments; in addition, dosages are imprecise.

An emulsion based system to deliver anti-fungals seems to have great advantages over many current suppository formulations. It is a "multi-phase" liquid, or semi-solid and it does not seep from the vagina. The system is designed to give controlled delivery for 3 or more hours.

Pessaries or tablets

Pessaries can be either tablets or suppositories designed for vaginal application. They are usually designed to either dissolve or melt and which utilize a variety of materials. Tablets are often modifications of suppositories used for rectal drug delivery.

Intravaginal inserts consisting of a polyester resin plug or sponge have been tried[13], but traumatic manipulation of the sponge, use during menstruation or the puerperium, and prolonged retention of the sponge may increase toxic shock syndrome risk[14]. The use of osmotic pumps has also been investigated[15].

Vaginal rings

Vaginal ring delivery systems are usually based upon silicone elastomers with an inert inner ring which is coated with another layer of elastomer containing drug. A third, outer rate controlling elastomer layer may be added to prevent an initial burst release which could be observed with newly applied rings.

The rings are approximately 6 cm in diameter with a circular cross-section diameter of 4-7 mm. They are positioned in the vagina around the cervix. For most contraceptive applications, the rings are left in place for 21 days then removed for 7 days to allow menstruation. The main challenge is to deliver enough drug to prevent conception, whilst not producing bleeding irregularities. Since their development in 1970, they have been used to deliver medoxyprogesterone acetate, chlormadinone acetate, norethindrone, norgestrel and levonorgestrel, among others. A low dose oestradiol vaginal ring has been found to be significantly more acceptable than creams for the treatment of urogenital atrophy[16]. Recently, a contraceptive ring has been developed containing oestrogen and progestin particles dispersed in aqueous polyethylene glycol throughout the ring. It successfully delivers both drugs, at a consistent ratio with approximately zero-order kinetics.

Bioadhesive delivery systems

Bioadhesive tablets and microparticles in particular hydrogels such as poly(acrylic acid) and celluloses are currently being utilised for sustained and controlled delivery[17]. The first bioadhesive tablets contained hydroxypropylcellulose and polyacrylic acid and were used to treat cancerous lesions with bleomycin.

A bioadhesive polycarbophil gel, a lightly cross-linked polyacrylic acid, used to retain moisture and lubricate the vagina has recently been introduced onto the market (Replens, Columbia Laboratories). Clinical assessment of local tissue pH, in postmenopausal women, shows the polycarbophil gel produces a reduction in pH from about 6 to 4 and maintains the acidic pH for about 3-4 days after the last dose. Hydration of the vaginal tissue occurs through an increase in vaginal blood flow as determined by a laser Doppler measurement. In patients with a history of breast cancer who experienced vaginal dryness, vaginal irritation, or dyspareunia, the polycarbophil gel produced a statistically significant reduction in mean vaginal pH and an improvement in vaginal moisture, mucosa secretions, and elasticity scores, as well as significant improvement in vaginal health measures[18].

The polycarbophil gel has been shown to remain on vaginal tissue for 3-4 days and hence has the potential to serve as a platform for drug delivery[19]. It appears to be an effective delivery system for the spermicidal/antiviral agent nonoxynol-9.

Intrauterine Devices

Intrauterine devices (IUDs) have been used for many years as a method of contraception. They are first described in 1909 by Richter[20] who used a ring made of silkworm gut. In 1930, Graefenberg also used silkworm gut but added an alloy of copper, nickel and zinc[21].

As a result of the long history of using IUDs, it is not surprising, therefore that intrauterine delivery has focused upon the use of medicated intrauterine devices. Newer IUDs have been constructed which contain copper or progesterone. Copper containing IUDs release some copper continuously whilst in situ. There was some concern about systemic absorption of copper with long term use, however this was not found to occur. The copper remains mainly in the uterine fluid which is thought to render it unabsorbable and only small quantities are found in the endometrium. Itching or allergic dermatitis, possibly due to absorption of copper into the circulation has been reported some months after insertion of the device. The concept of using conventional IUDs for the long-term delivery of contraceptive steroids is also being researched. The Progestasert IUD delivers progesterone at about 65 μg.day^{-1} over 1 year. The drug reservoir contains 38 mg of progesterone dispersed in silicone oil surrounded by a release rate controlling mechanism composed of ethylene-vinyl acetate copolymer. The greatest advantage of this system is that it eliminates the need for oestrogen which is required in oral contraceptives. Progesterone's half-life is only a few minutes since the endometrium metabolizes progesterone rapidly and the local delivery allows reduction of the dose and reduction in side effects.

The uterine wall is permeable to negatively charged molecules, high molecular weight drugs and its permeability is not affected by the degree of ionization of the compound[22]. This observation has lead to speculation that the tight junctions in the uterine wall are more permeable than those in other tissues. The size of the tight junctions in the uterus is between 400 and 700 Å, which is about twice that in the intestine or nasal mucosa. Absorption is facilitated by the exceptionally rich blood and lymph supply to the uterus. One possible drawback is that the constant outward flow of cervical secretion can dilute and cause a loss of drug delivered into the uterus.

Intrauterine delivery of insulin, calcitonin and erythrpoietin has been investigated in rats, but no human data is yet available[22]. It has been suggested that this route may be useful for delivering drugs to treat conditions such as osteoporosis.

Introduction of a foreign body into the uterine cavity results in increased vascular permeability, oedema and stromal infiltration of leucocytes, including neutrophils, mono-nuclear cells and macrophages. The foreign-body reaction should not be confused with endometritis which is bacterial in origin. Complications which have arisen from IUD use include uterine perforation, abortion of unsuspected pregnancies, uterine cramp and bleed-ing, menorrhagia and pelvic infections.

CONCLUSION

Vaginal delivery has the advantage that self-insertion and removal of delivery de-vices is possible. This route does avoid first-pass metabolism, but the mucosa is not as permeable as the uterus to peptides and proteins and the variability in bioavailability is too high to be used clinically. In contrast, the uterus appears to be very permeable to a wide variety of substances, but insertion and removal of devices has to be performed by medi-cally qualified personnel. Possible consequences of pregnancy occurring whilst the de-vices are in situ have to be studied thoroughly since the local concentration of the drug is likely to be high. Drugs absorbed from the uterus also avoid first-pass metabolism.

REFERENCES

1. Hanna NF, Taylor-Robinson D, Kalodiki-Karamanoli M, Harris JR, McFadyen IR. The relation between vaginal pH and the microbiological status in vaginitis. *Br. J. Obstetr. Gynaecol.* 1985;92:1267-1271.
2. Gleeson RP, Elder AM, Turner MJ, Rutherford AJ, Elder MG. Vaginal pH in pregnancy in women delivered at and before term. *Br. J. Obstetr. Gynaecol.* 1989;96:183-187.
3. Haukkamaa M, Stranden P, Jousimies Somer H, Siitonen A. Bacterial flora of the cervix in women using different methods of contraception. *Am. J. Obstetr. Gynaecol.* 1986;154:520-524.
4. Blackwell RE. Detection of ovulation. *Fertil. and Steril.* 1984;41:680-681.
5. Aref I, El-Sheikha Z, Hafez ESE. *Absorption of drugs and hormones in the vagina.* New York: North Holland Publishing Co., 1978.
6. Richardson JL, Illum L. Routes of delivery: case studies. The vaginal route of peptide and protein drug delivery. *Adv. Drug Deliv. Rev.* 1992;8:341-366.
7. Mizutani T, Nishiyama S, Amakawa I, Watanabe A, Nakamuro K, Terada N. Danazol concentra-tions in ovary, uterus, and serum and their effect on the hypothalamic-pituitary-ovarian axis during vaginal administration of a danazol suppository. *Fertil. and Steril.* 1995;63:1184-1189.
8. Kullander S, Svanberg X. On resorption and the effects of vaginally administered terbutaline in women with premature labour. *Acta Obstet. Gynecol. Scand.* 1985;64:613-616.
9. Bulletti C, De Ziegler D, Giacomucci E, Polli V, Rossi S, Alfieri S, Vaginal drug delivery: the first uterine pass effect. *Ann. N. Y. Acad. Sci.* 1997;828:285-290.
10. Richardson JL, Illum L. The vaginal route of peptide and protein drug delivery. *Adv. Drug Deliv Rev.* 1992;8:341-366.
11. Durrani MJ, Kusai A, Ho NFH. Topical vaginal drug delivery in the guinea pig. I. Effect of estrous cycle on the vaginal membrane permeability of vidarabine. *Int. J. Pharmaceut.* 1985;24:209-218.
12. Bassol S, Recio R, de la Cruz DL. Comparative trial between two soft jelly capsules containing Nonoxynol as spermicidal contraceptives. *Contraception* 1989;39:409-418.
13. Ahmad M, Asch RH. Study of the intravaginal insert (IVI): Acceptability, side effects, and post-coital spermicidal activity. *Acta Europaea Fertilitatis* 1984;15:369-376.

14. Faich G, Pearson K, Fleming D. Toxic shock syndrome and the vaginal contraceptive sponge. *J. Am. Med. Assoc.* 1986;255:216-218.

15. Amkraut A, Eckenhoff JB, Nichols K. Osmotic delivery of peptides and macromolecules. *Adv. Drug Deliv. Rev.* 1989;4:255-276.

16. Ayton RA, Darling GM, Murkies AL, Farrell EA, Weisberg E, Selinus I. A comparative study of safety and efficacy of continuous low dose oestradiol released from a vaginal ring compared with conjugated equine oestrogen vaginal cream in the treatment of postmenopausal urogenital atrophy. *Br. J. Obstetr. Gynaecol.* 1996;103:351-358.

17. Knuth K, Amiji M, Robinson JR. Hydrogel delivery systems for vaginal and oral applications. formulation and biological considerations. *Adv. Drug Deliv. Rev.* 1993;11:137-167.

18. Gelfand MM, Wendman E. Treating vaginal dryness in breast cancer patients: Results of applying a polycarbophil moisturizing gel. *J. Women's Health* 1994;3:427-434.

19. Robinson JR, Bologna WJ. Vaginal and reproductive system treatments using a bioadhesive polymer. *J. Cont. Rel.* 1994;28:87-94.

20. Richter R. Ein Mittel zur Verhutung der Konzeption (A means of preventing pregnancy). *Dtsch. Med. Wochenschr.* 1909;35:1525-1527.

21. Graefenberg AE. An intrauterine contraceptive method. *In: The practice of contraception.* Proc. 7th Int. Birth control conference, Zurich, Switzerland, Sept 1930, Williams and Wilkins, Baltimore 1930:33-47.

22. Golomb G, Shaked I, Hoffman A. Intrauterine administration of peptide drugs for systemic effect. *Adv. Drug Deliv. Rev.* 1995;17:179-190.

Glossary

A

α **-amylase** Enzymes which hydrolyses starch. α-amylases found in animals, ß-amylases found in plants.

α **-fucosidase** Enzyme which metabolises fucose, a mucopolysaccharide present in blood group substances and human milk.

α **-galactosidase** Enzyme which catalyses the metabolism of galactosides.

Acetazolamide Carbonic anhydrase inhibitor. Used as an anti-epileptic and to treat glaucoma. Has antidiuretic properties.

Acetominophen Also known as Paracetamol.

Acetylsalicylic acid Also known as Aspirin.

Achalasia Failure of muscles to react. Often refers to discordant oesophageal peristalsis leading to swallowing disorders.

Achlorhydria Absence of hydrochloric acid in the lumen of the stomach.

Acid phosphatase One of a group of enzymes which catalyse the hydrolysis of phosphoric acid esters. Acid phosphatase has an optimum pH of between 4.0 and 5.4. Present in kidney, serum, semen and prostate gland. It is associated with resorption of bone and teeth.

Acute myeloid leukaemia Malignant disease of leucopoietic tissue i.e. tissue which produces white blood cells.

Adrenocorticosteroids. A group of hormones secreted by the adrenal cortex. See also steroids.

Aerosol A dispersion of solid or liquid particles in a gas stream.

Air embolism A bubble or bolus of gas in the bloodstream. A sufficiently large embolism can be fatal.

Albumin One of the major serum proteins.

Albuterol See salbutamol.

Aldehyde dehydrogenase This enzyme catalyses the conversion of primary aldehydes to the corresponding carboxylic acid.

Aldolase Enzyme present in skeletal and heart muscle and liver. Converts glycogen to lactic acid.

Aldosterone Mineralocorticoid hormone secreted by the adrenal cortex. Regulates metabolism of sodium, chloride and potassium.

Alizapride A prokinetic agent. Synchronises and accelerated disturbed motility of the gut.

Alkaline phosphatase Phosphatase with an optimum pH of 9. Its function is in the mineralization of bone.

Alkaline tide Occurrence of alkaline urine during gastric digestion.

Alkanes Any saturated aliphatic hydrocarbon with the general formula C_nH_{2n+2}. Also called paraffins.

Alveolar-capillary membrane The one cell thick membrane through which gaseous exchange occurs in the lung.

Alzheimers disease A chronic, organic mental disorder characterised by presenile dementia.

Amberlite resin Trade name for a series of polyelectrolyte ion-exchange resins widely used for chromatography.

Amenorrhoea Absence or suppression of menstruation.

Aminophylline A mixture of theophylline and ethylenediamine used in acute asthma.

Aminosalicyclic acid An anti-tuberculosis drug.

Amitryptiline An antidepressant drug.

Amoxycillin A semi-synthetic penicillin.

Amylase A class of enzymes that split or hydrolyse starch.

Amylopectin The insoluble component of starch.

Amylose A groups of carbohydrates that includes starch cellulose and dextrin.

Anaerobes Able to live without oxygen.

Anaesthetics Drugs which reduce or eliminate certain sensory functions.

Angina pectoris Severe pain and a sensation of constriction of the heart. Caused by deficiency of oxygen to heart muscle.

Angiotensin A vasopressin substance produced when renin is released from the kidney.

Anorexia nervosa Psychiatric disorder with a fear of becoming obese. Weight loss may be extreme.

Anthracene An aromatic molecule consisting of 3 fused benzene rings. It is strongly carcinogenic.

Anthraquinones A class of laxative agents.

Anti-reflux agents Agents which react with gastric acid to form a floating foam on the gastric contents. These suppress gastro-oesophageal reflux.

Antibiotics A variety of natural and synthetic substances which destroy microorganisms.

Anticonvulsants An agent which prevents or relieves convulsions.

Antiemetics Agent which relieves or prevents nausea and vomiting.

Antigens A protein marker on the surface of a cell which identifies type of cell and whether it is "self" or "non-self".

Antihistamines Agents which oppose the effect of histamine.

Antihypertensives Agents which control or reduce high blood pressure.

Antimicrobials Destructive to or preventing the development of microorgamisms.

Antipyrine An analgesic and antipyretic drug.

Antisense oligonucleotide An oligonucleotide complementary to a specific gene sequence which binds to mRNA and prevents transcription.

Antivirals Opposing the actions of a virus.

Appendices epiploicae Pouches of peritoneum. Filled with fat and attached to the colon.

Appendix A short blind pouch arising near the junction of the small and large intestines.

Aqueous humor Transparent liquid contained in the anterior and posterior chambers of the eye.

Arachidonic acid An essential fatty acid formed from unsaturated acids of plants. It is a precursor of prostaglandins.

Arachis oil Ground-nut or peanut oil. Used as a faecal softener.

Areolar relating to the areola, which is a small space or cavity in tissue. Areolar tissue – loose connective tissue which occupies the interspaces of the body.

Aspirin Acetylsalicylic acid. A derivative of salicylic acid. A widely used analgesic and antipyretic.

Asthma Disease which causes increased responses of the tracheobronchial tree to various substances. The result is constriction of the airways.

Atopy Genetic predisposition to hypersensitivity or allergic reaction. Hayfever and asthma are common inherited allergies.

Atropine Alkaloid obtained from bella donna. It is a parasympathetic agent.

Auerbach plexus A plexus of sympathetic nerve fibres located between the circular and longitudinal layers of the stomach and small intestine.

Azelastine Topical preparations of an antihistamine used to treat seasonal allergic conjunctivitis.

B

ß-blockers Also known as ß-adrenoceptor blocking drugs. Agents which act on sympathetic nerves to block the action of adenaline and noradrenaline.

ß-cyclodextrins see Cyclodextrins.

ß-glucosidase An enzyme that catalyses the hydrolysis of a glucoside.

ß-glucuronidase An enzyme that splits glycosidic linkages in glucuronides.

B cells Lymphoid stem cels from the bone marrow which migrate to and become antigen specific cells in the spleen and lymph nodes.

B lymphocytes Cells which identify foreign antigens and can differentiate into antibody producing plasma cells or memory cells.

Bacteroid Resembling bacteria.

Bartholin's glands A small compound mucous gland situated one in each lateral wall of the vestibule of the vagina.

Basal lamina Bottom most layers of cells of a membrane. Gives structural integrity.

Basement membrane See Basal lamina.

Bauhin's valve Ileocaecal valve.

Beclomethasone A corticosteroid drug.

Benzalkonium chloride An antibacterial preservative.

Benzocaine A local anaesthetic used topically.

Benzoic acid Compound used in keratolytic ointments.

Betaxolol A ß-blocking drug.

Bethanechol Cholinergic drug used to treat paralytic ileus and urinary retention not caused by organic disease.

Bidisomide A sodium channel blocker used as a cardiovascular anti-arrhythmic.

Bifidobacterium A soil-borne bacterium commonly colonizing the gastrointestinal tract.

Bile A secretion of the liver. A thick viscid fluid that has a bitter taste. Used to emulsify dietary fats and oils prior to absorption.

Bioadhesion Adhesion of a substance to a biological substrate.

Bladder A membranous sac or receptacle for secretions.

Bleomycin Any one of a group of antitumour agents produced by *Streptomyces verticillus.*

Blood-brain barrier A barrier membrane between circulating blood and the brain preventing damaging substances from reaching the brain and cerebrospinal fluid.

Bowman's membrane Membrane separating corneal epithelium from corneal substance.

Bromisoval (Bromisovalum) A sedative and hypnotic drug

Bronchiectasis Chronic dilatation of a bronchus or bronchi.

Bronchitis Inflammation of mucous membrane of the bronchial tubes.

Brunner's glands Compound gland of the duodenum and upper jejunum. They secrete a clear alkaline mucinous fluid.

Budesonide Corticosteroid used to treat asthma.

Bulimia nervosa Disorder which is characterised by binge eating and vomiting to control weight.

Buprenorphine Opioid with both agonist and antagonist properties. Used as an adjunct in opioid dependence, premedication and analgesia.

Buserelin Gonadorelin analogue used to treat prostate cancer.

Butorphanol Anti-migraine drug.

C

Caffeine Alkaloid present in tea, coffee, chocolate and other food and over the counter medications. Actions include stimulation of the central nervous system, decreases total sleep time and increases gastric acid production.

Calcitonin Hormone released from the thyroid gland and important in bone formation and calcium metabolism.

Calcium Metallic element which must be carried in solution by the blood in order to be available for bone growth and metabolism. It is also of great importance in blood coagulation.

Calcium channel blockers A group of drugs which slow the influx of calcium into a cell. Used to treat angina, hypertension and supraventricular tachycardia.

Calveolated cells. See tuft cells

Candida A genus of yeastlike fungi which is part of the normal flora of the mouth, skin, intestinal tract and vagina. One of the most common causes of vaginitis in women of reproductive age.

Carbamazepine Drug used to treat temporal lobe epilepsy.

Carbohydrates A group of chemicals which include sugars, glycogen, starches, dextrins and celluloses that contain only carbon, oxygen and hydrogen. Basic source of energy for the body.

Carbomers Synthetic high molecular weight polymers of acrylic acid cross-linked with either allyl ethers of sucrose or allyl ethers of pentaerithrityl. Used to treat dry eye.

Carbon dioxide Colourless gas expelled from the lungs. It is the final metabolic product of carbon compounds present in food.

Carbonic anhydrase Enzyme which catalyses the union of water and carbon dioxide to form carbonic acid or reverses the action. Present in red blood cells.

Carbonic anhydrase inhibitors Inhibitor of the carbonic anhydrase enzyme used to treat glaucoma.

Carbopol Trade name for a series of poly-(acrylic acid) polymers used as bioadhesives due to their polyelectrolyte properties.

Carboxylesterase Any enzyme which hydrolylses an ester at the carboxyl linkage.

Carboxymethylcellulose A chemically modified cellulose polymer used as a thickening agent and rheological modifier in many formulations.

Carbromal Very little used sedative-hypnotic drug.

Caries Gradual decay and disintegration of soft or bony tissue or tooth.

Carteolol A ß-blocker used as a eye drop to reduce intra-ocular pressure.

Castor oil Oil expressed from the plant *Ricinus communis*. Used externally as an emollient and internally as a cathartic.

Cells of Cajal Located in oesophagus. Precise function not known.

Cellulose A structural polysaccharide abundant in plants

Cellulose acetate phthalate An acid-insoluble polymer used for enteric coatings

Cementum Thin layer of calcified tissue formed by cementoblasts which covers the tooth root.

Ceramides Class of lipids which do not contain glycerol.

Cerebrospinal fluid A water cushion which protects the brain and spinal cord from impact.

Cervix Neck or part of an organ resembling a neck.

Charcoal Soft powder prepared from soft charred wood.

Chewing gum A substance made for chewing such as polyvinyl acetate. Drugs may be delivered in this form.

Chief cells Cells which line the gastric glands and secrete pepsinogen.

Chitosan A biopolymer derived from chitin, a major component of animal exoskeletons.

Chloramphenicol An broad-spectrum antibiotic originally isolated from *Streptomyces venezuelae*, but is not made synthetically.

Chlorhexidine A topical anti-infective agent.

Chlormadinone acetate Orally active progestin.

Chlorobutol Pharmaceutical preservative.

Chlorofluorocarbon (CFC) A volatile liquid or gas used as an aerosol propellant, now banned due to its environmental ozone-damaging properties. Medical devices have exemption from the ban but CFC's are rapidly being replaced in most formulations.

Cholecystokinin Also known as cholecystokinin-pancreozymin. A hormone secreted intio the blood by the mucosa of the upper intestine. Stimulates gall bladder contraction.

Cholera An acute infection which involves the entire small bowel. It is characterised by a watery diarrhoea and vomiting resulting in acute dehydration.

Cholesterol A sterol widely distributed in animal tissues. It can be synthesised in the liver and it is a normal constituent of bile.

Cholinergic agonists These have their action on autonomic effector cells innervated by post-ganglionic parasympathetic nerves.

Chondroitin Polysaccharide present in connective tissue.

Choroid plexi Network of blood vessels between the sclera and retina.

Chylomicrons Small globule of fat in the fat after digestion and absorption.

Chyme Food which has been processed by the stomach. The particle size is reduced, it is hydrated and optimised for delivery to the small intestine where it can be absorbed.

Chymotrypsin A proteolytic enzyme present in the intestine. Hydrolyses proteins.

Ciliogenesis Formation of cilia.

Cilioinhibition Inhibiting the movement of cilia.

Ciliotoxicity Toxic to cilia, influencing or stopping the ciliary beat.

Cimetidine One of the first H receptor antagonists, for several years the world's no. 1 selling drug. Used to reduce gastric acid production.

Cinnarizine Antihistamine used to treat vertigo and nausea associated with Ménière's disease and middle ear surgery.

Citrate Anion of the tribasic citric acid, commonly found in fruit juice, and part of the citric acid cycle, a major energy-utilizing metabolic pathway.

Clara cells Secreting cells in the surface epithelia of bronchioles.

Clonazepam An anticonvulsant drug.

Clonidine An antihypertensive drug.

Codeine An alkaloid analgesic obtained from opium. Methylmorphine.

Collagen The predominant structural protein in animals.

Colloidal delivery The use of colloidal particles as drug delivery systems.

Colloid A small particle, generally smaller than 1 micrometre in size.

Conjunctiva mucus membrane that lines eyelids and is refelected onto the eyeball.

Connective tissue Noncellular tissue composed of fibrous proteins having a structural role in many organs.

Constipation Difficult defaecation. Infrequent defaecation with hard dry faecal matter.

Corticosteroids See steroids.

Cotransport A transport process for a molecule which depends on the simultaneous transport of another molecule.

Creams Viscous emulsions used to retain and deliver topically applied drugs. Despite their ubiquitous nature the structure of many creams is poorly understood.

Crohn's disease Regional inflammation of the ileum (ileitis).

Crypt Small sac or cavity extending into an epithelial surface or a tubular gland particularly those found in the intestine.

Crypts of Lieberkühn A tubular gland in the intestine which secretes intestinal fluid. Its wall is composed of columnar epithelium with aneth cells at the base. The crypts open between the bases of the villi.

Crystal suspension A suspension of crystalline drug in a vehicle, usually oil, often used for intramuscular delivery.

Cryptococcus A genus of pathogenic yeastlike fungi.

Cushing's syndrome Condition resulting from hypersecretion of pituitary corticosteroids, or from prolonged administration of adrenocortical hormones. Symptoms include adiposity, fatigue, impotence, skin discolouration and excess hair growth.

Cyanoacrylate microspheres Colloidal (q.v.) microspheres made from cyanoacrylate polymers. This material has the advantage of being degraded by esterases *in vivo*, thus forming a biodegradable colloid.

Cyclacillin A semisynthetic penicillin antibiotic.

Cyclic AMP A cyclic nucleotide participating in the activities of many hormones.

Cyclodextrins Cyclic polysaccharides with a tubular cylindrical structure which can enclose and solubilize a small hydrophobic molecule in their interior.

Cyclosporin A An immunosuppressive agent derived from a micro-organism.

Cystic fibrosis An inherited disease affecting exocrine glands. It is characterised by chronic respiratory infection, pancreatic insufficiency and increased electrolytes in sweat.

Cystic fibrosis transmembrane conductance regulator The apical or luminal membrane of crypt epithelial cells contain a cyclic AMP-dependent chloride channel known also as the cystic fibrosis transmembrane conductance regulator or CFTR because mutations in the gene for this ion channel result in the disease cystic fibrosis.

Cytosis the uptake of materials outside the cell by invagination and enclosure of a portion of the cell membrane.

Cytosol the aqueous liquid medium inside the cell, excluding the organelles.

D

Danazol Drug which inhibits pituitary gonadotrophins.

Decongestant sprays Nasal aerosols which unblock the congested nasal airways.

Decylmethyl sulphoxide A powerful hydrophobic solvent used as a transdermal penetration enhancer.

Defaecation The expulsion of faeces.

Deltoid muscle Triangular muscle which covers the shoulder.

Deoxycorticosterone A hormone from the adrenal gland which controls salt and water metabolism.

Dermis The inner layer of the skin, lying beneath the epidermis.

Descemet's membrane A fine membrane which lies between the endothelial layer of the cornea and the substantia propria.

Desmopressin A synthetic vasopressin analogue used as an antidiuretic.

Desmosomes Small spot-like structures joining adjacent cells.

Dexamethasone A synthetic glucocorticoid drug.

Dextran A polysaccharide used as a viscosity enhancer, and as a hydrophilic macromolecular marker.

Dextropropoxyphene Propoxyphene - an analgesic which can cause addition.

Diabetes insipidus Disease caused by insufficient secretion of vasopressin. Characterised by excessive thirst and urine production.

Diabetes mellitus A chronic disorder of carbohydrate metabolism. There are two-types, insulin dependant and non-insulin dependant diabetes.

Diarrhoea Liquid or watery faeces, often caused by lower gastrointestinal disturbances.

Diazepam Anti-anxiety and sedative drug, Trade name is Valium.

Diazoxide Drug used in treating hypertension emergencies.

Dichlorodiphenyltrichloroethane (DDT) An early insecticide, now ubiquitous throughout the animal and plant kingdom due to overuse.

Diclofenac Non-steroidal anti-inflammatory drug used to treat pain and inflammation in rheumatic disease.

Diffusion coefficient Constant of proportionality in Fick's law, a measure of the speed with which a molecule diffuses in a specified environment.

Diflunisal Non-steroidal anti-inflammatory drug used to treat pain and inflammation in rheumatic disease.

Digoxin A cardiac glycoside derived from the foxglove.

Dimethyl sulphoxide A powerful hydrophobic solvent used as a transdermal penetration enhancer.

Dipalmitoyl lecithin A phospholipid in which both acyl chains are derived from palmitic acid.

Disaccharides Small carbohydrates formed by linking two simple sugar molecules, the best-known example being sucrose.

Disodium cromoglycate Sodium cromoglycate. Mast cell stabilizer used to treat asthma, food allergies and allergic rhinitis.

Disopyramide Drug used to treat ventricular arrhythmia.

DNA Deoxyribonucleic acid, the nuclear component carrying the genetic code.

Domperidone An anti-nausea drug.

Dopamine A catecholamine synthesized by the adrenal gland It is the the precursor of noradrenaline. Also a neurotransmitter or brain messenger.

Dorzolamide A carbonic anhydrase inhibitor used in the treatment of glaucoma.

Doxycycline A broad-spectrum tetracycline antibiotic.

Duodenal receptors Receptors located in the duodenum, sensing the calorific load delivered to the small intestine.

Duodenogastric reflux Reflux of duodenal contents (often containing bile) into the stomach.

Duodenum The short length of gastrointestinal tract situated between the lower gastric pylorus and the small intestine.

Dyspepsia Vague term applied to a variety of upper gastrointestinal symptoms, often associated with food consumption and acid secretion.

E

Eccrine sweat glands Gland distributed over the entire skin surface which secrete sweat and are essential for regulation of body temperature.

EDTA Ethylene diaminetetracetic acid. A powerful chelating agent which binds many metal cations

Eicosanoids All of the products of metabolism of arachidonic acid.

Elastin An extracellular connective tissue protein that is principal component of elastic fibres.

Electroosmosis The movement of solvent to balance the osmotic pressure due to movement of ions in an electric field.

Electropermeabilization See electroporation.

Electroporation The permabilization of cell membranes by brief high voltage electric pulses.

Embolism A blockage in a blood vessel caused by a solid particle, gas bubble, blood clot, or oil droplet.

Emphysema A chronic pulmonary disease characterised increase in the size of air spaces and destructive changes to the wall.

Emulsions Codispersions of two immiscible liquids, normally requiring an emulsifier to remain stable.

Endocrine An internal secretion. Endocrine gland secretes directly into the bloodstream.

Endocytosis Ingestion of foreign substances by a cell.

Endometriosis Ectopic endometrium located in various sites throughout the pelvis or in the abdominal wall. It causes pelvic pain and can cause infertility.

Endometrium Mucous membrane lining the inner surface of the uterus.

Endoscopy The use of a viewing device such as a miniature camera or fibre optic probe to view inside the body.

Endotoxins Bacterial toxin confined within the body of a bacterium and is released only when the bacterium is broken down.

Enprofylline A phosphodiesterase inhibitor of the xanthine type

Enterocele Hernia of the intestine through the vagina or posterior vaginal hernia.

Enterocytes Intestinal cell.

Enteroglucagon Hormone release from the small intestinal endocrine cells.

Enterohepatic recirculation Bile acids are poorly absorbed in the proximal small intestine, but are absorbed by an active process in the terminal ileum. After absorption, bile acids have a high hepatic clearance and are re-secreted in the bile.

Enterokinase Previous term used for enteropeptidase.

Enteropeptidase Enzyme occurring in the mucosa of the duodenum essential for the activation of the trypsinogen to trypsin.

Enuresis Involuntary discharge of urine.

Eosinophilia Presence of an unusual number of eosinophils in the blood.

Ephelides Freckles.

Epidermis The outer layer of skin cells.

Epimysium Outermost sheath of connective tissue that surrounds a skeletal muscle.

Ergotamine tartate A alkaloid derived from ergot. Stimulates smooth muscle of blood vessels and the uterus inducing vasoconstriction and uterine contractions.

Erythema Redness of the skin.

Erythrocyte ghost The cell membrane of an erythrocyte emptied of its intracellular contents.

Erythromycin An antibiotic from *Streptomyces erythreus*. It is active against many gram positive and some gram negative bacteria.

Erythropoeitin A hormone which stimulates red blood cell production.

Escherichia coli One of the most common faecal bacteria .

Esterase An enzyme which degrades an ester, usually into an alcohol and a carboxylic acid.

Esters Compounds formed by reaction between an alcohol and a carboxylic acid.

Ethinylestradiol Synthetic oesotrogen.

Ethmoid bone Spongy bonewhich forms the roof of the nasal fossae.

Ethyl oleate An oil commonly used as a pharmaceutical excipient.

Ethylcellulose A chemically modified cellulose used as a pharmaceutical excipient.

Ethylenediaminepentaacetic acid A powerful chelating agent which binds many metal cations.

Eudragit Trade name for a series of wax-based pharmaceutical excipients.

Extravasation The escape of fluids into the surrounding tissue.

F

Faraday crispations Fluctuations in the surface of a liquid induced by ultrasound, leading to the production of aerosol droplets.

Fatty acids Carboxylic acid derivatives of higher alkanes, generally 4-24 carbon atoms long, often unsaturated.

Fenoterol Adrenoceptor stimulant used to treat reversible airways construction.

Ferrireductase A cytochrome P450 reductase which

converts ferric to ferrous iron.

Fibrinogen A protein present in the blood plasma essential for clotting.

Fibronectin A group of proteins present in blood plasma and extracellular matrix.

Fick's law Fundamental relation between diffusion rate and concentration gradient.

First-pass metabolism Blood from the small intestine goes directly to the liver where nutrients and some drugs are metabolised substantially. This can result in the loss of a large proportion of active drug before it can reach its target site.

Flunisolide Corticosteroid used in the prophylaxis and treatment of allergic rhinitis.

Fluorescein Strongly fluorescent dye often used as a biochemical marker.

Fluorocarbons Organic molecules in which a substantial fraction of the hydrogen atoms have been replaced by fluorine. If all the hydrogen has been replaced they are termed perfluorocarbons. These molecules dissolve substantial amounts of respiratory gases and have been widely studied for the formulation of blood substitutes.

Folds of kerckring Folding of the epithelium to increase surface area.

Formaldehyde The simplest aliphatic aldehyde, CH_2O, used as a preservative. It denatures proteins and is highly toxic.

Foveola A minute pit of depression.

Frenulum linguae Fold of mucous membrane which runs from the floor of the mouth to the inferior surface of the tongue.

Fundus The larger part, base or body of a hollow organ or the portion of the organ furthest from the opening. The fundus of the stomach is closest to the oesophagus.

G

GALT See gut-associated lymphoid tissue.

Gamma scintigraphy The use of gamma emitting radionuclides to study behaviour of drug formulations within the body for research. It is s routine technique in nuclear medicine for diagnosis. Requires a gamma camera.

Ganciclovir Antiviral drug.

Gastric glands cardiac, fundic or oxyntic and pyloric glands of the stomach.

Gastric inhibitory peptide (GIP) A polypeptide in the cells of the duodenum and jejunum which acts to inhibit secretion of gastric acid.

Gastrin A hormone secreted by the pyloric area of the stomach and duodenum to stimulate gastric secretion.

Gastritis Inflammation of the stomach.

Gastro-oesophageal junction Region where the stomach and oesophagus meet. Gastric tissue lines the first few centimetres of the oesophagus to protect it from acid damage.

Gastro-oesophageal reflux Reflux of gastric contents into the oesophagus where it can cause oesophagitis. Causes the classic symptom of "heartburn".

Gastrocolic reflex Peristaltic wave in the colon initiated by the intake of food into the stomach.

Gelatinase Enzyme which breaks down gelatin.

Gellan gum A polysaccharide used as a rheological modifier in pharmacy and as a food additive.

Gelling polymers Polymers which form gels in solution.

Gels Solutions which have become rigid due to a linked polymer network.

Gentamicin Aminoglycoside used in the treatment of serious infection.

Giant unilamellar vesicles Large (several micrometres) single-layered liposomes.

Gingiva The gum and tissue that surrounds the neck of the teeth.

Gingivitis Inflammation of the gums.

Glands of Kraus Small glands in the conjunctiva of the eyelids.

Glands of Manz Small glands which secrete the mucoid layer or tears.

Glands of Wolfring Produces the watery lacrimal secretion of tears.

Glands of Zeis Large sebaceous glands found in the eyelids.

Glaucoma Elevation of intraocular pressure.

Globulin One of a group of Simple proteins insoluble in water but soluble in neutral solutions of salts and strong acids.

Glucagon Polypeptide hormone which increases the concentration of glucose in the blood.

Glucocorticoids A general classification of hormones produced by the adrenal cortex and are primarily active in protecting against stress.

Glucose-6-phosphate dehydrogenase (G-6-PD) An enzyme which dehydrogenates glucose-6-phosphate to form 6-phopshoglucon. This is the initial step in the pentose phosphate pathway of glucose catabolism.

Glucuronic acid Important acid in human metabolism by virtue of its detoxifying action.

Glucuronosyltransferases Liver enzymes responsible for blucuronidation of xenobiotics.

Glutamine The monoamide of aminoglutaric acid. It is present in the juices of many plants and is essential in the hydrolysis of proteins.

Glutamic oxaloacetic transaminase A metabolic enzyme found in liver and heart tissue which is released into the bloodstream by tissue damage, and hence used as a therapeutic indicator.

Glutamic pyruvic transaminase see glutamic oxaloacetic transaminase.

Glutathione A tripeptideof glutamic acid, cysteine and glycine. Important in cellular respiration.

Glycerol A simple polyhydric alcohol, propane 1,2,3-triol.

Glyceryl trinitrate. See nitroglycerin.

Glycine The simplest amino-acid.

Glycocalyx A thin layer of glycoprotein and polysaccharide which covers the surface of some cells such as muscle.

Glycofurol A polar solvent used mainly in cosmetics and creams.

Glycogen A polysaccharide commonly called animal starch. The conversion of glycogen to glucose is called glycogenolysis. Glycogen is the form by which carbohydrate is stored in the body.

Glycolipids Lipids with an attached sugar molecule.

Glycoprotein A protein with an attached polysaccharide chain, often membrane-resident and conferring antigenic properties.

Glycosaminoglycan A mucopolysaccharide found in cell walls and mucus.

Goblet cells Secretes mucus in the gastrointestinal and respiratory tracts.

Gradient-charged system A controlled release system in which the concentration of drug varies throughout its thickness in order to achieve a specified release profile.

Gramicidin D An antibiotic.

Greenhouse gases Gases which absorb solar infrared radiation, causing an elevation in the Earth's temperature.

Griseofulvin An antifungal agent. It's poor water solubility led to its being used as a model drug for a wide range of formulation studies.

Guar gum A plant polysaccharide used as a viscosity modifier, pharmaceutical excipient, and food additive.

Guinea pig Small furry animal so widely used for experimental studies that it has given its name idiomatically to anyone or anything who is the subject of a novel experiment or trial.

Gut associated lymphoid tissue (GALT) term applied to all lymphoid tissue associated with the gastrointestinal tract incluuding tonsils, appendix and Payer's patches. It is responsible for controlling the entry of organisms via the gastrointestinal tract.

H

H⁺/K⁺ ATPase The active transporter system responsible for pumping acid (H^+) into the gastric lumen.

H₁ receptors Histamine receptors found in the cells of the bronchiole muscle.

H₂ receptors Histamine receptors found in the cells that secrete gastric acid.

Haemoglobin The mammalian oxygen transport protein located in the erythrocytes.

Haemolysis Disintegration of red blood cells with the release of haemoglobin.

Haemorrhoidal plexus The network of blood vessels surrounding the anal canal.

Haustra Sacculated pouches of the colon.

Hayfever Hypersensitivity of the eye and upper respiratory tract to inhaled pollens.

Heartburn See gastro-oesophageal reflux.

Helicobacter pylori An organism which lives beneath the mucus layer in the stomach and is associated with gastritis.

HEMA See hydroxyethyl methacrylate.

Hemidesmosomes See desmosomes.

Heparin A polysaccharide which inhibits blood coagulation.

Hepatic flexure The junction of the ascending and transverse colon.

Hepatic portal vein See also first pass metabolism. Only main vein in the body which does not go directly to the heart. It links the gastrointestinal tract to the liver.

Hexose transporter system An active transport system which transfers hexoses across the cell membrane.

HFAs See hydrofluoroalkanes.

Histamine A substance produced from the amino acid histidine. It is released from injured cells. Histamine increases gastric secretion, dilatation of capillaries and contraction of bronchial smooth muscle.

Histidine An amino acid obtained by hydrolysis from tissue proteins, necessary for tissue repair and growth.

Histiocytes A macrophage present in all loose connective tissue.

HIV infection Human immunodeficiency virus also known as AIDS (acquired immune deficiency syndrome).

Horseradish peroxidase Used to study aqueous pathways between cells.

Housekeeper contractions See migrating myoelectric complex.

Humidification saturation of air with water, esp. in the nose, so that the airflow does not dehydrate deeper tissues

Hyaluronic acid An acid mucopolysaccharide found in the ground sustance of connective tissue that acts as a binding and protective agent. Also found in the synovial fluid and aqueous and vitrous humors.

Hyaluronidase Enzyme found in the testes and is present in the semen. It depolymerises hyaluronic acid and acts to disperse cells of the ovum thus facilitating entry of sperm.

Hydrochloric acid HCl, the acid secreted in the stomach.

Hydrochlorthiazide A diuretic.

Hydrocortisone A corticosteroid hormone produced by the adrenal cortex.

Hydrocyanic acid HCN, the acid from which cyanides are derived.

Hydrodynamically balanced system A drug delivery device designed to have the same density as the gastric contents.

Hydrofluoroalkanes Alkanes in which a number of hydrogen atoms have been replaced by fluorine, replacing chlorofluorocarbons as aerosol propellants since they do not damage the ozone layer.

Hydrogels Hydrophilic gels fomed from a range of polymers, esp. polyions such as hydroxyethyl methacrylate.

Hydrogen sulphide H₂S, a toxic and malodorous gas commonly formed during digestion of sulphur-containing foods.

Hydrolases An enzyme that causes hydrolysis.

Hydroxyethyl methacrylate A hydrophilic gel-forming polymer.

Hydroxyethylcellulose A chemically modified cellulose used as a pharmaceutical excipient.

Hydroxyproline An amino-acid.

Hydroxypropylcellulose A chemically modified cellulose used as a pharmaceutical excipient.

Hydroxypropylmethylcellulose A chemically modified cellulose used as a pharmaceutical excipient.

5-Hydroxytryptamine See Serotonin.

Hypogonadism Excessive secretions of the sex glands.

I

IgA See Immunoglobulins.

IgG See Immunoglobulins.

Ileocaecal junction Junction between the small intestine and ascending colon.

Iliac fossa One of the concavities of the iliac bones of the pelvis.

Immunoglobulins One of a family of closely related proteins capable of acting as antibodies.

Impotence Absence of sexual power.

Indomethacin Anti-inflammatory drug used extensively to treat rheumatoid arthritis.

Infertility Inability of reduced ability to have children.

Inflammatory bowel disease Associated with pain, constipation or diarrhoea.

Insulin A hormone secreted by the islets of Langerhans of the pancreas. Essential for the metabolism of blood sugar.

Integument A covering or skin.

Interferon A group of proteins released by white blood cells and fibroblasts in response ti viral invasion. They inhibit the production of the virus within infected cells.

Intrinsic factor of Castle A substance present in the gastric juice that makes absorption of vitamin B .

Inulin A polysaccharide found in plants. It is used to study renal function.

Ion exchange resins Polymer resins with numerous ionized sites which can reversibly bind a number of ions; commonly used for separation and purification purposes.

Iontophoresis The process of forcing an ionized drug to pass into a tissue using an electric current.

Ipratropium bromide Anticholinergic drug used to control asthma.

Isomaltase A membrane protein involved in carbohydrate metabolism.

Isoprenaline An inotropic sympathomimetic used to treat heart block and severe bradycardia.

Ispaghula Bulk-forming laxative.

IUDs See intrauterine devices.

J

Jet nebulizer A nebulizer in which a liquid stream is dispersed by a jet of air under high pressure.

K

Kanamycin Aminoglycoside antibiotic now superceded by other aminoglycosides

Keratinocytes Any one of the cells in the skin that synthesize keratin.

Kerkring's folds See Folds of Kerkring.

Ketobemidone An opiate analgesic.

Kupffer cells A variety of macrophage cells found in the liver.

L

L-tryptophan An aromatic amino-acid

Labrafil WL A waxy material used as a pharmaceutical excipient

Lactase An intestinal enzyme which splits lactose into dextrose and galactose.

Lactate dehydrogenase An enzyme which is important in the oxidation of lactate.

Lacteal Pert. To milk or an intestinal lymphatic that takes up chyle and passes it to the lymphatic system.

Lactic acid Formed during muscular activity by the breakdown of glycogen.

Lactic dehydrogenase See Lactate dehydrogenase.

Lactobacillus A genuis of gram positive, nonmotile rod shaped bacteria. They are responsible for the souring of milk as they produce lactic acid from carbohydrates.

Lactobacillus acidophilus Organism which produces lactic acid by fermenting sugars in milk. Found in the faeces of bottle-fed infants and adults. Also present in carious teeth and the human vagina.

Lactose Disaccharide that hydrolyses to yield glucose and galactose.

Lactulose A synthetic disaccharide that is not digested or absorbed in humans. It is metabolised by colonic bacteria.

Lamina cribrosa Cribriform plate of the ethmoid bone.

Lamina propria Thin layer of fibrous connective tissue that lies immediately below the surface epithelium of mucous membranes.

Langerhans Islets of Special cells scattered through the pancreas which secrete insulin.

Langmuir trough An apparatus which allows surface-active molecules to be studied as films on the surface of a liquid.

Lanolin A wax derived from sheep fat used in a number of topical formulations.

Lanthanum A rare-earth element used in colloidal form as a marker.

Laryngectomy Removal of the larynx.

Lateral diffusion Transverse diffusion of a solute in a 2-dimensional system such as a lipid membrane.

Laureth-9 Non-ionic detergent.

LCFA See long-chain fatty acids

Lecithins Generic name for a wide range of natural phospholipids, generally implying a heterogenous mixture of headgroups and acyl chains.

Lectins Plant protein which causes stimulation of lymphocytes to proliferate.

Leucine animopeptidase A proteolytic enzyme present in the pancreas, liver and small intestine.

Leucotrienes A group of arachidonic acid metabolites which function as chemical mediators for inflammation. Leucotrienes C4, D4 and E4 constitutes what was formally known as slow-releasing substance of anaphylaxis (SRS-A).

Leucotriene inhibitors Used in the prophylaxis and treatment of asthma.

Levonorgestrel A steroid hormone used as a contraceptive.

Lidocaine A local anaesthetic.

Limbus The edge or border of a part.

Lipases Enzymes which degrade lipids

Lipids A generic name for a wide variety of fatty materials.

Liposomes hollow vesicular structures formed when phospholipids (lecithins) are dispersed in water. They contain an enclosed aqueous space which can be use to entrap and deliver hydrophilic molecules.

Lithium The smallest alkali metal, used in the treatment of certain mental disorders.

Locust bean gum A plant gum used as a food additive and excipient.

Long-chain fatty acids Fatty acids in which the alkane chain is generally longer than 12-14 carbon atoms.

Loperamide Antimotility drug used to treat diarrhoea.

Lorazepam Benzodiazepine used to treat anxiety, status epilepticus or insomnia.

Lotion Liquid applied to the skin.

Lower oesophageal sphincter Also known as the cardia. Sphincter which is located between the stomach and oesophagus and serves to prevent gastro-oesophageal reflux.

Loxiglumide Highly potent cholecystokinin receptor antagonist. It inhibits postprandial gall bladder contraction and causes accelerated gastric emptying.

Lozenge A drug delivery system designed to dissolve slowly in the mouth.

Lymphocytes Cell present in the blood and lymphatic tissue. These cells travel from the blood the the lymph and back again. They provide the main immune capability of the body.

Lymphoglandula Lymph gland.

Lypressin A posterior pituitary hormone obtained from pigs and used as an antidiuretic.

Lysine An amino-acid.

Lysosome Part of an intracellular digestive system that exists as separate particles in the cell. Inside their limiting membrane they are capable of breaking down and certain carbohydrates.

Lysozyme Enzyme now called muramidase. Found in blood cells.

M

Macrophages They have the ability to recognise and ingest all foreign antigens through receptors on the surface of their cell membranes. 50% of all macrophages are found in the Kupffer cells of the liver.

Malic acid Found is some fruits such as apples. Active in aerobic metabolism of carbohydrates.

Maltase A salivary and pancreatic enzyme that acts on maltose hydrolysing it to glucose.

Maltose A disaccharide present in malt, malt products and sprouting seeds. Maltase hydrolyses it to glucose.

Maltotriose A small carbohydrate produced by the action of salivary Amylase on starch.

Mast cells Cells which are located in the connective tissue just below epithelial surfaces, serous cavities and around blood vessels. They synthesize and store histamine. When stimulated they release all mediators of inflammation including leukotrienes. They produce the signs of hypersensitivity reactions.

Matrix-diffusion controlled system A controlled release device whose release rate is determined by the diffusion rate of the drug through a polymer matrix.

M-Cells these cells are located in the small intestine where they play an important part in the immune system. They lack fully developed microvilli, but are pinocytic and contain many vesicles.

MDR See multi-drug resistance.

Medoxyprogesterone acetate A progestational agent used intramuscularly.

Meibomian glands One of the sebaceous glands between the tarsi and conjunctiva of eyelids.

Meissner plexus Small aggregations of ganglion cells located in the intestinal submucosa.

Menopause Cessation of menstruation which occurs usually between the ages of 35 and 58.

Menthol An alcohol obtained from oil of peppermint or other mint oils. Has antispasmodic and antipruritic properties.

Mercaptans Ony organic chemical that contains the –SH radical. It is formed when the oxygen of an alcohol is replaced by sulphur.

Mesalazine An aminosalicylate used in the treatment of mild to moderate ulcerative colitis.

Mesentery A peritoneal fold circling most of the small intestine holding to the posterior wall.

Metaplasia Conversion of one kind of tissue into a form which is abnormal for that tissue type.

Met-enkephalin Polypeptide produced in the brain. It acts as opiates and produces analgesia by binding to opiate receptor sites involved in pain perception.

Metaproterenol A ß2 adrenergic stimulant.

Metered dose inhalers Used to deliver a controlled amount of drug to the lungs.

Methacrylate copolymer Any copolymer containing repeat methacrylate units. Due to the negative charge on acrylic acid, it is a polyanion.

Methadone A synthetic analgesic drug with potency equal to that of morphine, but the narcotic action is weaker than morphine. It is habit-forming.

Methane An inflammable gas. It is produced as a result of putrefaction and fermentation of organic matter.

Methohexital Very short acting barbiturate. Used in anaesthesia.

Methotrexate A folic acid antagonist. Used for treating acute lymphoblastic leukemia in children, choriocarcinoma and psoriasis.

Methylcellulose Pharmaceutical excipient used as a bulking agent. It also has adhesive or emulsification properties.

Methylene blue An antiseptic dye sometimes used in urinary infections often with hexamine. An intramuscular injection can be used as a renal function test.

Methylmethacrylate The monomer from which

poly(methacrylates) are derived, e.g poly(methyl methacrylate), more commonly called perspex.

Methylmorphine An alternative name for codeine.

Methylxanthines See xanthines.

Metoclopramide A prokinetic agent. Only enhances disordered and not normal motility of the gut.

Metronidazole Drug used to treat infections due to *Trichomonas vaginalis* or *Giardia lamblia* and in treating amoebiasis.

Micelles Aggregates of surfactant molecules in solution.

Microfold cells See M-cells.

Microparticle Any particulate system with a size less than approximately 1 millimetre. The term nanoparticulates is often applied to particles smaller than 1 micrometre.

Microsphere A spherical microparticle.

Midazolam A benzodiazepine used to produce sedation for brief periods e.g. for endoscopy or other diagnostic procedure which involves some discomfort to the patient.

Migraine Paroxysmal attacks of headache. Initially unilateral, accompanied ny disordered vision and gastrointestinal disturbances. Thought to be due to vasodilation of the extracerebral cranial arteries.

Migrating motor complex See Migrating myoelectric complex.

Migrating myoelectric complex Motility of the stomach and small intestine which occurs in the fasted state. Starts out a build up of contractions into the stomach to produce a powerful contraction which sweeps out undigested food. Transit through the small intestine is approximately 2 hours, since absorption of nutrients is not necessary.

Mitomycin An antibiotic with antineoplastic action.

Monozygotic twins Identical twins i.e. both derived from a single fertilized egg.

Montelukast sodium A leucotriene inhibitor used to treat asthma.

Morphine Main alkaloid found in opium. Used as an analgesic and sedative. Addictive.

Motilin Potent autocoid found in the enterochromaffin system, the function of which is not certain.

Mucoadhesion Adhesion to mucous membranes.

Mucoid cells Cells which produce mucoid which is a glycoprotein similar to mucus.

Mucolytics drugs which soften mucus to reduce its viscosity in the respiratory tract.

Mucopolysaccharides Polysaccharides which form chemical bonds with water. They contain hexosamine and sometimes protein. It is a thick gelatinous substance found in many places within the body. It forms intercellular ground substance and the basement membrane of cells. It is in mucous secretions and synovial fluid.

Mucostasis Stopping mucus secretion.

Multi-drug resistance (MDR) Resistance to a wide range of unrelated drugs which occurs after resistance has developed to one drug.

Multilamellar vesicles Vesicles (usually liposomes) with several concentric onion-like layers.

Multiparticulates Dosage forms such as pellets.

Muscle Tissue which is composed of contractile cells or fibres. The ability of the muscle to contract and relax allows the body movement.

Muscularis externa Muscular outer layer of an organ or tubule.

Muscularis mucosae Unstriated muscular tissue layer of the mucous membrane.

Myometrium Muscular wall of the uterus.

N

Na⁺/K⁺ ATPase The membrane protein responsible for maintaining the sodium/potassium imbalance in cells.

NAD⁺-dependent -hydroxyprostaglandin dehydrogenase An enzyme involved in prostanoid synthesis.

NAD⁺-dependent formaldehyde dehydrogenase An enzyme which detoxifies formaldehyde by binding it to glutathione.

Nadolol ß adrenoceptor blocking drug

Nafarelin Gonadorelin analogue used to treat endometriosis, infertility, anaemia due to interuterine fibroids, prostate cancer and before uterine surgery.

Nanoparticle A small particulate in the colloidal size range, generally smaller than 1 micrometre.

Nanosphere A spherical nanoparticle.

Nebulizers A device which converts a liquid into a fine spray. An atomiser.

Neurotensin A 13-amino-acid peptide having a range of hormonal activities.

Neutrophilia Increase in the number of neutrophilic leucocytes in the blood.

Nicotine A poisonous alkaloid found in all parts of the tobacco plant.

Nifedipine Calcium channel blocker used in the prophylaxis of angina and hypertension.

Nitrates A salt of nitric acid. Nitrates are useful for the management of stable angina. Potent vasodilators.

Nitroglycerin used in the prophylaxis and treatment of angina and left ventricular failure.

Non-steroidal anti-inflammatory drugs A group of drugs which have analgesic, anti-inflammatory and anti-pyretic actions. They are similar to aspirin and have been used extensively to treat arthritis, dysmenorrhea and general inflammation.

Non-ulcer dyspepsia Indigestion which is not caused by ulceration.

Nonoxynol-9 A surfactant with antibacterial and cytotoxic properties, commonly used as a spermicide in contraceptive formulations.

Norethindrone Progestogen belived to suppress the gonadotropin production by the pituitary. Used for dysmenorrhea and premenstrual tension

Norgestrel Also known as Levonorgestrel. It is a contraceptive agent released into the uterine cavity via an interuterine device.

NSAIDs See non-steroidal anti-inflammatory drugs.

Nystatin An anti-fungal drug.

O

Oedema Abnormal infiltration of tissues with fluid.

Oestradiol A steroid produced by the ovary.

Oestrogen Any natural or artificial substance that induces oestrogenic activity.

Oil A greasy liquid not miscible with water. Can be mineral vegetable or animal in origin.

Ointments A medicated fatty soft substances for external application to the body. Usually its base is petroleum jelly or lanolin.

Oleic acid A colourless oily liquid prepared from tallow and other fats, the salts of which are oleates.

Oligosaccharides A compound made up of a number of monosaccharide units.

Olsalazine Drug used to treat ulcerative colitis.

Opiates Any drug containing or derived from opium.

Opioids Non-opium derived synthetic narcotics. It may also refer to substances such as endorphins or enkephalins occurring naturally in the body to decrease the sensation of pain.

Osmotic delivery device A drug delivery system in which the release of active component is controlled by the osmotic uptake of solvent from its surroundings.

Osteoporosis Loss of bone density due to excessive absorption of calcium and phosphorous from the bone.

Oxidoreductases An enzyme that catalyses oxidation-reduction reactions.

Oxprenolol A ß adrenergic blocking drug.

Oxyntic cells cells which produce or secrete acid.

Oxyquinolone Alternative name for 8-hydroxyquinoline, and antiseptic and chelating agent.

Oxytocin A pituitary hormone which which stimulates the uterus to contract. Used to induce labour.

P

P-aminoclonidine Used in the prophylaxis of migraine.

P-glycoprotein P-glycoprotein is an ATP-dependent transporter which is capable of transporting an extremely wide variety of drugs out of the cell. P-glycoprotein is expressed in a variety of normal human tissues including the liver, brain, adrenal gland, kidney and intestinal tract epithelia. This suggests a common role as a protective mechanism. In the small intestine it is localised in the apical membranes of the cell, but is not detectable in crypt cells.

Palate Horizontal structure separating the nasal cavity and the roof of the mouth.

Palmitic acid A fatty acid found in palm oil, solid fats and some waxes and many fatty acids.

Paneth cells Large secretory cells containing course granules found at the blind end of the crypts of Lieberkühn in the small intestine.

Paracetamol A non-opioid analgesic used to control mild to moderate pain and pyrexia.

Parietal cells Large cells on the margin of the peptic glands in the stomach.

Partition coefficient The ratio of the concentration of drug in two equilibrated immiscible solvents, usually given the symbol P. The partition coefficient between n-octanol and water is a widely quoted indicator of the hydrophobic nature of a drug. Since partition coefficients vary from below 1 to several thousand, their logarithm to base 10 (Log P) is normally quoted.

Pectins purified carbohydrate obtained from the peel of citrus fruits or apple pulp. It forms a gel when heated with sugar.

Pectoral muscle Chest muscle.

Penbutolol A ß adrenergic blocking drug.

Penetration enhancers Compounds which promote absorption of drugs. Usually their action is non-specific.

Penicillin One of a group of antibiotics biosynthesized by several species of mold.

Pepsin Chief enzyme of gastric juice which converts proteins into proteoses and peptones. It is formed by the chief cells of the gastric glands.

Pepsinogen Pepsin precursor.

Peptides Building blocks of proteins formed from amino acids.

Perfusion Passing of fluid through spaces.

Perimysium Connective tissue sheath which envelops each bundle of muscle fibres.

Periodontal disease Disease of the supporting structures of the teeth.

Periodontitis Inflammation or degeneration or both of the dental periostium, alveolar bone, cementum and adjacent gingiva.

Periodontosis Any degenerative disease of the periodontal tissues.

Peritoneum The serous membrane reflected over the viscera and lining of the abdominal cavity.

Persorption Sloughing off of cells from the tips of villi in the small intestine leaves a gap through which particles can enter the blood stream.

Pessaries drug delivery device or supporting structure inserted into the vagina.

Pethidine Also known as Peridine. Opioid analgesic used for moderate to severe pain.

Petrolatum A purified semisolid mixture of hydrocarbons obtained from petroleum.

Petrolatum based jelly A purified semisolid mixture of hydrocarbons obtained from petroleum which is decolourised and stabilized.

Peyer's patches An aggregation of lymph nodules found chiefly in the ileum near to its junction with the colon. They are circular or oval and about 1 cm wide and 2-3 cm long.

pH Measurement of acidity and alkalinity ranging from 0(acid) to 14 (alkaline). pH 7 is neutral. . Formula is pH=-log[H+]. As the scale is logarithmic, there is a 10 fold difference between each unit.

pH-partition hypothesis The principle that drug passage through a membrane is controlled by the ph of the environment since this controls the ionization of thedrug, which can only be absorbed in its unionized state.

Phagocytosis Ingestion and digestion of bacteria and particles by phagocytes.

Pharmacokinetics Study of the metabolism and

action of drugs with particular emphasis on the time required for absorption, duration of action, distribution in the body and method of excretion.

Phenobarbital A hypnotic drug.long-acting sedative and anti-convulsant.

Phenol red A dye used an a pH indicator.

Phenylalanine An aromatic amino-acid.

Phenylephrine Vasoconstrictor and pressor drug similar to adrenaline, but more stable.

Phlebitis Irritation of a blood vessel.

Phonation Speaking; the act of making a sound.

Phosphatidylcholine (PC) One of the commonest phospholipids, consisting of a glycerol backbone in which the 1- and 2-alcohol groups are esterified to fatty acids, while the 3- alcohol is esterified to a phosphate group. The phosphate is in turn joined to a *headgroup*, which is choline in the case of phosphaticylcholine.

Phosphatidylethanolamine (PE) A phospholipid in which the headgroup is ethanolamine. See phosphatidylycholine.

Phosphatidylinositol (PI) A phospholipid in which the headgroup is inositol. See phosphatidylycholine.

Phosphatidylserine (PS) A phospholipid in which the headgroup is serine. See phosphatidylycholine.

Phosphoglucomutase An enzyme which interconverts glucose-1 phosphate and glucose-6-phosphate.

Phospholipid; stealth A phospholipid carrying an ethylene oxide chain attached to the headgroup, which forms a heavily hydrated outer layer when the phospholipid is formed into liposomes. This reduces the extent which the liposomes are recognised by the reticuloendothelial system.

Pilocarpine Alkaloid which is used to cause contraction of the pupil.

Pituitary hormones Hormones secreted from the pituitary gland which regulate many body processes. These include growth hormone, adrenocorticotropic hormone which regulates functional activity of the adrenal cortex, thyrotropic hormone which regulates activity of the thyroid gland and gonadotrophic hormone amongst others.

Plaque A patch on the skin or on a mucous surface. A blood platelet. Dental plaque is a gummy mass of microorganisms that grows on the crowns and spreads along the roots of teeth. These are the forerunner of caries.

Plasma membrane The outer membrane of the cell, composed of phospholipids, proteins, etc.

Platelets A round or oval disk 2 to 4 µm in diameter found in the blood. They are important for coagulation.

Plicae semilunares Transverse fold of mucosa of the large intestine lying between sacculations.

Pluronic® Trade name for a range of poly(ethylene oxide)-poly(propylene oxide)-poly(ethylene oxide) triblock copolymers widely used in drug formulation and delivery.

pMDI See pressurized metered dose inhalers.

Polyacrylic acid A copolymer of acrylic acid.

Polyalkylene glycols Block copolymers of the form HO-(R-O)-H where R is any alkyl group. Polyethylene glycol and polypropylene glycol are the most commonly encountered.

Polycarbophil Generic name for crosslinked acrylic acid copolymers used as thickening agents and bioadhesives.

Polyethylene One of the earliest polymers, consisting of a long alkyl chain, formed by polymerizing ethylene.

Polyps A tumor with a pedicle. Commonly found in vascular organs such as the nose, uterus and rectum.

Polysaccharides Biopolymers formed from chains of carbohydrate (sugar) molecules.

Polysorbates Complicated surfactants formed by esterifying sorbitol with fatty acids to render it hydrophobic, and conjugating poly(ethylene oxide) to provide hydrophilic groups. Available commercially as the Tween® series of surfactants.

Polyurethane A polymer widely used in medical devices such as catheters.

Polyvinyl alcohol A water soluble polymer made by polymerizing vinyl alcohol, commonly used as a surfactant and viscosity enhancer in drug delivery systems.

Polyvinylpyrrolidone A polymer used as a swelling agent and binder in formulation.

Positron emission tomography (PET) Reconstruction imaging of various organs by using various positron emitting isotopes.

Prazosin A drug used in treating hypertension.

Prednisolone A glucocorticosteroid drug.

Preservatives Compounds added to a formulation to enhance stability. They include antibacterials, antioxidants, and chelating agents.

Pressurized metered dose inhalers Miniature aerosols which use a metering valve to eject a fixed dose of drug for inhalation therapy.

Progesterone A steroid hormone obtained from the corpus luteum and placenta. It is responsible for the changes in the endometrium in the second half of the menstrual cycle.

Progestin A corpus luteum hormone which prepares the endometrium for implantation of the fertilized ovum.

Prolapse A falling or dropping of an organ or internal part e.g. uterus or rectum.

Proline An amino-acid.

Promethazine An anti-histamine.

Propranolol A ß adrenergic blocking drug.

Propylene glycol Propane(1,2 diol), a solvent widely used in the forulation of creams and injectables.

Prostaglandins A large group of biologically active unsaturated fatty acids. They are short range autocoids which have a wide range of actions including lipolysis, fluid balance, platelet aggregation, blood flow, gastrointestinal function, neurotransmission, pancreatic endocrine function and corpus luteum regression.

Prostap A morphiate narcotic antagonist.

Proteoglycans Structural polysaccharides found in cartilage.

Ptyalin Salivary enzyme which hydrolyses starch

and glycogen to maltose and a small amount of glucose.

Pylorectomy Surgical removal of the pylorus.

Pyloroplasty Operation to repair the pylorus especially one to increase the diameter of the pylorus by stretching.

Pyrogens Any substance which induces fever.

Q

Quinine An alkaloid derived from cinchona bark, one of the first successful antimalarials.

R

Racemose glands Glands which resemble a bunch of grapes.

Radiolabelling the act of making a drug or formulation radioactive to facilitate its tracking in vivo or the study of its metabolism.

Radiotelemetry capsule A capsule containing a small transmitter which can be swallowed or implanted, and transmits the value of a physiological variable, commonly pH or pressure.

Ranitidine H receptor antagonist used to reduce acid secretion.

Rectocele protrusion or herniation of the posterior vaginal wall with anterior wall of the rectum through the vaginal.

Reserpine Drug which lowers blood pressure and acts as a tranquiliser.

Respiration Interchange of oxygen and carbon dioxide by breathing.

Reticulin An albuminoid or scleroprotein substance in the connective tissue framework or reticular tissue.

Reticuloendothelial system The collection of immune cells such as macrophages which identify and remove foreign materials.

Rhinitis Inflammation of the nasal mucosa.

Rhinorrhea Thin watery discharge from the nose.

Riboflavin Vitamin B essential for tissue repair.

Rivinus's gland A sublingual gland.

Rivotril Trade name for Clonazepam, a benzodiazepine.

Ryle's tube A small bore gastric tube, weighted at the tip and generally inserted through the nose.

S

Saccharin Artificial sweetener.

Salbutamol ß adrenoceptor agonist used to treat asthma. Also called Albuterol.

Salicylates Salts of salicylic acid.

Salicylazosulphapyridine See sulphasalazine.

Salicylic acid o-hydroxybenzoic acid, one of the earliest analgesics, derived from willow bark.

SCFA See short-chain fatty acids.

Sebum Fatty secretion of sebaceous glands of the skin.

Secretin A hormone which stimulates pepsinogen secretion by the stomach and inhibits the secretion of acid by the stomach.

Sennosides Anthraquinone glucosides present in senna and used as cathartics.

Sephadex® Trade name for a polymeric gel with pores of controlled sizes, commonly used for size exclusion (gel filtration) chromatography, in which macromolecules are separated on the basis of their molecular weight.

Serotonin Also known as 5-hydroxytryptamine, a chemical present in platelets, gastrointestinal mucosa, mast cells and carcinoid tumors. It is also believed t be important in sleep and sensory perceptions.

Shellac A natural resin derived from the dried secretions of the lac insect.

Short-chain fatty acids Fatty acids with an acyl chain of less than 5-6 carbon atoms.

Sialase An enzyme which degrades sialic acid.

Sialic acid An amino-sugar widely found in mucus polysaccharides

Silicones Polymers based on silicon rather than carbon.

Silicones elastomers Highly flexible and elastic cross-linked silicone polymers used for medical devices such as catheters.

Silicones oil medium-chain silicone polymers widely used as viscosity standards.

Single photon emission computed tomography (SPECT) An imaging method which allow reconstructions of cross-sections through the body of a radiotracer.

Sinusitis Inflammation of the sinuses.

Skene's glands Glands lying just inside and on the posterior of the female urethra.

Slow-reacting substance of anaphylaxis See Leucotrienes.

Smallpox Acute contagious disease, which is regarded to have been eradicated in the modern world.

Smoking Inhalation of cigarette or cigar smoke. Persons indulging in this habit are at risk of extreme damage to their lungs.

Sodium alginate A viscous carbohydrate biopolymer derived from various seaweeds. Used in oral controlled release devices and to form a floating gastric 'raft' in antireflux agents.

Sodium azodisalicylate See olsalazine.

Sodium caprate Salt of capric acid, a short-chain fatty acid.

Sodium cromoglycate See Disodium cromoglycate

Sodium deoxycholate A surfactant with a steroid nucleus found in bile, whose purpose is to emulsify and transport fats during digestion. Used as a solubilizing agent and emulsifier in some drug formulations.

Sodium glycocholate A surfactant similar to sodium deoxycholate (q.v.).

Sodium hyaluronate A polysaccharide used to treat osteoarthritis of the knee. It is injected intra-articularly to supplement natural hyaluronic acid.

Sodium laurate Sodium salt of dodecanoic acid, used as a surfactant.

Sodium lauryl sulphate An anionic surface active agent used in pharmaceutics.

Sodium taurocholate A surfactant similar to sodium deoxycholate (q.v.).

Sodium valproate An anti-epileptic drug.

Sodium-potassium exchange pump An alternative name for the Na⁺/K⁺ ATPase.

Solution A liquid containing a dissolved substance. The liquid into which the substance is dissolved is called the solvent. The solute is the substance which is dissolved.

Solvent drag Proposal that the amount of water present in the small intestine affects paracellular drug absorption and may affect the absorption of small and hydrophilic drugs.

Somatostatin A hormone which inhibits the release of somatotropin. It is a hypothalmic peptide that also inhibits the secretion of insulin and gastrin.

Sonophoresis The use of ultrsound to increase the absorption of drugs through the skin.

Spacer devices These are used with pressurised inhalers. They provide a space between the device and the mouth reducing the velocity of the aerosol and the subsequent impaction on the oropharynx. They also allow greater evapration of the propellant so a larger proportion of the drug can be inhaled into the lung.

Span Trade name for a family of hydrophilic surfactants produced by esterifying fatty acids with a hydrophilic sorbitol nucleus.

Splenic flexure Junction of the transverse and descending colon.

Squalane An unsaturated carbohydrate present in shark-liver oil and some vegetable oils. It is an intermediate in the biosynthesis of cholesterol.

Squamous epithelia Flat form of epithelial cells.

SRS-A See Leucotrienes.

Starch Carbohydrate of the polysaccharide group found in plants. And includes pectins, dextrins and gums. All are reduced to simple sugars before being absorbed.

Status epilepticus A type of epileptic seizure.

Stem cells Cell which gives rise to a specific type of cell.

Stensen's duct Excretory duct of the parotid gland.

Stercobilin Brown pigment derived from bile. Gives the colour to faeces.

Steroid A Term applied to a large group of substances chemically related to sterol. Includes sterols, D vitamins, bile acids and certain hormones.

Sterol A group of substances related to fats and belonging to the lipoids. They are found in both plants and animals.

Stilboestrol A synthetic preparation possessing oestrogenic properties. It is several times more potent than the natural compound and may be given orally.

Stomach Sac-like distensible portion of the gut. It lies between the oesophagus and small intestine. It acts as the initial receptacle for ingested food where it processes it to chyme (q.v.).

Stokes' law The relationship between settling rate, particle size, and viscosity in a particle supension.

Stratum basale Innermost layer of the uterus.

Stratum compactum Superficial layer of the endometrium.

Stratum corneum Outermost horny layer of the epidermis.

Stratum germinativum Innermost layer of the epidermis.

Stratum spongiosum Middle layer of the uterus.

Stroma Formation supporting tissues of an organ.

Subclavian vein Large vein draining arm.

Subcutaneous delivery drugs introduced beneath the skin.

Subcutaneous fat Layer of fat beneath the skin.

Sublingual tablet Tablets which are designed to be placed under the tongue.

Substance P An 11-amino acid polypeptide believed to be important as a neurotransmitter in the pain fibre system.

Succinic dehydrogenase An enzyme involved in the Krebs'cycle which converts succinate to fumarate.

Succus entericus See intestinal juice.

Sucrase Enzyme found in the intestinal juice which splits cane sugar into glucose and fructose.

Sucrose Sugar found in sugar cane and sugar beet. Split into glucose and fructose in the small intestine by sucrase.

Sufentanil An analgesic opiate analogue.

Sulphotransferases Enzymes responsible for sulpation of xenobiotics in the liver

Sulphapyridine A sulphonamide used to treat dermatitis herpetiformis.

Sulphasalazine Drug used to treat ulcerative colitis, Crohn's disease and rheumatoid arthritis.

Sulphomucins Sulphated mucin.

Sulphur dioxide An irritating gas. Used in refrigerators and as a bactericide.

Sumatriptan An antimigrane drug.

Superioris alaeque Muscle which raises upper lip and flares nostrils.

Suppository A semi-solid substance which is used to deliver drug to the rectum, vagina or urethra.

Surfactant An agent which lowers surface tension.

Suspension Solid particles which are suspended in, but not dissolved in, a liquid.

Symphysis pubis Junction of the pubic bones on midline in front.

T

T cells Lymphoid cells from the bone marrow that migrate to the thymus gland, where they develop into mature differentiated lymphocytes that migrate between the blood and lymph. Mature T cells are antigen specific i.e. each responds to different antigens.

T lymphocytes See T cells.

Tachycardia Abnormal rapid heartbeat.

Talin A sweet-tasting protein extracted from *Thaumatococcus danielli*, approximately 100,000 times sweeter than sucrose. Also known as Thaumatin.

Technetium-99m (^{99m}Tc) A gamma emitting radioisotope with a half-life of 6 h. Used as a diagnostic agent for diagnostic gamma imaging. It is also used in research to follow the behaviour of formulations in the body. It can be complexed in many ways e.g. with diethylenetriaminepentaacetic acid (DTPA), hexakis (t-butyl isonitrile), hexamethylpropyleneamine oxidase, HIDA or with tannous phytate.

Teflon (polytetrafluorethylene) A white thermoplastic material with a waxy texture. It is non-flammable, resists chemical action and radiation and has a low coefficient of friction.

Terbutaline A synthetic sympathomimetic anime used for treating asthma.

Terpenes Any member of the family of hydrocarbons with the formula C_nH_n. There are found in the essential oil of many plants especially conifers.

Testosterone Androgen produced by the testes. The hormone is also produced by the adrenal cortex in both males and females.

Tetracyclines Broad spectrum antibiotics.

Tetrahydrozoline A vasoconstrictor used as a nasal decongestant.

Theophylline Bronchodilator drug used for reversible airway constriction.

Thermogram A graphic record of variation in the amount of heat required to cause a change in temperature; the heat capacity as a function of temperature.

Thermophoresis The movement of small particles toward a warm surface as a result of differences indiffusion rate.

Thiomersal An organomercurial used as a pharmaceutical antibacterial and preservative.

Thrombosis Formation, development of existence of a blood clot or thrombus. Life-saving during haemorrhage, but life threatening if it occurs at any other time since it can occlude blood supply to a vessel.

Thymidine A nucleoside present in deoxyribonucleotide.

Timolol A ß adrenergic blocking drug.

Titanium dioxide Used to protect the skin from the sun.

Total parenteral nutrition (TPN) Intravenous nutrition which provides total nourishment to a patient.

Tragacanth Dried gum exuded from the plant *Astragalus gummifer*. Used as a mucilage for greaseless lubrication and as an application for chapped skin.

Transferrin Blood globulin which binds and transports iron.

Transfersomes Liposomes made from a blend of phospholipids which have a high degree of flexibility, allowing them to pass through small gaps in the lipid structure of the epithelium.

Transition temperature (lipids) The temperature at which a phospholipid bilayer undergoes a phase transition from an ordered to a disordered state.

Transitional epithelium Epithelium which shows a gradation in type at the boundary between different organs, for example between the oesophagus and the stomach.

Tributyrase An enzyme which hydrolyses tributyrin to glycerol and butyric acid.

Triceps muscle Extends forearm and arm.

Tricyclic antidepressants Drugs used to treat moderate to severe endogenous depression.

Trypsin Proteolytic enzyme formed in the intestine.

Trypsinogen Proenzyme of inactive form of trypsin.

Tuberculin A soluble cell substance prepared from the tubercle bacillus used to determine the presence of a tuberculosis infection.

Tuft cells An intestinal epithelial cell of uncertain function.

Turbinates Bones which project from the lateral nasal wall.

Tween Trade name for a family of hydrophilic surfactants produced by conjugating ethylene oxide and fatty acids to a sorbitol nucleus.

Tyrosine An amino acid.

U

Ulcer An open sore or lesion of the skin or mucous membrane.

Ulcerative colitis Inflammation and ulceration in the colon.

Urea The diamine of carbonic acid found in the blood lymph and urine. It is formed in the liver from ammonia derived from amino acids by deamination. It is the main constituent in urine.

Urobinin A brown pigment formed from the oxidation of urobilinogen, a decomposition product of bilirubin.

Uveal tract The portionof the eye consisting of the iris, ciliary body, and choroid.

Uvula Small soft structure hanging from the free edge of the soft palate.

V

Vaccines A suspension of infectious agents or part of them administered for the purpose of establishing resistance to an infection.

Vagus The 10th cranial nerve. It is a mixed nerve with both motor and sensory functions.

Valium Trade name of diazepam.

Vasoactive intestinal peptide (VIP) Peptide present in the mucosa of the gastrointestinal tract with the main function of inhibiting gastric function and secretion.

Vasopressin Hormone formed in the hypothalamus. It has an antidiuretic effect and pressor effect that elevates blood pressure.

Vastus One of three muscles of the thigh.

Verapamil Calcium channel blocker used to treat hypertension and angina.

Villi Pl. of Villus. Short filamentous processes found on certain cells, generally to increase absorptive area.

Vinca alkaloids Drugs such as vincristine and vinblastine derived from periwinkles. Antineoplastic drugs.

Virus A minute organism not visible with ordinary light microscopy. It is parasitic and relies entirely on nutrients in host cells. They consist of a strand of DNA or RNA but not both.

Viscolyzers Agents used to enhance the viscosity of solutions or suspensions.

Viscosity modifiers See Viscolyzers.

Vomer The bone which forms the lower and posterior portion of the nasal septum.

W

Wharton's duct Duct of the submandibular salivary glands opening into the mouth at the side of the frenulum linguae.

Witepsol Trade name for a series of surfactants used in some oral dose forms.

X

X-ray studies x-rays are high energy electromagnetic waves varying in length from 0.05 to 100 Å. They can penetrate solid matter to differing degrees and act on photographic film. Hence they are used for diagnosis and therapy. They were used to study the behaviour of drug formulations within the body, but the radioopaque materials adulterated the formulations nd the radiation dosimetry limited the number of x-rays which could be taken.

Xanthines drugs such as caffeine, theophylline and theobromine which are stimulants and diuretics.

Xerostomia Dryness of the mouth caused by reduction in the normal production of saliva.

Xylan An anticoagulant poysaccharide similar to heparin.

Xylometazoline A vasoconstrictor drug used to treat nasal congestion.

Z

Zeta potential The electrical potential of a charged particle at its hydrodynamic plane. This is similar to the potential at the particle surface but takes into account the fact that the particle normally moves carrying a layer of adsorbed solvent. It is the zeta potential which is calculated from the drift velocity in an electrophoresis experiment.

Zonulae adherens See desmosomes.

Zonulae occludens See tight junctions.

Zymogen A substance that develops into a chemical ferment or enzymes. Zymogen granules are secretory granules of a pre-enzyme substance seen in cells of organs such as salivary glands or the pancreas.

Index